HOARDING DISORDER
A Comprehensive Clinical Guide

HOARDING DISORDER
A Comprehensive Clinical Guide

Carolyn I. Rodriguez, M.D., Ph.D.
Randy O. Frost, Ph.D.

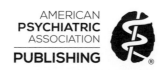

AMERICAN
PSYCHIATRIC
ASSOCIATION
PUBLISHING

Note: The authors have worked to ensure that all information in this book is accurate at the time of publication and consistent with general psychiatric and medical standards, and that information concerning drug dosages, schedules, and routes of administration is accurate at the time of publication and consistent with standards set by the U.S. Food and Drug Administration and the general medical community. As medical research and practice continue to advance, however, therapeutic standards may change. Moreover, specific situations may require a specific therapeutic response not included in this book. For these reasons and because human and mechanical errors sometimes occur, we recommend that readers follow the advice of physicians directly involved in their care or the care of a member of their family.

Books published by American Psychiatric Association Publishing represent the findings, conclusions, and views of the individual authors and do not necessarily represent the policies and opinions of American Psychiatric Association Publishing or the American Psychiatric Association.

If you wish to buy 50 or more copies of the same title, please go to www.appi.org/specialdiscounts for more information.

Copyright © 2023 American Psychiatric Association Publishing

ALL RIGHTS RESERVED

First Edition

Manufactured in the United States of America on acid-free paper
26 25 24 23 22   5 4 3 2 1

American Psychiatric Association Publishing
800 Maine Avenue SW, Suite 900
Washington, DC 20024-2812
www.appi.org

Library of Congress Cataloging-in-Publication Data
A CIP record is available from the Library of Congress.

British Library Cataloguing in Publication Data
A CIP record is available from the British Library.

Contents

About the Authors. vii

Preface ix

Acknowledgments xi

PART I
Phenomenology

1 Introduction and History. .3

2 Diagnosis and Comorbidity 27

3 Assessment 47

4 Insight and Motivation 69

PART II
Etiology

5 Cognitive-Behavioral Model 89

6 Neurobiology 109

PART III
Interventions

7 Cognitive-Behavioral Therapy 127

8 Pharmacotherapy. 149

9 Harm Reduction. 165

10 Community. 179

PART IV
Challenges

11 Elders. 199

12 Animal Hoarding 215

13 Squalor. 233

14 Conclusion and Future Directions 253

APPENDICES

APPENDIX A
Structured Interview for Hoarding Disorder (SIHD). 267

APPENDIX B
Clutter Image Rating (CIR) 281

APPENDIX C
Saving Inventory—Revised (SI-R) 285

APPENDIX D
Hoarding Rating Scale (HRS). 289

APPENDIX E
Activities of Daily Living—Hoarding Scale (ADL-H). 293

Index 295

About the Authors

Carolyn I. Rodriguez, M.D., Ph.D., is associate chair and associate professor and director of the Translational Therapeutics Lab in the Department of Psychiatry and Behavioral Sciences at Stanford University School of Medicine in Stanford, California. Dr. Rodriguez received her B.S. in computer science from Harvard University, followed by an M.D. from Harvard Medical School–M.I.T. and a Ph.D. in neuroscience and genetics from Harvard Medical School. Born in San Juan, Puerto Rico, she now lives with her husband and three children in Palo Alto, California.

Randy O. Frost, Ph.D., is Harold Edward and Elsa Siipola Israel Professor Emeritus of Psychology at Smith College in Northampton, Massachusetts. Dr. Frost received his Ph.D. in clinical psychology from the University of Kansas. He lives with his wife in Northampton, Massachusetts, and Bonita Springs, Florida. He has two children and three grandchildren.

Preface

Written for psychiatrists, psychologists, human service and other mental health professionals, peer support counselors, community advocates, and professionals in training, this book presents in detail the diagnosis, phenomenology, neurobiology, and pharmacotherapeutic and psychotherapeutic treatments for hoarding disorder. In addition, health science and basic science students may benefit from advancing their knowledge on the topic to further contribute interdisciplinary approaches to our understanding of hoarding behaviors. This book draws on the authors' extensive experience in mental health treatment (psychiatry/psychology) as well as reviews and compiles published research findings. This book will improve a clinician's knowledge and skill in treating patients with hoarding disorder—those with straightforward presentations as well as those with complicated ones. This is a practical guide and essential resource for treatment planning. Each chapter includes key clinical points that reflect the latest thinking in each topic area. The final chapter describes future directions that are possible because of advances that have occurred in the field and increased awareness of the disorder. The book's appendices contain useful symptom rating scales. This book represents a unique compilation, bringing together a wealth of information not otherwise available in a single source.

The authors have made every effort to provide accurate and up-to-date information at the time of publication. That said, clinical standards evolve as knowledge continually changes—informed by both research and regulation. Furthermore, the authors' understanding of this field is informed by their mental health background and represents only one of many possible views.

In this spirit, we humbly invite the reader to point us toward new information or additional information that should be included in future editions. Readers are encouraged to seek detailed information from the manufacturer of any drugs they plan to use. They can also access the hoarding disorder resource pages curated by the American Psychiatric Association (https://www.psychiatry.org/patients-families/hoarding-disorder) and the International OCD Foundation (www.iocdf.org/hoarding) to gain more information on training, referrals, and educational materials.

Acknowledgments

From Carolyn

I am indebted to many individuals who have supported the genesis of this book. I want to thank my patients, their families, and the many research study participants who have helped me understand the profound impact of this illness on their lives. Laura Roberts, chair of Stanford's Department of Psychiatry and Behavioral Sciences, encouraged the development of this book and has been an inspiration and stalwart advocate from our first meeting. Lorrin Koran, professor emeritus and founder of the Stanford OCD Clinic, has been a fierce champion, thoughtful mentor and collaborator, and model for going the extra mile for patients. Alan Schatzberg, former Chair of Stanford's Department of Psychiatry and Behavioral Sciences, has been a long-time sponsor and visionary collaborator, and I am thankful our paths crossed early in my career. I am grateful to my lab, students, and collaborators who continue to push the envelope.

It has been an honor to coauthor this book with my mentor and research collaborator, Randy Frost, who not only pioneered the hoarding disorder field but also has fostered a culture of collaboration and inclusion within its academic, clinical, advocacy, and community components. His efforts—alongside the efforts of numerous esteemed and newly engaged hoarding disorder colleagues—have enabled researchers and clinicians to create new research, treatments, advocacy, and hope. Lee Shuer and Becca Belofsky have imparted wisdom about the importance of language, stigma, and intention, which helped to shape my research, partnerships, and approach to care; I am grateful for their partnership. I also wish to give a special thanks to Becky Fullmer for her skillful editing, thoughtful feedback, and kind support on this project from beginning to end. I greatly appreciate the assistance of the staff of American Psychiatric Association Publishing.

This book is dedicated to individuals and their loved ones impacted by hoarding disorder and in loving memory of Karen Million. I wish to express my gratitude to my treasured friend Christina for her compassion and steadfast support. My brother Walter, sister-in-law Masami, nephews Oliver and Elliott, sister-in-law Elizabeth, and brothers-in-law Evan and Erik have been a constant source of encouragement and warmth. My parents, Walter and Melba, sacrificed greatly to give my brother and me educational opportunities; they were my first and most valuable teachers. I am above all grateful for the love and unwavering support of my husband, Ryan, and my children, Ryan, Alex, and Marisa.

From Randy

I owe much to my wife, Sue; my daughters, Erica and Olivia; and their families, whose love and support have sustained me through the writing of this book. The landscape of this work is populated by three groups of people: the professionals who study and treat the problem, the people who live with it, and the family and friends who often bear a great deal of the burden. There are hundreds of people from each of these groups who deserve my thanks for helping me develop an understanding of this problem. The sharing of information by these three groups has allowed us to detail what we know about hoarding in this volume. A special thanks is due to the people who work tirelessly to bridge the gaps between these groups. The International OCD Foundation and its staff provide a forum for education and training that has advanced the field tremendously. Lee Shuer and Becca Belofsky have been wonderful colleagues and friends from whom I have learned a great deal about the lived experience of hoarding. Gail Steketee, my close friend and colleague in research for more than 30 years, has been a constant source of support and inspiration. Thanks are also due to Becky Fullmer, who has been adept at editing much of our prose. A special thanks to my students, who have stimulated much of my thinking about the development of attachments to possessions over the 30-plus years that I have been studying hoarding. Finally, it has been a special treat for me to work with my coauthor, Carolyn Rodriguez, on this book. She has been a joy as well as a source of many new ideas for paths forward in the study of hoarding.

PART I
Phenomenology

CHAPTER 1
Introduction and History

In 2013, the American Psychiatric Association adopted hoarding as one of the new disorders, including it in the fifth edition of the *Diagnostic and Statistical Manual of Mental Disorders* (DSM-5; American Psychiatric Association 2013). The latest revision of the World Health Organization's *International Classification of Diseases* (ICD-11; World Health Organization 2018) also includes hoarding disorder as a new diagnosis. Before these additions, hoarding was considered an infrequent symptom of obsessive-compulsive disorder (OCD) or a symptom of obsessive-compulsive personality disorder (OCPD). However, neither of these designations fits what has been discovered over the last three decades about this troublesome behavior.

Although hoarding was mostly ignored in the psychiatric literature prior to the mid-1990s, it has been a topic of interest in literature for centuries. The word *hoard* derives from the Old English word *hord*, which means "treasure," while in Proto-Germanic the word denotes "hidden treasure." While some early descriptions of hoarding behaviors took the form of collections of actual treasures, references to hoarding of everyday objects date as far back as 319 B.C.E. to Theophrastus, a student of Aristotle, who attempted to catalog all forms of human behavior. Two negative character types he described were the Penurious Man and the Avaricious Man. He believed people with these character types collected and saved material possessions excessively. Centuries later in the 1300s, Dante Alighieri referred to hoarding in *The Inferno* (Ciardi 1954). In the story, Dante is led through each of the nine circles of hell by his guide, the shade Virgil. When they enter the fourth circle, they see two groups of people at war heaving great stones against each other with their chests, overseen by Plutus, the god of wealth. Virgil explains that these are "hoarders" and "wasters" in life, Avarice and Prodigia. These people spent their life pursuing wealth and failed to use it with moderation. By doing so, they became blind to the real value of possessions and were thus shielded from God's light. In punishment, they are forever doomed to do battle, with one group crashing against the other with the cry "Why do you hoard?" and the other reciprocating with "Why do you waste?" Their possessions become the heavy stones they are forced to heave for eternity.

Other descriptions of hoarding behaviors dot the landscape of literature. The Russian writer Nikolai Gogol's epic novel *Dead Souls*, published in 1842, describes a classic hoarding character named Plyushkin: "He wandered about the streets of his village every day looking under the bridges, under the planks thrown over puddles, and everything he came across, an old sole, a bit of a peasant woman's rag, an iron nail, a piece of broken earthenware, he carried them all to his room and put them on the heap. 'There goes the fisherman angling again!' the peasants used to say when they saw him going in search of booty" (Gogol 1842/1996, p. 126). In Russian slang, *Plyushkin* is a term used to describe someone who collects useless things. In Russian psychiatry, the behavior is called *Plyushkin syndrome*.

Charles Dickens' *Bleak House*, written in 1852–1853, described Krook, a rag and bottle man who collected documents even though he could not read and for whom "everything seemed to be bought, and nothing to be sold" (Dickens 1852–1853/2002, p. 48). Other examples can be found in George Eliot's novel *Silas Marner* (Eliot 1861) and Sir Arthur Conan Doyle's Sherlock Holmes stories, written in the 1890s. Doyle describes Sherlock Holmes as having "a horror of destroying documents," and as a result "his papers accumulated, until every corner of the room was stacked with bundles of manuscripts which were on no account to be burned, and which would not be put away save by their owner" (Doyle 1970, p. 386).

In popular media, perhaps the most recognizable hoarding case is that of the Collyer brothers of New York City (Frost and Steketee 2010). With a phone call to the Harlem police station in 1947, their story started to publicly unfold. The anonymous caller told police that there was a dead body in the Collyer mansion on Fifth Avenue, a once fashionable section of Harlem. The brothers, Homer and Langley, belonged to one of the long-distinguished families of New York. Their father was a physician, and their mother was a member of the high society. The brothers were both highly intelligent and well educated. Langley was an engineer and Homer a lawyer, though neither had much of a work history. Both graduated from Columbia University. They lived in the three-story, 12-room brownstone home that the family acquired in 1909. All appeared normal until after their parents' death in the 1920s, when Homer and Langley grew increasingly reclusive.

There had been numerous calls to the police about the Collyers over the years, mostly suggesting that one or both of the brothers were dead or seriously injured. Each call was dutifully investigated by the police, much to the annoyance of Langley, who most often dealt with them. Homer had not been seen outside the house in a number of years. He was blind and suffered from rheumatism. Langley cared for him with a strict diet of 100 oranges each week, which he believed would help restore Homer's sight. Many locals believed that Homer had been dead for some time. When the police arrived to check on the brothers after the last call, there was no answer at the front door. The police tried banging on the drainpipes, a technique that had successfully roused Langley in the past. This time there was no answer. Believing the report was credible enough to require a closer inspection, police forced open the iron grille door to the basement. Behind the door was a solid wall of bound newspapers so thick that they could not force their way in. Other doors and windows on the first floor were also barricaded. After several frustrating hours, they called the fire department for a ladder truck. Most of the upper-story windows were impassable as well, but after a few hours of searching, a patrolman was finally able to squeeze through the top of a second-floor window.

Inside he found a house packed with everything imaginable—newspapers, magazines, old stoves, books, a horse-drawn carriage, bicycles, 14 pianos, and much more. Most rooms were stacked to the ceiling and virtually impossible to navigate. After some searching, officers discovered a series of tunnels that the brothers used to move through the house. Some were dead ends or apparent dead ends that required removing items to continue. Some had booby traps designed to collapse on an unwanted intruder. The searchers never discovered the way Langley entered or exited the home to get food and other necessities.

After fighting his way over the mountain of stuff blocking the window, a patrolman found the body of 65-year-old Homer Collyer, clad only in a tattered bathrobe, in a small clearing in the center of the room. He had been dead for not more than 12 hours. His emaciated body was in a sitting position with his head resting on his knees. His death was ruled a heart attack, possibly brought on by starvation. Police had to lower Homer's body down the ladder since they could not navigate through the house. There was no sign of Langley. Within hours of the discovery of Homer's body, the police issued a missing person's report. The authorities became concerned that Langley was either hiding, lying injured, or dead elsewhere amid the hoard.

The next day, the headline of the *New York Daily News* read: "The Palace of Junk." All of the New York newspapers led with the story about the dead body in the "Ghost House." The news made the Collyer brothers household names. Thousands of people turned out to watch as authorities slowly unpacked the house in search of Langley. After starting in the basement, engineers realized that removing the stuff on the lower levels of the house destabilized the upper floors, since the empty lower floors would no longer be able to support the weight of the material above. The clearing process moved to a room on the top floor, where workers extracted objects through a hole cut in the roof. At times the process was interrupted by reports of sightings of Langley. Once the transit authority stopped a subway train before reaching a station to check out the report of a Langley sighting. The search—both inside the house and throughout the greater New York area—continued for 3 weeks until Langley's body was discovered in the mansion less than 10 feet from where Homer was found. Langley had apparently tripped a booby trap in one of the tunnels and was crushed to death by baled newspapers and a heavy chest. He appeared to have died before Homer. His body lay hidden there so long that it had been partially eaten by rats. In the end, over 170 tons of material was removed from the home, along with 30 feral cats and thousands of roaches and rats. Because of the condition of the house, it had to be demolished, but it was replaced with a small park named after the brothers—Collyer Brothers Park. The Collyer brothers' story is a familiar one to most New Yorkers. Among firefighters, a home filled with clutter is officially referred to as a "Collyer residence" and marked for the extreme danger involved in fighting a fire in it.

The Collyer brothers' story is not unusual. Most cities have similar stories, such as that of Edmund Trebus, a Londoner whose difficulties with the local council over his hoarding behavior were memorialized in a television documentary series called *A Life of Grime*. In the United States, as described by Cappelletti et al. (2019), a 75-year-old woman died of traumatic and confined space asphyxia after a large number of objects collapsed on her in her apartment. In China, the mother of the well-known contemporary artist Song Dong struggled with difficulty parting with possessions most of her life. She adhered to the Chinese virtue of fully using and not wasting anything, and consequently saved everything that might be of use. After the death of her husband, her hoarding intensified as she saved everything reminding her of him. Her small one-room house was stuffed with over 10,000 objects. Increasingly worried about his mother and desperate to find a way to help her, Song Dong took advantage of her beliefs about waste and utility. He convinced her to let him use her possessions in an art installation. He called the installation, created in 2005, *Waste Not* (Wu 2009). It consisted of all of her belongings carefully arranged around her small house. The organization of objects into categories with careful placement—such as bars of partially used soap arranged by size—stood in stark contrast to the chaos she lived with inside her home. In 2009, *Waste Not* was installed in the atrium of the Museum of Modern Art in New York City (Alcon et al. 2011; Wu 2009).

Though the story of hoarding has had a long history in literature, its existence in the mental health world has been a short one. It was not until 1993 that the first systematic account of hoarding behavior appeared in the scientific literature (Frost and Gross 1993). A series of research articles that followed demonstrated the impairment associated with hoarding, elucidated the nature of abnormal attachments that people form to their possessions, and hinted at the staggering prevalence. Just a short 20 years after the 1993 publication, hoarding entered DSM as a separate disorder. By the time the first theoretical model was published in 1996 (Frost and Hartl 1996), there had been only 10 scientific articles written about hoarding. Just over 20 years later, there were hundreds. Research laboratories have since been established around the world to study the phenomenon.

Three features characterize the complexity of hoarding symptoms: excessive acquisition, difficulty discarding or letting go of possessions, and cluttered living spaces (Frost and Hartl 1996). Difficulty discarding or letting go of possessions is the hallmark behavior of the disorder, while clutter is the consequence. The vast majority of individuals with hoarding disorder acquire excessively, which intensifies the impact of the difficulty discarding and clutter. To understand the nature of hoarding disorder, we need to understand the underlying motivation for these behaviors. Individuals with hoarding disorder have rationales for the decisions they make in acquiring and saving the possessions in their homes. The attachments that they form to their possessions are the driving force behind the reluctance to let go of them. These attachments will be explored in more detail in Chapter 5. A number of associated features have been identified as well, including indecisiveness, perfectionism, attention deficits, distress intolerance, and problems with planning and organization. These features may not be central to the disorder, but they are certainly relevant to understanding its phenomenology. They will also be delved into in Chapter 5. Other major features include a number of information processing deficits that appear to contribute to the development of hoarding. They will be examined in Chapter 5 as well.

Ownership

At its core, hoarding is about ownership of objects. But what does it mean to "own" something? This question has interested philosophers for centuries. In her review of the meaning of possessions, Lita Furby, a well-known authority on the psychology of ownership, concluded that to own something is fundamentally to have control over it (Furby 1978). Control means the power to determine where it is located, who has access to it, and how it is used. Ownership is also defined by the role it plays in the life of the owner. For Plato, ownership was a vice leading to degradation and was something to be avoided. In contrast, Aristotle believed ownership was instrumental to the development of moral character. Later, religious philosophers spoke of ownership differently—as a temporary state akin to stewardship. Still others, like French philosopher Jean-Paul Sartre, believed that possessions allowed people to develop a sense of identity. More recent theorizing about ownership has come from the social and biological sciences. In the late nineteenth century, psychologist William James posited that "acquisitiveness" was instinctual. Ascribing human behavior to instincts was in vogue at that time and has made a resurgence with the development of neuroscience. James suggested that accumulated possessions contributed to the sense of self—a sort of fusing of self with possessions (James 1890, pp. 291–292).

In the middle of the twentieth century, philosopher Erich Fromm developed a theory of character in which acquiring and saving possessions played a central role (Fromm 1947). He believed that acquiring things was a way for people to connect with the world around them and each other. He went further to suggest that when acquiring and saving were done in excess, they amounted to a "hoarding orientation," which he believed to be one of four types of nonproductive character. For people with a hoarding orientation, collecting and saving things were necessary in order to feel secure. He went on to suggest two aspects of human existence that defined one's relationship to the world: having and being. A having-oriented person derives meaning in life from collecting and saving possessions, while a being-oriented person derives meaning from experiences rather than possessions. Fromm believed that the having orientation was a dangerous form of avarice and the most destructive form of human existence.

Sigmund Freud had little to say about the hoarding of possessions. However, he described a trio of traits he believed to derive from an anal fixation: orderliness, parsimony, and obstinacy. In his view, the parsimony leg of this anal triad included stinginess, miserliness, and the hoarding of money (Freud 1908/1960). Ernest Jones (1913) developed this idea further, suggesting that objects as well as money could serve as copro-symbols. These ideas were the roots of theorizing about the existence of an anal personality that in turn formed the basis for the current DSM criteria for OCPD, including the criterion of difficulty discarding worn-out and worthless items with no sentimental value.

Collecting vs. Hoarding

Everyone experiences ownership of possessions. So how does this normative experience differ from the experience of people with hoarding disorder? One way to answer this question is to compare people with hoarding disorder to people who engage in normative behavior but own a large number of possessions, such as collectors (Nordsletten et al. 2013a). Luckily, there is a lot of literature on collectors and collecting behavior. Broadly speaking, most scholars who study collecting define it as building a collection of objects that have some sort of theme or are related in some way. Collectors, by and large, actively acquire with a process that is typically organized, intentional, and targeted. Once acquired, the items are removed from normal usage but are subject to being organizing, admired, and displayed to others. Often the collecting behavior follows a roughly defined sequence involving fantasizing about acquiring a particular object, planning for acquisition of it, hunting for it, actually acquiring it, cataloging it, and finally displaying it. Then the object is often used in communicating with others, especially other collectors. Communication through possessions comes in the form of sharing information about the objects, as well as more subtle messaging to others about one's success in the world, one's competence at creating something of interest, or demonstrations of one's worthiness. These behaviors differ markedly from what we know about the collecting behaviors of people with hoarding problems. Acquisition of objects in people who hoard is largely impulsive (Frost et al. 2009). There is little active planning of acquiring episodes. The acquisition is usually triggered by the sight of an object that could be owned—either seeing it in a store or noticing it at the curb. Excessive levels of acquisition are much more common in hoarding than in collecting. Although up to half of people with hoarding describe themselves as "collectors," their collections are more accidental than planned, and they include a much wider variety of objects. The idea of acquiring a particular item does not begin before an acquiring episode in hoarding cases (i.e., there is no fantasizing about or hunting for the treasure). The emotional experience of acquiring may be quite similar between the two groups, including intense euphoria and a sense of well being. However, the objects acquired by people with hoarding lack a consistent theme, whereas those of collectors are narrowly focused on a particular topic. People who hoard seldom let go of any of their possessions, whereas collectors often cull their collections, trading items with others or eliminating duplication. In contrast to the objects of a collector, once acquired, objects of people who hoard are not cataloged but rather placed somewhere amid the piles of things in the living areas of the person's home. There may be limited attempts at organizing objects, but they are largely unsuccessful. Objects typically stay in their place in the pile, and there is little interaction with them going forward. Also, in contrast to collectors, people who hoard go to great lengths to prevent anyone from seeing or interacting with them about the object.

People with hoarding disorder differ from collectors on a number of demographic variables as well (Nordsletten et al. 2013a). They are more likely to live alone and are less likely to be married or partnered. Collecting is more often done by men, but hoarding appears with equal frequency in men and women. People who hoard tend to have fewer rooms in their home, as well as a smaller number of bedrooms, and they have completed fewer years of education. There is evidence that they are more likely to suffer from OCD and be taking psychiatric medicines. In terms of diagnostic criteria, most collectors may meet the DSM-5 "difficulty discarding and distress when discarding" criterion. However, very few of them meet criteria for the amount of clutter and impairment that are required for diagnosis. A further distinction is that the presence of excessive acquisition of free things is much more common in people who hoard.

Despite these differences, in many respects hoarding disorder closely resembles normative ownership, particularly regarding motivations for saving. The reasons given for saving items generally are the same for people with and without hoarding behaviors (Frost and Gross 1993; Nordsletten et al. 2013a). The difference is that in people who hoard, these reasons are applied to a wider range of objects and applied more rigidly. Perceived usefulness and avoidance of waste appear to be the strongest motivations for saving (Dozier and Ayers 2014; Frost et al. 2015; Nordsletten et al. 2013a).

Severity

Severity of hoarding symptoms ranges from mild to severe and even life-threatening. At the mild end of the spectrum, hoarding creates minor difficulties with finding things. In more serious cases, it can interfere with the ability to complete basic activities of daily living, including preparing food, using appliances, moving around inside the home, and even sitting on sofas and chairs (Frost et al. 2013). At the more severe end, it can be life-threatening. A study examining residential fires over a 10-year period by the Metropolitan Fire Brigade of Melbourne, Australia, revealed that although hoarding-related fires were infrequent (representing less than 0.25% of fires), they represented 24% of fires involving loss of life (Lucini et al. 2009).

Hoarding has been shown to interfere in a host of other aspects of life. In a study of the economic and social burden of hoarding, Tolin et al.

(2008a) surveyed 861 people who reported having hoarding problems. Those judged to have serious problems described serious impairments due to their hoarding. Nearly 6% had been fired from a job because of the hoarding. Those who were employed lost an average of seven workdays a month because of hoarding. This was significantly higher than the reported work impairment days of people with major depressive disorder, social phobia, PTSD, or alcohol and drug disorders, as reported in the National Comorbidity Study (Kessler et al. 2001). Over 75% of participants had problems finding things at work because of the clutter. Other studies have replicated higher levels of unemployment and work disability among hoarding participants (Archer et al. 2019; Diefenbach et al. 2013; Landau et al. 2011; Mathes et al. 2019; Pertusa et al. 2008).

The ability to manage finances can be affected by hoarding as well. Among the participants in the Tolin et al. (2008a) study, 22% had failed to file a tax return for at least 1 of the last 5 years. Findings from other studies suggest that the failure to file taxes may be related to the inability to locate important financial documents (Frost et al. 2013). Numerous other studies have reported that those with hoarding are less likely to be employed and more likely to receive income assistance and to be at lower socioeconomic levels (Spittlehouse et al. 2016). In addition to the financial burden, Tolin et al. (2008a) reported that 8% of hoarding participants in their sample had been evicted or threatened with eviction because of the hoarding. Echoing that finding, nearly a quarter of the people who seek help from an eviction intervention agency in New York City suffer from hoarding problems (Rodriguez et al. 2012).

People with hoarding appear to suffer from poor health, including greater frequencies of chronic illnesses such as arthritis, asthma, tuberculosis, visual impairments, hypertension, diabetes, heart disease, severe kidney and liver disease, lupus, multiple sclerosis, epilepsy, ulcers, cancer, chronic fatigue syndrome, and stroke (Ong et al. 2015a; Saxena et al. 2011; Spittlehouse et al. 2016; Tolin et al. 2008a, 2019). There are reports of disturbed sleep patterns associated with hoarding severity as well (Mahnke et al. 2020; Raines et al. 2015).

Not surprisingly, several studies have found significantly lower quality of life among people with hoarding problems (Ong et al. 2015a; Saxena et al. 2011; Tolin et al. 2019), as these problems affect their functioning in the areas of psychosocial, emotional, occupational, family, and general health. Most of these deficits remained after the effects of emotional problems were controlled.

The financial costs of hoarding are not limited to those with the problem. The general community in which the individual with hoarding behaviors lives can be severely affected as well. Health departments often get involved in trying to resolve hoarding problems. Frost et al. (2000) found that nearly 80% of hoarding cases reported by health departments also involved extra costs because of work by multiple agencies requiring multiple home visits. The estimated cost to the community for these efforts can be quite high. For instance, the annual cost of hoarding to landlords and social service agencies in San Francisco was estimated to be over $6 million (San Francisco Task Force on Compulsive Hoarding 2009). The Metropolitan Fire Brigade study mentioned earlier reported that the cost of fighting residential fires in hoarded units and the subsequent repairs was eight times the cost of fires not attributable to hoarding (Lucini et al. 2009). Just one such apartment fire in Toronto in 2010 injured 17 and displaced more than 1,000 people for several weeks. The cost of the damage was estimated to be over $1 million.

The burden shouldered by family members is also substantial. Social service agencies often remove children, elders, and pets from the homes of those afflicted with hoarding disorder. Tolin et al. (2008b) found such removals in 4% of cases studied. Drury et al. (2014) found a significantly greater care burden than was observed with relatives of collectors. A consistent pattern among adult children of hoarding individuals is decades of frustration and conflict, followed by resentment and abandonment of the parent(s) by the adult children (Tolin et al. 2008b). Growing up in a hoarded home affects the quality of childhood, and the aftereffects persist into adulthood. Growing up in a hoarded home is associated with a less happy childhood, greater difficulty making friends, more embarrassment about the home, inability to have friends over to play, and more family strain (Tolin et al. 2008b). If the child lives with the parent with hoarding behaviors when they are younger than 10 years, the effects are particularly powerful. Severe hoarding is also associated with high levels of frustration, rejection, and hostility by family members toward the hoarding relative (Tolin et al. 2008b). Even more striking is that the interpersonal conflicts extend to the clinicians who are treating people with hoarding problems (Tolin et al. 2012). Clinicians report more frustration with hoarding clients than with nonhoarding ones. They are more often irritated by the client's behavior and relieved when the client misses a session, and have frequent feelings of wanting the client to transfer to another therapist.

Prevalence

The chances are very high that you know someone with a hoarding problem. Estimates of the prevalence of hoarding behavior range widely depending on how it is defined and measured and on what population is being examined. Probably the best estimate is that hoarding occurs in 1.5%–6% of the general population.

Several large epidemiological studies of mental disorders have included questions about OCD and OCPD symptoms, including hoarding. Ruscio et al. (2010) used data from the OCD portion of the World Health Organization Composite International Diagnostic Interview administered to participants in the National Comorbidity Survey Replication (2001–2003; N=9,282). Hoarding was the second most frequently reported symptom and was endorsed by a surprising 14.4% of the sample. In contrast, Fullana et al. (2010) relied on data from the European Study of the Epidemiology of Mental Disorders, which included more than 21,000 interviewed participants. Interviewers asked about the existence of hoarding "compulsions" among the questions about OCD symptoms. Hoarding was reported in 2.6% of the sample. Rodriguez et al. (2013) examined data from more than 43,000 participants in the National Epidemiologic Survey on Alcohol and Related Conditions. In this study, interviewers used the single-item OCPD hoarding criterion (i.e., difficulty discarding worn-out or worthless items with no sentimental value) to determine prevalence. Remarkably, difficulty discarding was reported by 20.6% of the sample. Data from 742 participants in the Hopkins Epidemiology of Personality Disorder Study were used to establish hoarding based on the OCPD criterion of difficulty discarding worn-out and worthless items with no sentimental value. The estimated weighted prevalence rate was 5.3% (Samuels et al. 2008). Dong et al. (2012) reported prevalence rates of hoarding and self-neglect among a population-based sample of elderly people in Chicago. Hoarding was assessed by questions about clutter rather than by difficulty discarding or impairment. Based on interviews with over 4,500 participants, 4.1%–5.4% of men and 2.3%–5.0% of women displayed significant hoarding, with men showing increasing prevalence with age and women showing decreasing prevalence. These rates for hoarding varied widely, from 2.6% to over 20%. This variability probably results from the unreliability of the hoarding measures used. Also, hoarding in these studies was inferred from responses to questions about OCD symptoms or the OCPD difficulty discarding criterion, which do not mirror current definitions or established measures of hoarding or hoarding severity. Consequently, these rates may not reflect the true prevalence.

More recent studies have relied on validated assessment procedures or the DSM-5 criteria for hoarding disorder to establish prevalence rates. Nordsletten et al. (2013c) conducted a two-wave epidemiological study in London using the DSM-5 diagnostic criteria. In the first wave, 1,698 adults were recruited and responded to a screening question regarding the experience of problems with clutter in the home. Follow-up interviews were solicited from the 191 individuals who responded affirmatively and consented to be recontacted. Ninety nine of those individuals were successfully interviewed using the Structured Interview for Hoarding Disorder, an interview developed to establish a diagnosis of hoarding disorder based on DSM-5 criteria (see Appendix A). The weighted prevalence following their interviews was 1.5%, substantially lower than the prevalence rates from other studies. However, as the authors note, their recruitment strategy of door-to-door canvasing for participation may have led to underdetection of hoarding cases. People with hoarding problems are typically very reticent to open their door to strangers and may be overrepresented among the participants who never answered their door.

Other investigations have relied on one of two widely used measures of hoarding: the Saving Inventory—Revised (SI-R; see Appendix C) and Hoarding Rating Scale (HRS; see Appendix D). The SI-R is a well-validated self-report measure that gives an indication of the severity of hoarding and three subscales: excessive acquisition, difficulty discarding, and clutter. Cutoff scores for clinically significant hoarding have been established by examining the sensitivity and specificity in identifying known hoarding cases (see Chapter 3). The HRS is a five-item scale used either as an interview or for self-report. Cutoff scores for clinically significant hoarding have been empirically established for the HRS as well (see Chapter 3). The five items correspond to clutter, difficulty discarding, excessive acquisition, distress, and impairment. These items were used as a basis for the DSM-5 criteria for hoarding disorder.

Three studies have examined prevalence rates using the SI-R with large samples. Mueller et al. (2009) used the SI-R with a representative sample of 2,300 German citizens. In this sample, 4.6% scored more than 2 standard deviations above the mean. Using a more stringent criterion of 3 standard deviations above the mean lowered the prevalence rate to 1.5%. Prevalence rates in two studies in Italy that used the recommended severity criteria from the SI-R ranged from 3.7% (n=462) to 6.0% (n=1,012) (Bulli et al. 2014). In a random sample of New Zealand residents (N=404), Spittlehouse et al. (2016) reported a prevalence of 2.5% based on the SI-R (score>41), while another 4% of residents displayed subclinical hoarding.

Multiple studies have examined prevalence rates using the HRS with large samples. Iervolino et al. (2009) examined hoarding behavior in participants in an adult twin registry in the United Kingdom. Hoarding caseness was determined using an HRS cutoff score that was more conservative than the established cutoff (17 vs. 14). Prevalence in the sample of 5,000 cases was 2.3%. Timpano et al. (2011) used the same conservative HRS cutoff to establish hoarding prevalence in Germany. In a representative sample of more than 2,500 German citizens, they found a prevalence rate of 6.7%.

However, since the HRS includes an item about excessive acquisition—which is a specifier and not a diagnostic criterion in DSM-5—this rate may be an overestimate. When this item was dropped and only items mapping onto DSM-5 criteria were used, the rate was lower (5.8%). Using established HRS cutoffs to determine prevalence with the Australian Twin Registry, López-Solà et al. (2014) reported a hoarding prevalence between 1.6% and 3.3% in a sample of more than 6,900 participants. In a similar study that included over 15,000 people from the Netherlands Twin Register, Mathews et al. (2014) reported a prevalence of 6.8% using the same more conservative criterion cutoff employed by Iervolino and Timpano.

Cath et al. (2017) surveyed a random sample of over 15,000 people from the Netherlands Twin Register regarding the presence of hoarding and OCD symptoms. Using individual items from the HRS selected to map onto the DSM-5 criteria, they found an overall prevalence rate of 2.12%. The prevalence rate was lowest (below 2%) among younger participants and increased with age beginning at around age 35 years. For those older than 70 years, the prevalence rate was over 6%. Severity of hoarding symptoms increased more rapidly for older males than for older females. Among the hoarding symptoms measured (difficulty discarding, clutter, impairment), the increase in severity with age was driven mostly by difficulty discarding.

In a review and meta-analysis of studies involving more than 53,000 cases, Postlethwaite et al. (2019) reported a pooled point prevalence estimate of 2.6% (95% CI: 1.7–3.7). The lifetime pooled prevalence rate was 1.7% (95% CI: 0.4–6.8), and the overall pooled prevalence rate was 2.5% (95% CI: 1.7–3.6). This review provides the best estimate to date of the true prevalence of hoarding disorder. However, it should be noted that there are reasons to think these rates may be an underestimate. The shame, self-criticism, and limited insight that are frequently experienced by people with hoarding symptoms (Chou et al. 2018; Kim et al. 2001; Tolin et al. 2010) may affect people's willingness to admit hoarding problems, especially to strangers conducting surveys.

Several studies have examined the prevalence of hoarding in childhood and adolescence. Ivanov et al. (2013) examined the prevalence of clinically significant hoarding in a population-based sample of 15-year-old twins in Sweden ($N=3,974$). Using the DSM-5 criteria derived from the HRS-Self-Report, they found a prevalence rate of 2%. A complication with diagnosing children and adolescents is that they frequently do not have control over the amount of clutter in their home or even, in some cases, bedroom. When the authors excluded the clutter criterion from consideration, the prevalence rate was significantly higher (3.7%).

Alvarenga et al. (2015) examined OCD symptom dimensions, including hoarding, in a population-based sample of school-age children (6–18 years old) and their parents in Brazil (total sample N=29,459). They used a single-item question from the Dimensional Yale Brown Obsessive Compulsive Scale (DY-BOCS) asking participants if anyone in the family "needed to collect or store MANY things or useless objects." More than 9% of the children said yes.

Beyond the community prevalence rate, there are subpopulations that appear to vary with respect to hoarding prevalence. In a sample of people seeking assistance to maintain housing and at risk for eviction in New York City, 22% met criteria for hoarding using the HRS interview and 23% met criteria using the SI-R (Rodriguez et al. 2012). Online classified advertisement networks that list items for sale are likely to attract individuals who may be predisposed to hoarding. In a large survey of network users, 12.3% of participants met criteria for hoarding on the SI-R (Turna et al. 2018).

Among people with psychiatric problems, the prevalence for hoarding appears to be quite high. In a study of 200 randomly sampled adult psychiatric inpatients in New York—none of whom had been previously diagnosed with hoarding—33% met criteria for clinically significant hoarding (Basu et al. 2019). Hoarding cases existed across all age groups, races, and genders, with no differences in frequency. The highest frequency of hoarding occurred among patients with a primary diagnosis of depression (42%). Twenty-six percent of patients with psychotic spectrum disorders had clinically significant hoarding. Other primary diagnoses were too infrequent to draw conclusions. Similarly, among 500 treatment-seeking psychiatric outpatients in Singapore, 30.2% scored above the cutoff for clinically significant hoarding on the SI-R (Ong et al. 2015b). When DSM-5 criteria were employed by eliminating the acquisition questions from the SI-R, 13.8% had significant difficulty discarding and clutter, while 12.9% met criteria for all three symptoms (difficulty discarding, clutter, and excessive acquisition). Tolin et al. (2011) found that a large percentage of clients seeking outpatient treatment for anxiety disorders displayed clinically significant hoarding behaviors (12.3%) despite the fact that none of the clients reported hoarding as a presenting problem. The frequency varied across disorders, with 29% of generalized anxiety disorder patients scoring above the clinical cutoff but none of the panic disorder patients doing so. Similarly, in another study, among children ages 7–13 years seeking help for anxiety disorders, 22% had elevated hoarding levels on the child version of the SI-R (Hamblin et al. 2015).

Culture

The extent to which possessions are viewed as central to life varies across cultures. For the Manusians of Papua New Guinea, lost objects are grieved over as much as one would grieve over the loss of a loved one. On the other hand, some cultures, such as the Tasaday of the Philippines, place little importance on possessions. Just how much culture plays a role in the prevalence of hoarding is not clear. Most of the research on hoarding has been conducted in Western Europe and the United States (Fernández de la Cruz et al. 2016). Although limited, the studies that do exist from other parts of the world reveal similar prevalence rates, core symptoms, and associated features.

In Asia, Subramaniam and colleagues (2014) reported a 2% prevalence rate for hoarding in a population based in Singapore. Prevalence was based on a single question about difficulty discarding. Despite this fact, the study showed a prevalence rate similar to those found in the West. Other research in Singapore suggests the rate may be higher. Lee et al. (2016) found that over 30% of psychiatric outpatients seeking psychiatric treatment met criteria for clinically significant hoarding on the SI-R. Recognition of this problem goes beyond the psychiatric community in Singapore. In 2014, for instance, a national Hoarding Task Force was established with representatives from a variety of governmental agencies in order to cope with problems associated with hoarding (Choo et al. 2015).

A cross-cultural comparison of hoarding in Chinese and American students revealed stronger endorsement of hoarding symptoms on the SI-R among the Chinese students (Timpano et al. 2015). While the reason for this difference is not entirely clear, what is clear is that hoarding exists in China and looks similar in symptoms and beliefs about possessions to the phenomena seen elsewhere. Several differences with respect to beliefs about saving showed up in this study as well. In China, much greater emphasis was placed on the usefulness of possessions and the importance of avoiding waste as reasons for saving. These beliefs are consistent with the observation from Wang et al. (2016) that Chinese culture puts an emphasis on "making the best use of everything" and "avoiding waste" (p. 104). They also mirror the motivations of Song Dong's mother as depicted in the *Waste Not* exhibit (Wu 2009).

In a different part of Asia, researchers in Japan have reported that as many as 32% of OCD patients display significant hoarding behavior (Matsunaga et al. 2010), a figure that is similar to those observed in Western countries using comparable methodologies (i.e., single-item hoarding question). Kuwano et al. (2020) also found the clinical characteristics of those with hoarding disorder in Japan to be similar to the clinical characteristics of those with hoarding disorder in other countries. In one of the few actual cross-cultural comparisons, Nordsletten et al. (2018) found that hoarding symptoms, cognitions, and associated features in Japan were similar to those found in the United Kingdom, Spain, and Brazil.

Among OCD patients in India, 10% had scores above the cutoff score on the SI-R, indicating clinically significant hoarding (Chakraborty et al.

2012). Although this percentage is smaller than the 30% or higher seen in studies like Matsunaga et al.'s (2010), the methodology in the Chakraborty et al. study is more precise, relying on an empirically validated measure of hoarding rather than a single question. Jaisoorya et al. (2021) reported a hoarding prevalence rate of 1.02% among a sample of primary care patients in India using the HRS interview cutoff score.

Studies of hoarding phenomena exist in Iran and Turkey as well, and the phenomena are similar to those seen around the world, although to date none of these studies have established prevalence rates (Asadi et al. 2016; Tükel et al. 2005).

There is a relatively long history of conceptualizations of hoarding in Spanish- and Portuguese-speaking countries. In the 1970s, a Spanish psychiatrist, Juan Antonio Vallejo-Nágera, proposed a disorder that he described as the "mirror image" of phobias. Rather than fear of the target stimulus, he described an excessive attachment to it (Fontenelle 2016). He suggested that the condition he called "soteric neurosis" would lead to excessive accumulation of possessions. Several of the comorbidities and associated features he attributed to the disorder have since been confirmed by recent research, such as the association with obesity.

A few studies have reported on hoarding in Latin America. In a cross-cultural comparison, 33% of OCD patients in Costa Rica reported hoarding on the Yale-Brown Obsessive Compulsive Scale (Y-BOCS) checklist (Chavira et al. 2008). This figure was comparable to that found in the U.S. sample of OCD patients who reported hoarding (38%). Also, in Nordsletten and colleagues' (2018) transcultural study, hoarding in Brazil was similar in form and frequency to hoarding in the United Kingdom, Japan, and Spain. However, there were some differences in the extent of clutter, with less severe clutter occurring in the Brazilian sample.

Nordsletten et al. (2018) assessed hoarding symptoms, beliefs, and associated features across four countries (United Kingdom, Spain, Japan, and Brazil). Hoarding disorder diagnoses were established using the Structured Interview for Hoarding Disorder (Nordsletten et al. 2013b). The core features were consistent across all four countries. (There were some differences, however, in the amount of clutter reported. As noted above, Brazil hoarding participants reported less clutter than other participants.) Other cross-cultural comparisons indicate similar associated features for hoarding. For instance, the relationship between hoarding and impulsivity is nearly identical across U.S. and German samples (Timpano et al. 2013).

Very few studies have examined hoarding behavior in minority groups within the United States. Among Chinese Americans, Dong (2014) found that nearly 15% of older adults surveyed reported significant hoarding behavior. While this figure is difficult to interpret because it was not based on a standardized measure, it does suggest that a significant number of people have some concern about their hoarding behavior.

Only three studies have reported on the frequency of hoarding among African Americans. In all three studies the participants were people with OCD. Hoarding was established in each study by endorsement of either hoarding obsessions or hoarding compulsions on the Y-BOCS checklist using a single item (with a yes/no response). The frequency of hoarding in these studies ranged from 39% to 54% (Friedman et al. 2003; Williams et al. 2012, 2017). These percentages are in line with or slightly higher than what is observed with white OCD participants.

While research on hoarding is limited outside the West, there is growing recognition across the world about the seriousness of this problem. Efforts to understand and deal with hoarding problems have been concentrated in the health and housing sector, specifically public health, housing, elder services, and mental health. In the early 2000s, however, reality television brought hoarding to America's living rooms in the form of shows like *Hoarders* and *Hoarders: Buried Alive*. Although these shows have been criticized for being more sensational than educational, they have demonstrated for the public the seriousness of the disorder. They have also exposed the stereotypes that people who hoard are just lazy or that the classification of hoarding as a disorder just pathologizes poor housekeeping. The shows demonstrate the lack of control over acquisition and saving behavior that characterizes the behavior of people with hoarding disorder. They also demonstrate the impairment and suffering endured by those with the malady as well as their loved ones and others living nearby. On the other hand, they are highly sensationalized—emphasizing extreme cases, especially those characterized by squalid living conditions. Many people with hoarding disorder find these shows stigmatizing and degrading. Despite the benefits, the shows do little to elucidate the true nature of the problem, and, perhaps worse, they emphasize the clearing of clutter as the solution. Anyone who has dealt with a hoarding case knows that clearing the clutter only temporarily changes the living conditions. Without a change in the acquiring and saving behavior, the problem will resurface remarkably quickly, and when it does there is little motivation to cooperate further.

Conclusion

Hoarding has had a long history in literature but a relatively short one in psychiatry. The last 25 years have provided enough evidence of the severity and prevalence of problem hoarding to justify inclusion of a new diagnostic category in 2013. Although still limited, research on hoarding outside of Europe and the United States suggests that hoarding exists with similar frequency and appears to be similar in form and associated features worldwide. The cross-cultural comparisons that have been done do not reveal large differences in prevalence across different countries. The chapters in this book provide a guide to our existing knowledge of hoarding and hoarding disorder.

KEY CLINICAL POINTS

- Descriptions of hoarding have appeared in literature for centuries, but this behavior has only recently been addressed in the psychiatric world.

- Three features characterize hoarding symptoms: excessive acquisition, difficulty discarding or parting with possessions, and cluttered living spaces.

- Hoarding ranges from mild to severe and even life-threatening, with a wide variety of negative consequences.

- There are clear differences between hoarding and more normative collecting, with hoarding posing significant threats to the health and safety of the individual as well as those living nearby.

- The overall prevalence of hoarding disorder is approximately 2.6%, with higher rates for people older than 60 years and people with other psychiatric diagnoses, especially anxiety and depression.

- The prevalence and features of hoarding appear to be similar across countries and cultures.

References

Alcon J, Glazier K, Rodriguez C: From clutter to modern art: a Chinese artist's perspective on hoarding behaviors. Am J Psychiatry 168(12):1248, 2011 22193669

Alvarenga PG, Cesar RC, Leckman JF, et al: Obsessive-compulsive symptom dimensions in a population-based, cross-sectional sample of school-aged children. J Psychiatr Res 62:108–114, 2015 25702286

American Psychiatric Association: Diagnostic and Statistical Manual of Mental Disorders, 5th Edition. Arlington, VA, American Psychiatric Association, 2013

Archer CA, Moran K, Garza K, et al: Relationship between symptom severity, psychiatric comorbidity, social/occupational impairment, and suicidality in hoarding disorder. J Obsessive Compuls Relat Disord 21:158–164, 2019

Asadi S, Daraeian A, Rahmani B, et al: Exploring Yale-Brown Obsessive Compulsive Scale symptom structure in Iranian OCD patients using item-based factor analysis. Psychiatry Res 245:416–422, 2016 27620324

Basu A, Goel N, Puvvada S, Jacob T: Prevalence of hoarding in an adult inpatient population and its association with Axis I diagnoses. Am J Geriatr Psychiatry 27(5):564–568, 2019 30773455

Bulli F, Melli G, Carraresi C, et al: Hoarding behaviour in an Italian non-clinical sample. Behav Cogn Psychother 42(3):297–311, 2014 23286647

Cappellctti S, Cipolloni L, Piacentino D, Aromatario M: A lethal case of hoarding due to the combination of traumatic and confined space asphyxia. Forensic Sci Med Pathol 15(1):114–118, 2019 30535912

Cath DC, Nizar K, Boomsma D, Mathews CA: Age-specific prevalence of hoarding and obsessive compulsive disorder: a population-based study. Am J Geriatr Psychiatry 25(3):245–255, 2017 27939851

Chakraborty V, Cherian AV, Math SB, et al: Clinically significant hoarding in obsessive-compulsive disorder: results from an Indian study. Compr Psychiatry 53(8):1153–1160, 2012 22796017

Chavira DA, Garrido H, Bagnarello M, et al: A comparative study of obsessive-compulsive disorder in Costa Rica and the United States. Depress Anxiety 25(7):609–619, 2008 17823962

Choo KW, Lee WL, How CH, Ng BY: Hoarding in Singapore. Singapore Med J 56(9):484–486, quiz 487, 2015 26464529

Chou CY, Tsoh J, Vigil O, et al: Contributions of self-criticism and shame to hoarding. Psychiatry Res 262:488–493, 2018 28939393

Ciardi J (trans): The Inferno by Dante Alighieri. New Brunswick, NJ, Rutgers University Press, 1954

Dickens C: Bleak House (1852–1853). New York, Modern Library, 2002

Diefenbach GJ, DiMauro J, Frost R, et al: Characteristics of hoarding in older adults. Am J Geriatr Psychiatry 21(10):1043–1047, 2013 23567383

Dong X: Self-neglect in an elderly community-dwelling U.S. Chinese population: findings from the Population Study of Chinese Elderly in Chicago study. J Am Geriatr Soc 62(12):2391–2397, 2014 25439674

Dong X, Simon MA, Evans DA: Prevalence of self-neglect across gender, race, and socioeconomic status: findings from the Chicago Health and Aging Project. Gerontology 58(3):258–268, 2012 22189358

Doyle AC: The adventure of the Musgrave ritual, in The Complete Sherlock Holmes, Vol 1. New York, Doubleday, 1970

Dozier ME, Ayers CR: The predictive value of different reasons for saving and acquiring on hoarding disorder symptoms. J Obsessive Compuls Relat Disord 3(3):220–227, 2014 32670784

Drury H, Ajmi S, Fernández de la Cruz L, et al: Caregiver burden, family accommodation, health, and well-being in relatives of individuals with hoarding disorder. J Affect Disord 159:7–14, 2014 24679383

Eliot G: Silas Marner: The Weaver of Raveloe. Edinburgh, Blackwood & Sons, 1861

Fernández de la Cruz L, Nordsletten A, Mataix-Cols D: Ethnocultural Aspects of Hoarding Disorder. Curr Psychiatry Rev 12:115–123, 2016

Fontenelle LF: Vallejo-Nágera (1926–1990) and the concept of "soteric neurosis": a forgotten sketch of hoarding disorder in the obsessive-compulsive spectrum literature. J Med Biogr 24(1):85–89, 2016 24658218

Freud S: Character and anal eroticism (1908), in The Standard Edition of the Complete Psychological Works of Sigmund Freud, Vol 9. Translated and edited by Strachey J. London, Hogarth Press, 1960, pp 167–176

Friedman S, Smith L, Halpern B, et al: Obsessive-compulsive disorder in a multiethnic urban outpatient clinic: Initial presentation and treatment outcome with exposure and ritual prevention. Behav Ther 34:397–410, 2003

Fromm E: Man for Himself: An Inquiry Into the Psychology of Ethics. New York, Rinehart, 1947

Frost RO, Gross RC: The hoarding of possessions. Behav Res Ther 31(4):367–381, 1993 8512538

Frost RO, Hartl TL: A cognitive-behavioral model of compulsive hoarding. Behav Res Ther 34(4):341–350, 1996 8871366

Frost RO, Steketee G: Stuff: Compulsive Hoarding and the Meaning of Things. Boston, MA, Houghton Mifflin Harcourt, 2010

Frost RO, Steketee G, Williams L: Hoarding: a community health problem. Health Soc Care Community 8(4):229–234, 2000 11560692

Frost RO, Tolin DF, Steketee G, et al: Excessive acquisition in hoarding. J Anxiety Disord 23(5):632–639, 2009 19261435

Frost RO, Hristova V, Steketee G, Tolin DF: Activities of Daily Living Scale in hoarding disorder. J Obsessive Compuls Relat Disord 2(2):85–90, 2013 23482436

Frost RO, Steketee G, Tolin DF, et al: Motives for acquiring and saving in hoarding disorder, OCD, and community controls. J Obsessive Compuls Relat Disord 4:54–59, 2015 25729641

Fullana MA, Vilagut G, Rojas-Farreras S, et al; ESEMeD/MHEDEA 2000 investigators: Obsessive-compulsive symptom dimensions in the general population: results from an epidemiological study in six European countries. J Affect Disord 124(3):291–299, 2010 20022382

Furby L: Sharing: decisions and moral judgments about letting others use one's possessions. Psychol Rep 43(2):595–609, 1978

Gogol NV: Dead Souls (1842). Translated by Pevear R, Volokhonsky L. New York, Pantheon Books, 1996

Hamblin RJ, Lewin AB, Salloum A, et al: Clinical characteristics and predictors of hoarding in children with anxiety disorders. J Anxiety Disord 36:9–14, 2015 26407051

Iervolino AC, Perroud N, Fullana MA, et al: Prevalence and heritability of compulsive hoarding: a twin study. Am J Psychiatry 166(10):1156–1161, 2009 19687130

Ivanov VZ, Mataix-Cols D, Serlachius E, et al: Prevalence, comorbidity and heritability of hoarding symptoms in adolescence: a population based twin study in 15-year olds. PLoS One 8(7):e69140, 2013 23874893

Jaisoorya TS, Thamby A, Manoj L, et al: Prevalence of hoarding disorder among primary care patients. Braz J Psychiatry 43(2):168–173, 2021 32876135

James W: The Principles of Psychology. New York, Henry Holt, 1890

Jones E: Papers on Psycho-analysis. New York, Wood, 1913

Kessler RC, Greenberg PE, Mickelson KD, et al. The effects of chronic medical conditions on work loss and work cutback. J Occup Environ Med 43(3):218–225, 2001 11285869

Kim HJ, Steketee G, Frost RO: Hoarding by elderly people. Health Soc Work 26(3):176–184, 2001 11531193

Kuwano M, Nakao T, Yonemoto K, et al: Clinical characteristics of hoarding disorder in Japanese patients. Heliyon 6(3):e03527, 2020 32181397

Landau D, Iervolino AC, Pertusa A, et al: Stressful life events and material deprivation in hoarding disorder. J Anxiety Disord 25(2):192–202, 2011 20934847

Lee SP, Ong C, Sagayadevan V, et al: Hoarding symptoms among psychiatric outpatients: confirmatory factor analysis and psychometric properties of the Saving Inventory—Revised (SI-R). BMC Psychiatry 16(1):364, 2016 27784281

López-Solà C, Fontenelle LF, Alonso P, et al: Prevalence and heritability of obsessive-compulsive spectrum and anxiety disorder symptoms: a survey of the Australian Twin Registry. Am J Med Genet B Neuropsychiatr Genet 165B(4):314–325, 2014 24756981

Lucini G, Monk I, Szlatenyi C: An Analysis of Fire Incidents Involving Hoarding Households. Report to Worcester Polytechnic Institute, Worcester, MA, 2009

Mahnke AR, Linkovski O, Timpano K, et al: Examining subjective sleep quality in adults with hoarding disorder. J Psychiatr Res 137:597–602, 2020 33309063

Mathes BM, Henry A, Schmidt NB, Norberg MM: Hoarding symptoms and workplace impairment. Br J Clin Psychol 58(3):342–356, 2019 30548281

Mathews CA, Delucchi K, Cath DC, et al: Partitioning the etiology of hoarding and obsessive-compulsive symptoms. Psychol Med 44(13):2867–2876, 2014 25066062

Matsunaga H, Hayashida K, Kiriike N, et al: Clinical features and treatment characteristics of compulsive hoarding in Japanese patients with obsessive-compulsive disorder. CNS Spectr 15(4):258–265, 2010 20414175

Mueller A, Mitchell JE, Crosby RD, et al: The prevalence of compulsive hoarding and its association with compulsive buying in a German population-based sample. Behav Res Ther 47(8):705–709, 2009 19457476

Nordsletten AE, Fernández de la Cruz L, Billotti D, Mataix-Cols D: Finders keepers: the features differentiating hoarding disorder from normative collecting. Compr Psychiatry 54(3):229–237, 2013a 22995450

Nordsletten AE, Fernández de la Cruz L, Pertusa A, et al: The Structured Interview for Hoarding Disorder (SIHD): development, usage and further validation. J Obsessive Compuls Relat Disord 2(3):346–350, 2013b

Nordsletten AE, Reichenberg A, Hatch SL, et al: Epidemiology of hoarding disorder. Br J Psychiatry 203(6):445–452, 2013c 24158881

Nordsletten AE, Fernández de la Cruz L, Aluco E, et al: A transcultural study of hoarding disorder: Insights from the United Kingdom, Spain, Japan, and Brazil. Transcult Psychiatry 55(2):261–285, 2018 29508639

Ong C, Pang S, Sagayadevan V, et al: Functioning and quality of life in hoarding: a systematic review. J Anxiety Disord 32:17–30, 2015a 25847547

Ong C, Sagayadevan V, Lee SP, et al: Hoarding among outpatients seeking treatment at a psychiatric hospital in Singapore. J Obsessive Compuls Relat Disord 8:56–63, 2015b

Pertusa A, Fullana MA, Singh S, et al: Compulsive hoarding: OCD symptom, distinct clinical syndrome, or both? Am J Psychiatry 165(10):1289–1298, 2008 18483134

Postlethwaite A, Kellett S, Mataix-Cols D: Prevalence of hoarding disorder: a systematic review and meta-analysis. J Affect Disord 256:309–316, 2019 31200169

Raines AM, Portero AK, Unruh AS, et al: An initial investigation of the relationship between insomnia and hoarding. J Clin Psychol 71(7):707–714, 2015 25760757

Rodriguez CI, Herman D, Alcon J, et al: Prevalence of hoarding disorder in individuals at potential risk of eviction in New York City: a pilot study. J Nerv Ment Dis 200(1):91–94, 2012 22210369

Rodriguez CI, Simpson HB, Liu S-M, et al: Prevalence and correlates of difficulty discarding: results from a national sample of the US population. J Nerv Ment Dis 201(9):795–801, 2013 23995036

Ruscio AM, Stein DJ, Chiu WT, Kessler RC: The epidemiology of obsessive-compulsive disorder in the National Comorbidity Survey Replication. Mol Psychiatry 15(1):53–63, 2010 18725912

Samuels JF, Bienvenu OJ, Grados MA, et al: Prevalence and correlates of hoarding behavior in a community-based sample. Behav Res Ther 46(7):836–844, 2008 18495084

San Francisco Task Force on Compulsive Hoarding: Beyond Overwhelmed: The Impact of Compulsive Hoarding and Cluttering in San Francisco and Recommendations to Reduce Negative Impacts and Improve Care. San Francisco, CA, The Mental Health Association of San Francisco, 2009

Saxena S, Ayers CR, Maidment KM, et al: Quality of life and functional impairment in compulsive hoarding. J Psychiatr Res 45(4):475–480, 2011 20822778

Spittlehouse JK, Vierck E, Pearson JF, Joyce PR: Personality, mental health and demographic correlates of hoarding behaviours in a midlife sample. PeerJ 4:e2826, 2016 28028484

Subramaniam M, Abdin E, Vaingankar JA, et al: Hoarding in an Asian population: prevalence, correlates, disability and quality of life. Ann Acad Med Singapore 43(11):535–543, 2014 25523857

Timpano KR, Exner C, Glaesmer H, et al: The epidemiology of the proposed DSM-5 hoarding disorder: exploration of the acquisition specifier, associated features, and distress. J Clin Psychiatry 72(6):780–786, quiz 878–879, 2011 21733479

Timpano KR, Rasmussen J, Exner C, et al: Hoarding and the multi-faceted construct of impulsivity: a cross-cultural investigation. J Psychiatr Res 47(3):363–370, 2013 23168138

Timpano KR, Çek D, Fu ZF, et al: A consideration of hoarding disorder symptoms in China. Compr Psychiatry 57:36–45, 2015 25483851

Tolin DF, Frost RO, Steketee G, et al: The economic and social burden of compulsive hoarding. Psychiatry Res 160(2):200–211, 2008a 18597855

Tolin DF, Frost RO, Steketee G, Fitch KE: Family burden of compulsive hoarding: results of an internet survey. Behav Res Ther 46(3):334–344, 2008b 18275935

Tolin D, Fitch K, Frost R, Steketee G: Family informants' perceptions of insight in compulsive hoarding. Cognit Ther Res 34:69–81, 2010

Tolin DF, Meunier SA, Frost RO, Steketee G: Hoarding among patients seeking treatment for anxiety disorders. J Anxiety Disord 25(1):43–48, 2011 20800427

Tolin D, Frost R, Steketee G: Working with hoarding vs non-hoarding clients: a survey of professionals' attitudes and experiences. J Obsessive Compuls Relat Disord 1:48–53, 2012

Tolin DF, Das A, Hallion LS, et al: Quality of life in patients with hoarding disorder. J Obsessive Compuls Relat Disord 21:55–59, 2019 31595215

Tükel R, Ertekin E, Batmaz S, et al: Influence of age of onset on clinical features in obsessive-compulsive disorder. Depress Anxiety 21(3):112–117, 2005 15965994

Turna J, Patterson B, Simpson W, et al: Prevalence of hoarding behaviours and excessive acquisition in users of online classified advertisements. Psychiatry Res 270:194–197, 2018 30261409

Wang Z, Wang Y, Zhao Q, Jiang K: Is the DSM-5 hoarding disorder diagnosis valid in China? Shanghai Jingshen Yixue 28(2):103–105, 2016 27605866

Williams MT, Elstein J, Buckner E, et al: Symptom dimensions in two samples of Africans Americans with obsessive-compulsive disorder. J Obsessive Compuls Relat Disord 1(3):145–152, 2012 22708117

Williams MT, Brown TL, Sawyer B: Psychiatric comorbidity and hoarding symptoms in African Americans with obsessive-compulsive disorder. J Black Psychol 43(3):259–279, 2017

World Health Organization: International Classification of Diseases, 11th Revision (ICD-11). 2018. Available at: https://icd.who.int/en/. Accessed September 14, 2021.

Wu H: Waste Not. Zhao Xiangyuan & Song Dong. Translated by Krischer O. Beijing, Tokyo Gallery and Beijing Tokyo Art Projects, 2009

CHAPTER 2
Diagnosis and Comorbidity

Hoarding Before DSM-5

Hoarding was first mentioned as a form of obsessive-compulsive disorder (OCD) in the "Differential Diagnosis" section in relation to obsessive-compulsive personality disorder (OCPD) in DSM-IV-TR (American Psychiatric Association 2000). DSM-IV-TR recommended that when hoarding is observed, "a diagnosis of OCD should be considered, especially when hoarding is extreme..." (p. 728). The reason for this recommendation is unclear but may have originated with the DSM-IV field trial for OCD, which relied on the Yale-Brown Obsessive Compulsive Scale (Y-BOCS). Among the more than 50 obsessions and compulsions itemized, the Y-BOCS checklist contains one item for hoarding obsessions and one for hoarding compulsions. The Y-BOCS checklist items went on to become the basis for research on symptom-based OCD subtypes. Numerous factor and cluster analyses of checklist items generated a relatively consistent pattern of four or five subtypes, the most consistent of which was hoarding (Mataix-Cols et al. 2010). As a result, hoarding came to be widely viewed as a subtype or symptom of OCD.

As more research became focused on this topic, however, it became increasingly clear that hoarding fit uncomfortably as a subtype of OCD (Mataix-Cols et al. 2010). Closer scrutiny of the phenomenological features of hoarding revealed important differences from OCD (Mataix-Cols et al. 2010). Perhaps most telling of these differences was that hoarding-related

27

thoughts are not experienced as intrusive or unwanted, as is required for an OCD diagnosis. Rather, they are ego-syntonic—part of the normal stream of thought (Frost and Hartl 1996, Steketee et al. 2003). They are also not repetitive the way that obsessions are, nor are they unpleasant or distressing. Distress in hoarding does not occur with the collecting or saving behavior; rather, it arises only with attempts to discard or curtail acquisition. The nature of the distress also differs from what is usually seen in OCD. Grief or anger characterizes attempts to let go of possessions just as often as anxiety, and perhaps more so. Also striking is that some hoarding behaviors, especially acquisition, are associated with positive emotional states. Many people with hoarding disorder describe their acquiring episodes as a "high," and often their only source of joy (Frost and Steketee 2010).

Neural correlates of hoarding are unlike those identified in OCD (Mataix-Cols et al. 2010), and other differences can be seen as well in prevalence, onset, course, and response to treatment. Clinically significant hoarding appears to be more prevalent than OCD, and while there is some overlap, only around 20% of hoarding cases involve comorbid OCD (Frost et al. 2011). Hoarding has an onset between ages 10 and 20 and a chronic course that accelerates after age 35, in contrast to OCD (Cath et al. 2017). Also, participants with primarily hoarding symptoms show poorer outcomes following OCD treatment than individuals with more classic OCD symptoms (Bloch et al. 2014).

Nevertheless, there are some similarities in the function that certain hoarding behaviors serve. Decisions to save possessions, like neutralizing or compulsive behavior, allow the individual to avoid or escape negative emotions that emerge when letting go of possessions. This functional relationship between the behavior and avoidance of negative emotion is common to all anxiety disorders and not specific to hoarding. What distinguishes hoarding from other anxiety disorders sharing this characteristic is that the underlying reason for the negative emotion in hoarding is not a catastrophic reaction to an intrusive thought or a fear stimulus, but rather an extreme attachment to a physical object that will be lost if the object is discarded. The nature of these attachments will be explored in more detail in Chapter 5.

Beginning with DSM-III-R in 1987, hoarding-like behavior appeared as a diagnostic criterion for OCPD, where it was described as "an inability to discard worn-out or worthless objects even when they have no sentimental value" (American Psychiatric Association 1987, p. 356). Unfortunately, while this might describe behaviors associated with some hoarding patients, it does not match well with what has been learned over the last 25 years about most hoarding behavior. First, this definition limits hoarding to problems with discarding, while research has clearly shown that hoarding involves difficulty letting go of items through donation, sale, lending, and recycling as well (Mataix-Cols et al. 2010). Second, research on the nature of saved items among hoarding patients does not support the restriction to worn-out or worthless objects. While people with hoarding problems often save things that other people would consider worn out or worthless, they also save things in excess that have value (Frost and Gross 1993). In other words, their saving behavior is not restricted to worn-out or worthless things as is implied by the OCPD criterion. People who hoard collect and save all types of possessions. Most homes of people with hoarding disorder contain numerous new items, such as appliances still in their unopened boxes or rooms full of never-worn clothes, many with the price tags still attached. Rankings of the most to least saved objects among people who hoard and those who don't are virtually the same (Frost and Gross 1993). The nature of the items saved does not distinguish people who hoard—only the volume does. Hoarding individuals simply save more of everything, including valuable as well as seemingly worthless items.

Finally, the OCPD criterion restricts difficulty discarding to items with "no sentimental value." The growing body of research on attachments to possessions indicates that sentimental and emotional reasons are some of the most prominent motives for saving among those with hoarding disorder (Frost et al. 2015; Steketee et al. 2003; Yap and Grisham 2019). Consequently, defining hoarding using the OCPD criteria risks misleading conclusions.

The OCPD difficulty discarding criterion may be a poor indicator of true hoarding, but it is related. Frost et al. (2011) found that when all criteria for OCPD were used, hoarding patients were significantly more likely to be comorbid for OCPD than were OCD patients (29.5% vs. 16.7%). However, when the OCPD difficulty discarding criterion was omitted, there was no significant difference in the percentage of cases comorbid for OCPD between hoarding patients and OCD patients (18.4% vs. 14.6%).

DSM-5 and Beyond

Based on the growing body of literature on hoarding and recognition of the serious impairments associated with it, hoarding became a new disorder in the fifth edition of DSM (American Psychiatric Association 2013). For similar reasons, the World Health Organization has recently included it as a separate condition in the latest (eleventh) revision of the *International Classification of Diseases* (ICD-11; World Health Organization 2018). With a few exceptions, the disorders are described similarly in both documents.

ICD-11 provides a description of hoarding disorder rather than diagnostic criteria:

> Hoarding disorder is characterised by accumulation of possessions that results in living spaces becoming cluttered to the point that their use or safety

is compromised. Accumulation occurs due to both repetitive urges or behaviours related to amassing items and difficulty discarding possessions due to a perceived need to save items and distress associated with discarding them. If living areas are uncluttered this is only due to the intervention of third parties (e.g., family members, cleaners, authorities). Amassment may be passive (e.g., accumulation of incoming flyers or mail) or active (excessive acquisition of free, purchased, or stolen items). The symptoms result in significant distress or significant impairment in personal, family, social, educational, occupational or other important areas of functioning. (World Health Organization 2018)

The DSM criteria for hoarding disorder (Box 2–1) were derived from the 1996 definition of hoarding, where it was described as 1) the acquisition of and failure to discard a large number of possessions that seem to be useless or of limited value, 2) living spaces sufficiently cluttered so as to preclude activities for which those spaces were designed, and 3) significant distress or impairment in functioning caused by the hoarding (Frost and Hartl 1996, p. 251).

Box 2–1.   DSM-5 diagnostic criteria for hoarding disorder

A. Persistent difficulty discarding or parting with possessions, regardless of their actual value.

B. This difficulty is due to a perceived need to save the items and to distress associated with discarding them.

C. The difficulty discarding possessions results in the accumulation of possessions that congest and clutter active living areas and substantially compromises their intended use. If living areas are uncluttered, it is only because of the interventions of third parties (e.g., family members, cleaners, authorities).

D. The hoarding causes clinically significant distress or impairment in social, occupational, or other important areas of functioning (including maintaining a safe environment for self and others).

E. The hoarding is not attributable to another medical condition (e.g., brain injury, cerebrovascular disease, Prader-Willi syndrome).

F. The hoarding is not better explained by the symptoms of another mental disorder (e.g., obsessions in obsessive-compulsive disorder, decreased energy in major depressive disorder, delusions in schizophrenia or another psychotic disorder, cognitive deficits in major neurocognitive disorder, restricted interests in autism spectrum disorder).

Specify if:

With excessive acquisition: If difficulty discarding possessions is accompanied by excessive acquisition of items that are not needed or for which there is no available space.

Specify if:
  With good or fair insight: The individual recognizes that hoarding-related beliefs and behaviors (pertaining to difficulty discarding items, clutter, or excessive acquisition) are problematic.
  With poor insight: The individual is mostly convinced that hoarding-related beliefs and behaviors (pertaining to difficulty discarding items, clutter, or excessive acquisition) are not problematic despite evidence to the contrary.
  With absent insight/delusional beliefs: The individual is completely convinced that hoarding-related beliefs and behaviors (pertaining to difficulty discarding items, clutter, or excessive acquisition) are not problematic despite evidence to the contrary.

Source. Reprinted from American Psychiatric Association: *Diagnostic and Statistical Manual of Mental Disorders*, 5th Edition. Arlington, VA, American Psychiatric Association, 2013. Copyright 2013, American Psychiatric Association. Used with permission.

Research on the acceptability of preliminary criteria and a field trial examining their utility led to some refinements. In DSM-5, there are four inclusion criteria and two exclusion criteria, along with two specifiers for hoarding disorder (excessive acquisition and level of insight). The first inclusion criterion and cardinal feature of hoarding disorder is "persistent difficulty discarding or parting with possessions, regardless of their actual value" (American Psychiatric Association 2013, p. 247). This includes any attempt to relinquish possessions—whether that involves selling, donating, or even loaning possessions to others. This difficulty must be persistent. That is, it must be long-standing and not simply a reaction to temporary events such as the sudden accumulation of meaningful possessions because of the death of a family member. The wording of this criterion was careful to distinguish hoarding from the "difficulty discarding" criterion in OCPD. The phrase "regardless of their actual value" was added in order to make it clear that hoarding is not restricted to "worn-out or worthless" items. Absent from the DSM-5 definition is any mention of the nature of the attachment to the owned objects to make it clear that hoarding is not restricted to items "without sentimental value."

The second DSM-5 criterion—"the difficulty is due to a perceived need to save the items and to distress associated with discarding them" (American Psychiatric Association 2013, p. 247)—was included to clarify that the behavior is not due to simple messiness or laziness, but rather an intentional behavior. Emphasis on the distress associated with discarding distinguishes this behavior from saving behavior that may be generated by more passive accumulation associated with other forms of psychopathology, such as depression, where there may be no distress if others remove the items.

The third criterion has to do with the consequences of difficulty discarding: "The difficulty discarding possessions results in the accumulation of possessions that congest and clutter active living areas and substantially compromises their intended use. If living areas are uncluttered, it is only because of the interventions of third parties (e.g., family members, cleaners, authorities)" (American Psychiatric Association 2013, p. 247). While clutter is the most visible feature of hoarding, it is a product of the dysfunctional behavior. It is included here because it represents the most substantial form of impairment. Emphasis is placed on the living areas of the home because severe clutter in these areas is most likely to produce interference with normal functioning, as well as health and safety risks. If the clutter is confined to other areas of the home, such as the basement, attic, or garage, this criterion would not be met. An exception to this criterion applies to situations in which the clutter is controlled by someone other than the patient, such as a spouse, parent, or authorities. This may require some investigation on the part of the diagnosing clinician. Cleaning or clearing interventions by others are common and a source of significant interpersonal strife and trauma. Following forced or unwanted cleanings, the clutter usually returns to previous levels in a short time, and the motivation to cooperate with subsequent attempts to help is greatly lessened. This clause is particularly relevant for children who hoard because they often do not have full control over the amount of clutter in their living spaces. In such cases, the dysfunction usually takes the form of intensely emotional reactions to others touching or removing their things.

The fourth inclusion criterion is that "the hoarding causes clinically significant distress or impairment in social, occupational, or other important areas of functioning (including maintaining a safe environment for self and others)" (American Psychiatric Association 2013, p. 247). This is the standard criterion for most mental health diagnoses in DSM-5—to distinguish an abnormal from a normal behavior state. Acquisition of possessions and decisions to save rarely generate distress. Attempts to curb acquisition or discard a cherished possession generate a wide variety of intense negative emotions, including sadness, anger, anxiety, and bitterness (Frost and Hartl 1996). Some people with hoarding disorder experience distress regarding the condition of their home yet are unable to change it. Impairment in hoarding cases can be widespread and range from mild impairment in the ability to carry out basic activities of daily living to life-threatening situations when the risk of fire is high.

There are two exclusion criteria for hoarding disorder. The first (Criterion E) is "The hoarding is not attributable to another medical condition (e.g., brain injury, cerebrovascular disease, Prader-Willi syndrome)" (American Psychiatric Association 2013, p. 247). Several medical conditions have been reported to result in excessive accumulation and difficulty discarding possessions. These include traumatic brain injury, cerebrovascular disease, and damage to the anterior ventromedial prefrontal and cingulate cortices (Anderson et al. 2005). In addition, Prader-Willi syndrome, a rare genetic condition, is frequently accompanied by hoarding behavior (Pertusa and Fonseca 2014).

The second exclusion criterion (Criterion F) has to do with other DSM disorders that might result in hoarding-like behavior: "The hoarding is not better explained by the symptoms of another mental disorder (e.g., obsessions in obsessive-compulsive disorder, decreased energy in major depressive disorder, delusions in schizophrenia or another psychotic disorder, cognitive deficits in major neurocognitive disorder, restricted interests in autism spectrum disorder)" (American Psychiatric Association 2013, p. 247). If the accumulation and difficulty discarding can be attributed to these disorders, then the diagnosis of hoarding disorder is not given. In OCD, accumulation and difficulty discarding can result from the experience of incompleteness or from the abandonment of rituals that are difficult, such as excessive checking and cleaning (Pertusa et al. 2010). If the hoarding-like behavior is due to OCD, it is more likely to involve the saving of bizarre items such as body products (e.g., feces and urine) or rotting food (Pertusa et al. 2008). In depression, clutter may accumulate because of a lack of motivation to clean and organize. In psychotic and neurocognitive disorders, clutter may accumulate due to delusional thinking or the inability to organize goal-directed cleaning behavior.

There are two specifiers in DSM-5 for hoarding disorder: insight and excessive acquisition. The insight specifier is standard across the DSM-5 obsessive-compulsive and related disorders, with three levels: good or fair, poor, and absent or delusional. Insight in hoarding cases is difficult to assess because of the defensiveness that develops in response to intense criticism by family and friends (Frost and Steketee 2010). See Chapter 4 for a more complete review of insight in hoarding disorder.

Although excessive acquisition was a primary feature in the early conceptualization of hoarding disorder (Frost and Hartl 1996), it is not necessary for a hoarding disorder diagnosis in DSM-5. Instead, once a diagnosis of hoarding disorder is made, the clinician must specify if difficulty discarding possessions is accompanied by excessive collecting or buying or stealing of items that are not needed or for which there is no available space (American Psychiatric Association 2013, p. 247).

A review of research on excessive acquisition suggests a closer look at the importance of acquiring as a component of hoarding. Findings from a number of studies indicate that a very high percentage of people with hoarding acquire excessively. Across samples of self-identified and carefully diagnosed hoarding cases, the overwhelming majority of people (80%–95%) do so, although excessive acquisition is much less common among children who hoard (30%–40%) (Ivanov et al, 2013). Compulsive buying and the excessive acquiring of free things are the most common forms, and roughly half of adults with hoarding behaviors do both (Frost et al. 2009, 2013; Mataix-Cols et al. 2013). A relatively small percentage of patients with hoarding behaviors acquire through stealing (5%–9%) (Frost et al. 2009; Mataix-Cols et al. 2013), though up to 20% experience urges to do so (Frost et al. 2013). Existing research suggests that it is important to assess each of these forms of acquisition when patients have hoarding problems, because both buying and free acquisition independently predict hoarding severity (Frost et al. 2009; Timpano et al. 2011).

Several things are noteworthy with respect to the assessment of excessive acquisition. First, the ability to recognize excessive acquisition in oneself, especially in the context of a hoarding problem, may be limited. Family members of people with hoarding problems identify excessive acquisition at a higher rate than people who self-identify with hoarding problems (Frost et al. 2009, 2013). This suggests that in some cases, a close outside observer may be better able to recognize excessive acquisition. Second, some people who present for treatment deny excessive acquiring, only to have the problem surface later during treatment (Frost et al. 2013; Steketee et al. 2010). Finally, people with hoarding problems frequently avoid their triggers for acquiring—such as stores, typical acquiring locations, and even whole cities—in an effort to control excessive acquisition (Frost et al. 2013) and as a result deny having a problem with acquiring. Patients with hoarding behaviors who deny excessive acquisition may fail to recognize it or may believe it is not a problem because they can temporarily control it by avoiding cues to acquire. Denial of acquiring problems among those with hoarding problems may reflect the belief that avoidance will solve the problem. Unfortunately, although avoidance may be effective in the short term, it is unlikely to work in the long run, since acquiring cues are ubiquitous in modern society. Consequently, very careful assessment of acquiring urges and avoidance is necessary to avoid treatment failure. It is common for patients who deny acquiring problems at the start of treatment to experience difficulties controlling acquiring urges later in treatment when they are unable to avoid acquiring cues. Continued monitoring of acquiring throughout treatment may be necessary.

These findings suggest that acquiring should be considered a core diagnostic feature of hoarding instead of a specifier. Several lines of evidence point to this conclusion. Multiple studies have found that measures of excessive acquisition are highly correlated with hoarding severity and level of impairment (Frost et al. 2009, 2013; Timpano et al. 2011). In fact, some studies have found that acquisition measures are stronger predictors of distress, general impairment, and social impairment in hoarding than difficulty discarding (Timpano et al. 2011). Furthermore, a multivariate twin study (Nordsletten et al. 2013) found that there was a substantial overlap between excessive acquisition and difficulty discarding and that both traits were heritable. Symptoms of excessive acquisition along with difficulty discarding and clutter have also been found to co-occur so strongly that they can be considered a unidimensional construct or a "cohesive hoarding phenotype" (Meyer et al. 2013). A recent network analysis of hoarding disorder symptoms and related features found that acquiring was part of a central node, although somewhat less important than difficulty discarding or clutter (Timpano et al. 2020). For these reasons, the World Health Organization included excessive acquisition as a central/core symptom of hoarding disorder in ICD-11 (Fontenelle and Grant 2014). ICD-11 defines hoarding disorder as the "accumulation of possessions due to excessive acquisition of or difficulty discarding possessions" (Burki 2018).

Onset and Course

Hoarding behaviors appear relatively early in life and then follow a chronic course. Most studies report onset between ages 15 and 19 years. A meta-analysis of all studies of hoarding onset found the average age at onset is 16.7 (Zaboski et al. 2019). Onset late in life has been reported only rarely. Since all onset studies of hoarding have been retrospective, however, these estimates vary according to the procedures used to establish them. Asking participants to "remember two significant events from each decade of their lives" before asking about hoarding symptoms during that time has produced significantly younger age-at-onset estimates—by about 10 years—than would be obtained by simply asking when the behaviors started (Ayers et al. 2010). However, only three studies of hoarding onset have used this approach (Ayers et al. 2010; Grisham et al. 2006; Tolin et al. 2010). All three concluded that onset is between ages 10 and 20 years.

Relatively few studies have examined the onset of specific features of hoarding (excessive acquisition, difficulty discarding, clutter). In these studies, a somewhat later onset has been observed for excessive acquisition compared with difficulty discarding or clutter (Frost et al. 2013; Grisham et al. 2006).

Despite a relatively early onset, the severity of hoarding symptoms increases with each decade of life and reaches moderate or greater severity by the person's late 30s or early 40s. The course of hoarding appears to be chronic. In a large sample of people with self-identified hoarding problems (*N*=751), 94% described an increasing or chronic course. Five percent reported a remitting and relapsing course, and less than 1% had a decreasing course of symptoms (Tolin et al. 2010). Hoarding increases in severity with each decade of life (Ayers et al. 2010), especially for clutter (Dozier et al. 2016), with few signs of remission (Grisham et al. 2006). Cath et al. (2017) found that the prevalence of hoarding disorder rose by 20% for every 5 years of age and that severity increased more sharply for subsequent years beginning around age 35. This increase was largely due to increases in difficulty discarding.

Life events can precipitate an increase in hoarding severity. Family and marital conflict over hoarding often result in family members moving out of their hoarding loved one's home. Once they are gone, they seldom return—not even to visit. The severity of clutter and disorganization increases dramatically when people with hoarding disorder live alone. Another inflexion point is when parents pass away, leaving the hoarding individual in possession of their parents' belongings. The sentimental valence of loved ones' possessions makes disposing of them difficult (Frost and Steketee 2010).

Trauma and other stressful life events also affect the onset, severity, and course of hoarding symptoms. Most studies show an association between trauma and hoarding symptom severity (see Shaw et al. 2016 for a review). Frost et al. (2011) found that twice as many patients with hoarding had experienced trauma as patients with OCD (49.8% vs. 24.4%), and significantly more patients with hoarding had experienced childhood trauma in particular (32.8% vs. 20.9%). Despite this difference in trauma experiences, there was no significant difference in the diagnosis of PTSD between these two groups. The relatively high percentage of patients with hoarding who experienced trauma and the relatively low percentage who developed PTSD suggest that the hoarding symptoms may have a protective effect against the development of full-blown PTSD. In one case study, PTSD symptoms only surfaced when decluttering started in the room where a sexual assault had occurred (Frost and Steketee 2010). Exposure to trauma has been found to result in greater emotional attachment to possessions (Chou et al. 2018), which is consistent with the suggestion that possessions may represent signals of safety (Frost and Hartl 1996; Gordon et al. 2013).

Stressful or traumatic events not only are associated with the severity of hoarding symptoms; there is also evidence that those events can precipitate onset of hoarding. Episodes of interpersonal violence have been found to occur more often during periods of hoarding onset and hoarding increase compared with periods of hoarding symptom stability or decrease (Tolin et al. 2010). Other commonly reported life events occurring prior to onset involve loss of possessions through fire or forced discarding (Hartl et al. 2005; Landau et al. 2011; Tolin et al. 2010). Several studies (Grisham et al. 2006; Tolin et al. 2010) have found that trauma around the time of onset is more characteristic of those with late-onset hoarding than of those with earlier onset of hoarding—suggesting a subgroup of individuals for whom trauma and stressful life events are more closely tied to hoarding symptoms. However, at least one study found traumatic life events to be more characteristic of individuals with an early onset of hoarding (Chou et al. 2018). Overall, these findings suggest that trauma may be a risk factor for the development of hoarding behaviors. Relatedly, however, several studies have failed to find an association between hoarding severity and early history of material deprivation (Frost and Gross 1993; Landau et al. 2011).

Demographics

The bulk of evidence suggests that hoarding occurs with equal frequency in men and women. Of the 10 major prevalence studies based on the current conceptualization of hoarding disorder, two found a higher prevalence in males (Iervolino et al. 2009; Mathews et al. 2014), three found a higher prevalence in females (Ivanov et al. 2013; López-Solà et al. 2014; Spittlehouse et al. 2016), and the rest found no difference (Bulli et al. 2014; Cath et al. 2017; Mueller et al. 2009; Nordsletten et al. 2013; Timpano et al. 2011). While Samuels et al. (2008) is often cited as demonstrating a higher prevalence in men, the study used the OCPD definition of difficulty discarding rather than the current conceptualization of hoarding disorder to determine hoarding status.

Despite the fact that there appears to be no clear gender difference, most of the research on the phenomena of hoarding and its treatment has relied on female participants (74%–78%). A higher percentage of men (40%–54%) are identified among community samples generated by health and human service agencies dealing with hoarding problems (Woody et al. 2020). This suggests that males are less likely to volunteer to participate in research on this topic and/or do not recognize hoarding as a problematic behavior.

People with hoarding disorder differ from those without hoarding problems on a variety of other important demographic features. Despite the early age at onset, most diagnosed cases of hoarding are among older adults. As mentioned, the severity of hoarding increases with age, particularly after age 35 (Cath et al. 2017). People with hoarding disorder are also more likely to be single, divorced, widowed, or never married than people who do not hoard (Kim et al. 2001; Nordsletten and Mataix-Cols 2012; Spittlehouse et al. 2016). This could reflect deficits in interpersonal attachment (Grisham et al. 2018; Medard and Kellett 2014) or situations in which loved ones have been driven away by the deteriorating conditions in the home. In any case, people with hoarding disorder are more likely to live alone (Archer et al. 2019). This is especially the case with severe hoarding. With no one else in the home and the accompanying reduction in visitors, the clutter gets worse and the Individual becomes more isolated (Frost and Steketee 2010).

Financial problems are also closely associated with hoarding. Although some people with hoarding disorder are wealthy, the negative correlation between hoarding severity and socioeconomic status is significant (Spittle-house et al. 2016; Tolin et al. 2008). Hoarding is associated with considerable work impairment as well as difficulties managing financial responsibility (Tolin et al. 2008). For instance, almost a quarter of people with hoarding disorder report not having filed tax returns in at least one of the previous five years (Tolin et al. 2008). The ability to find, organize, and manage documents is severely compromised in hoarding individuals. These difficulties un-doubtedly contribute to their economic woes.

Comorbidity

There is a great deal of comorbidity with other mental disorders among people with hoarding disorder (Archer et al. 2019). Comorbidity was nearly 75% for mood and/or anxiety disorders, similar to the rate in patients with OCD (Frost et al. 2011). The most closely associated disorder is major de-pressive disorder (MDD). In approximately 50% of hoarding cases, the hoarding is comorbid with MDD (Archer et al. 2019; Frost et al. 2011; Hall et al. 2013). Although in these studies hoarding did not result from the de-pression, the presence of depression influences the severity of hoarding and greatly complicates treatment, especially the motivation and activation that are necessary to overcome the disorder. In addition, there is some evidence that hoarding severity is associated with increased suicidality (Archer et al. 2019).

In a latent class analysis of a large number of people with hoarding prob-lems, Hall et al. (2013) found three patterns of diagnostic comorbidity: pure hoarding, hoarding with depression plus impulsivity, and hoarding with de-pression plus ADHD. The pure hoarding group did not have clinically sig-nificant levels of OCD, depression, or ADHD. However, this group still had more depressed mood and ADHD symptoms—as well as associated fea-tures such as indecisiveness—compared with nonclinical norms. The de-pression plus impulsivity group had high levels of depression, impulsivity, and acquiring behaviors along with poor emotion regulation strategies and higher levels of perfectionism and indecisiveness. It was suggested that this group would be more likely to use maladaptive emotion regulation strategies. The depression plus ADHD group had high levels of inattentiveness, inde-cisiveness, and cognitive failures. It also had higher levels of activities of daily living that were impaired by the clutter, suggesting that this group might be more seriously affected by their hoarding.

As suggested by the Hall et al. findings, ADHD is common in hoarding. A number of studies have confirmed the association, particularly with symptoms of inattention in adults (Frost et al. 2011; Hall et al. 2013; Hartl et al. 2005), but with children as well (Fullana et al. 2013; Hacker et al. 2016). Current—as well as childhood—inattentive symptoms of ADHD predict the core features of hoarding (difficulty discarding, excessive acquisition, clutter) in adults, while ADHD hyperactivity/impulsivity does not (Fullana et al. 2013; Tolin and Villavicencio 2011). Childhood ADHD appears to be a risk factor for later development of hoarding (Fullana et al. 2013).

A growing number of studies highlight the importance of screening all psychiatric patients for hoarding behavior. Up to a third of psychiatric inpatients have been found to display clinically significant hoarding (Basu et al. 2019). Several studies have examined the prevalence of hoarding within other disorders. Tolin et al. (2011) assessed hoarding symptoms in patients seeking treatment for anxiety disorders. Although none of the patients requested help for hoarding or mentioned hoarding during assessment, 12% of the anxious patients reported significant hoarding symptoms. Over 28% of generalized anxiety disorder (GAD) patients, nearly 17% of OCD patients, and 15% of social anxiety disorder patients scored above the clinical cutoff on the Saving Inventory—Revised (see Chapter 3 and Appendix C in this volume). Similarly, Novara et al. (2016) found significant hoarding in just over 7% of their anxiety disorder patients, despite the fact that none of these patients volunteered information about hoarding problems until specifically asked about them. It is not clear whether these patients did not report hoarding because they did not recognize it or rather because they were too embarrassed to do so.

Novara et al. (2016) found that nearly 23% of bulimia patients exceeded the hoarding symptom criterion score cutoff on the Saving Inventory—Revised, but none mentioned hoarding to their clinician. The relationship was driven primarily by the clutter dimension of hoarding. Other studies have also observed a relationship between hoarding and eating pathology, especially binge eating and obesity (Nicoli de Mattos et al. 2018; Raines et al. 2015; Tolin et al. 2008; Wheaton et al. 2008).

Although there have been reports of an association between hoarding and pathological gambling (Frost et al. 2001), more recent studies have failed to replicate this relationship (Frost et al. 2011). Only impulse-control disorders related to the acquisition of possessions (buying, acquiring free things, stealing) appear to be associated with hoarding (Frost et al. 2011). In each of these cases, the acquiring behavior is more prevalent in patients diagnosed with hoarding than in other psychiatric patients.

A substantial number of OCD patients have hoarding symptoms (Tolin et al. 2011). This overlap is difficult to interpret, however, since hoarding was considered a subtype of OCD when these estimates were obtained, and the overlap may be confounded by people whose OCD diagnosis was due to hoarding symptoms.

Comorbidity with personality disorders is common among hoarding disorder patients. Dozier et al. (2020) found at least one elevated score on the Millon Clinical Multiaxial Inventory–III (MCMI-III) in 89% of diagnosed hoarding disorder cases. More than half of the hoarding disorder participants had elevations in two or more scales. Hoarding severity in their sample predicted traits in 10 of 14 MCMI-III scales. For five of these scales (schizoid, compulsive, negativistic, masochistic, borderline), hoarding severity accounted for more than 15% of the variance.

Hoarding-Like Behaviors in Other Disorders

Hoarding-like behaviors have been observed as a direct result of other mental disorders. These are distinct from hoarding disorder in that the behavior is a direct result of the other disorder. The clearest example is the accumulation of clutter by depressed individuals due to the decrease in both their energy and their motivation to clean and organize. In such cases, the individual seldom offers objections to others managing or disposing of possessions. Likewise, cognitive deficits associated with neurocognitive disorders such as dementia or Alzheimer's disease may result in clutter and difficulty discarding, but these behaviors are a direct result of the other disorder and not considered hoarding disorder. Acquiring and saving behavior are sometimes seen in individuals with autism spectrum disorder, but the phenomenology is different in that the choice of saved items is more selective and less indiscriminate (Pertusa et al. 2012).

Confusingly, hoarding-like behaviors sometimes result from other OCD symptoms. One clear example is a person with contamination obsessions who cannot touch food containers after use. The containers may accumulate—not because of any attachment to them, but because of the fear of contamination. Several other obsessions are closely related to hoarding. Incompleteness or not-just-right experiences are often seen in both OCD and hoarding cases and can result in accumulation of possessions. These obsessions may represent overlapping phenomena and require both diagnoses (Mataix-Cols et al. 2010).

Mataix-Cols et al. (2010) have suggested questions to determine whether hoarding behavior should be considered OCD or hoarding:

1. Are the behaviors driven by prototypical obsessions such as fear of contamination or superstitions?
2. Is the hoarding unwanted or distressing? (In hoarding, the clutter may cause distress, but the decisions to save rarely do.)
3. Is there evidence of excessive acquisition, and what motivates it?

Excessive acquisition occurs in 80%–90% of hoarding cases but is seldom a factor in OCD. Also, OCD acquisition is driven by obsessions (e.g., acquiring a touched item to avoid contaminating others) and not by a genuine desire to own the specific object. In contrast, the urge to acquire in hoarding is driven by a desire for ownership.

The inclusion of hoarding disorder in DSM-5 has set the stage for major advances in research and treatment. With a standard definition and clear diagnostic criteria, research findings can be more clearly interpreted. In addition, treatment protocols can be more reliably developed and evaluated.

KEY CLINICAL POINTS

- Hoarding disorder was included as a new disorder in the most recent versions of DSM (DSM-5) and ICD (ICD-11).

- Hoarding disorder has a symptom profile, neural correlates, and associated features that differ from those of obsessive-compulsive disorder (OCD).

- Similar to OCD and other anxiety disorders, hoarding behavior is partially driven by the avoidance of distress.

- Excessive acquisition occurs in the vast majority of cases and, although not a core diagnostic feature, should be carefully monitored.

- Hoarding behavior begins relatively early in life and increases in severity with each decade.

- Hoarding disorder cases are characterized by high levels of comorbidity, including depression, ADHD, anxiety disorders, and the experience of trauma.

- Hoarding occurs with equal frequency in males and females.

- Hoarding behavior can occur in other disorders but is easily distinguishable from hoarding in hoarding disorder.

References

American Psychiatric Association. Diagnostic and Statistical Manual of Mental Disorders, 3rd Edition, Revised. Washington, DC, American Psychiatric Association, 1987

American Psychiatric Association: Diagnostic and Statistical Manual of Mental Disorders, 4th Edition, Text Revision. Washington, DC, American Psychiatric Association, 2000

American Psychiatric Association: Diagnostic and Statistical Manual of Mental Disorders, 5th Edition. Arlington, VA, American Psychiatric Association, 2013

Anderson SW, Damasio H, Damasio AR: A neural basis for collecting behaviour in humans. Brain 128 (Pt 1):201–212, 2005 15548551

Archer CA, Moran K, Garza K, et al: Relationship between symptom severity, psychiatric comorbidity, social/occupational impairment, and suicidality in hoarding disorder. J Obsessive Compuls Relat Disord 21:158–164, 2019

Ayers CR, Saxena S, Golshan S, Wetherell JL: Age at onset and clinical features of late life compulsive hoarding. Int J Geriatr Psychiatry 25(2):142–149, 2010 19548272

Basu A, Goel N, Puvvada S, Jacob T: Prevalence of hoarding in an adult inpatient population and its association with Axis I diagnoses. Am J Geriatr Psychiatry 27(5):564–568, 2019 3077345

Bloch MH, Bartley CA, Zipperer L, et al: Meta-analysis: hoarding symptoms associated with poor treatment outcome in obsessive-compulsive disorder. Mol Psychiatry 19(9):1025–1030, 2014 24912494

Bulli F, Melli G, Carraresi C, et al: Hoarding behaviour in an Italian non-clinical sample. Behav Cogn Psychother 42(3):297–311, 2014 23286647

Burki T: Hoarding disorder: a medical condition. Lancet 392(10148):626, 2018 30152334

Cath DC, Nizar K, Boomsma D, Mathews CA: Age-specific prevalence of hoarding and obsessive compulsive disorder: a population-based study. Am J Geriatr Psychiatry 25(3):245–255, 2017 27939851

Chou CY, Mackin RS, Delucchi KL, Mathews CA: Detail-oriented visual processing style: its role in the relationships between early life adversity and hoarding-related dysfunctions. Psychiatry Res 267:30–36, 2018 29883858

Dozier ME, Porter B, Ayers CR: Age of onset and progression of hoarding symptoms in older adults with hoarding disorder. Aging Ment Health 20(7):736–742, 2016 25909628

Dozier ME, Davidson EJ, Pittman JOE, Ayers CR: Personality traits in adults with hoarding disorder. J Affect Disord 276:191–196, 2020 32697698

Fontenelle LF, Grant JE: Hoarding disorder: a new diagnostic category in ICD-11? Br J Psychiatry 36 (suppl 1):28–39, 2014 25388610

Frost RO, Gross RC: The hoarding of possessions. Behav Res Ther 31(4):367–381, 1993 8512538

Frost RO, Hartl TL: A cognitive-behavioral model of compulsive hoarding. Behav Res Ther 34(4):341–350, 1996 8871366

Frost RO, Steketee G: Stuff: Compulsive Hoarding and the Meaning of Things. Boston, MA, Houghton Mifflin Harcourt, 2010

Frost RO, Meagher BM, Riskind JH: Obsessive-compulsive features in pathological lottery and scratch-ticket gamblers. J Gambl Stud 17(1):5–19, 2001 11705017

Frost RO, Tolin DF, Steketee G, et al: Excessive acquisition in hoarding. J Anxiety Disord 23(5):632–639, 2009 19261435

Frost RO, Steketee G, Tolin DF: Comorbidity in hoarding disorder. Depress Anxiety 28(10):876–884, 2011 21770000

Frost RO, Rosenfield E, Steketee G, Tolin DF: An examination of excessive acquisition in hoarding disorder. J Obsessive Compuls Relat Disord 2(3):338–345, 2013

Frost RO, Steketee G, Tolin DF, et al: Motives for acquiring and saving in hoarding disorder, OCD, and community controls. J Obsessive Compuls Relat Disord 4:54–59, 2015 25729641

Fullana MA, Vilagut G, Mataix-Cols D, et al: Is ADHD in childhood associated with lifetime hoarding symptoms? An epidemiological study. Depress Anxiety 30(8):741–748, 2013 23606213

Gordon OM, Salkovskis PM, Oldfield VB: Beliefs and experiences in hoarding. J Anxiety Disord 27(3):328–339, 2013 23602947

Grisham JR, Frost RO, Steketee G, et al: Age of onset of compulsive hoarding. J Anxiety Disord 20(5):675–686, 2006 16112837

Grisham JR, Roberts L, Cerea S, et al: The role of distress tolerance, anxiety sensitivity, and intolerance of uncertainty in predicting hoarding symptoms in a clinical sample. Psychiatry Res 267:94–101, 2018 29886277

Hacker LE, Park JM, Timpano KR, et al: Hoarding in children with ADHD. J Atten Disord 20(7):617–626, 2016 22923782

Hall BJ, Tolin DF, Frost RO, Steketee G: An exploration of comorbid symptoms and clinical correlates of clinically significant hoarding symptoms. Depress Anxiety 30(1):67–76, 2013 23213052

Hartl TL, Duffany SR, Allen GJ, et al: Relationships among compulsive hoarding, trauma, and attention-deficit/hyperactivity disorder. Behav Res Ther 43(2):269–276, 2005 15629755

Iervolino AC, Perroud N, Fullana MA, et al: Prevalence and heritability of compulsive hoarding: a twin study. Am J Psychiatry 166(10):1156–1161, 2009 19687130

Ivanov VZ, Mataix-Cols D, Serlachius E, et al: Prevalence, comorbidity and heritability of hoarding symptoms in adolescence: a population based twin study in 15-year olds. PLoS One 8(7):e69140, 2013 23874893

Kim HJ, Steketee G, Frost RO: Hoarding by elderly people. Health Soc Work 26(3):176–184, 2001 11531193

Landau D, Iervolino AC, Pertusa A, et al: Stressful life events and material deprivation in hoarding disorder. J Anxiety Disord 25(2):192–202, 2011 20934847

López-Solà C, Fontenelle LF, Alonso P, et al: Prevalence and heritability of obsessive-compulsive spectrum and anxiety disorder symptoms: a survey of the Australian Twin Registry. Am J Med Genet B Neuropsychiatr Genet 165B(4):314–325, 2014 24756981

Mataix-Cols D, Frost RO, Pertusa A, et al: Hoarding disorder: a new diagnosis for DSM-V? Depress Anxiety 27(6):556–572, 2010 20336805

Mataix-Cols D, Billotti D, Fernández de la Cruz L, Nordsletten AE: The London field trial for hoarding disorder. Psychol Med 43(4):837–847, 2013 22003395

Mathews CA, Delucchi K, Cath DC, et al: Partitioning the etiology of hoarding and obsessive-compulsive symptoms. Psychol Med 44(13):2867–2876, 2014 25066062

Medard E, Kellett S: The role of adult attachment and social support in hoarding disorder. Behav Cogn Psychother 42(5):629–633, 2014 24103104

Meyer JF, Frost RO, Brown TA, et al: A multitrait-multimethod matrix investigation of hoarding. J Obsessive Compuls Relat Disord 2(3):273–280, 2013 23814700

Mueller A, Mitchell JE, Crosby RD, et al: The prevalence of compulsive hoarding and its association with compulsive buying in a German population-based sample. Behav Res Ther 47(8):705–709, 2009 19457476

Nicoli de Mattos C, Kim HS, Lacroix E, et al: The need to consume: hoarding as a shared psychological feature of compulsive buying and binge eating. Compr Psychiatry 85:67–71, 2018 30005178

Nordsletten AE, Mataix-Cols D: Hoarding versus collecting: where does pathology diverge from play? Clin Psychol Rev 32(3):165–176, 2012 22322013

Nordsletten AE, Reichenberg A, Hatch SL, et al: Epidemiology of hoarding disorder. Br J Psychiatry 203(6):445–452, 2013 24158881

Novara C, Bottesi G, Dorz S, Sanavio E: Hoarding symptoms are not exclusive to hoarders. Front Psychol 7:1742, 2016 27891104

Pertusa A, Fonseca A: Hoarding behavior in other disorders, in The Oxford Handbook of Hoarding and Acquiring. Edited by Frost RO, Steketee G. Oxford, UK, Oxford University Press, 2014, pp 59–74

Pertusa A, Fullana MA, Singh S, et al: Compulsive hoarding: OCD symptom, distinct clinical syndrome, or both? Am J Psychiatry 165(10):1289–1298, 2008 18483134

Pertusa A, Frost RO, Mataix-Cols D: When hoarding is a symptom of OCD: a case series and implications for DSM-V. Behav Res Ther 48(10):1012–1020, 2010 20673573

Pertusa A, Bejerot S, Eriksson J, et al: Do patients with hoarding disorder have autistic traits? Depress Anxiety 29(3):210–218, 2012 22065544

Raines AM, Allan NP, Oglesby ME, et al: Specific and general facets of hoarding: a bifactor model. J Anxiety Disord 34:100–106, 2015 26210824

Samuels JF, Bienvenu OJ, Grados MA, et al: Prevalence and correlates of hoarding behavior in a community-based sample. Behav Res Ther 46(7):836–844, 2008 18495084

Shaw AM, Witcraft SM, Timpano KR: The relationship between traumatic life events and hoarding symptoms: a multi-method approach. Cogn Behav Ther 45(1):49–59, 2016 26895444

Spittlehouse JK, Vierck E, Pearson JF, Joyce PR: Personality, mental health and demographic correlates of hoarding behaviours in a midlife sample. PeerJ 4:e2826, 2016 28028484

Steketee G, Frost RO, Kyrios M: Cognitive aspects of compulsive hoarding. Cognit Ther Res 27:463–479, 2003

Steketee G, Frost RO, Tolin DF, et al: Waitlist-controlled trial of cognitive behavior therapy for hoarding disorder. Depress Anxiety 27(5):476–484, 2010 20336804

Timpano KR, Exner C, Glaesmer H, et al: The epidemiology of the proposed DSM-5 hoarding disorder: exploration of the acquisition specifier, associated features, and distress. J Clin Psychiatry 72(6):780–786, quiz 878–879, 2011 21733479

Timpano KR, Bainter SA, Goodman ZT, et al: A network analysis of hoarding symptoms, saving and acquiring motives, and comorbidity. J Obsessive Compuls Relat Disord 25:100520, 2020

Tolin DF, Villavicencio A: Inattention, but not OCD, predicts the core features of hoarding disorder. Behav Res Ther 49(2):120–125, 2011 21193171

Tolin DF, Frost RO, Steketee G, et al: The economic and social burden of compulsive hoarding. Psychiatry Res 160(2):200–211, 2008 18597855

Tolin DF, Meunier SA, Frost RO, Steketee G: Course of compulsive hoarding and its relationship to life events. Depress Anxiety 27(9):829–838, 2010 20336803

Tolin DF, Meunier SA, Frost RO, Steketee G: Hoarding among patients seeking treatment for anxiety disorders. J Anxiety Disord 25(1):43–48, 2011 20800427

Wheaton M, Timpano KR, Lasalle-Ricci VH, Murphy D: Characterizing the hoarding phenotype in individuals with OCD: associations with comorbidity, severity and gender. J Anxiety Disord 22(2):243–252, 2008 17339096

Woody SR, Lenkic P, Bratiotis C, et al: How well do hoarding research samples represent cases that rise to community attention? Behav Res Ther 126:103555, 2020 32044474

World Health Organization: International Classification of Diseases, 11th Revision (ICD-11). 2018. Available at: https://icd.who.int/en/. Accessed September 14, 2021.

Yap K, Grisham JR: Unpacking the construct of emotional attachment to objects and its association with hoarding symptoms. J Behav Addict 8(2):249–258, 2019 31112034

Zaboski BA III, Merritt OA, Schrack AP, et al: Hoarding: a meta-analysis of age of onset. Depress Anxiety 36(6):552–564, 2019 30958911

CHAPTER 3
Assessment

Highly reliable and readily obtainable instruments are available for assessing hoarding and its associated features. This chapter provides an overview of these instruments and a recommended assessment protocol for hoarding disorder. The decision to start a hoarding assessment protocol is based on requests for help or suspicion that a client is struggling with this issue. Informal observations might suggest that a more detailed assessment is warranted. If an assessment protocol is needed, it can be divided into four parts: assessing risk, conducting a diagnostic interview, assessing symptom severity, and assessing important attachments and beliefs about possessions.

Informal Observations

Informal observations can be helpful in deciding whether a more complete hoarding assessment is needed. Many people with hoarding go to great lengths to hide their symptoms, even from therapists they have engaged for other problems. Reluctance to admit a problem can hamper identification of serious hoarding conditions. Several simple observations may indicate the presence of a potential hoarding problem that deserves further assessment. Many—if not most—people with hoarding problems carry large numbers of "just-in-case" items with them (Frost and Gross 1993). Often these items require extra bags or extra-large purses, as well as extra time and effort to move from place to place. Similarly, automobiles owned by people with hoarding problems are typically cluttered, if not full to the point of not allowing passengers. Another clue that might indicate a problem is over-elaborate speech. People with hoarding problems often have trouble artic-ulating something without giving so much detail that the main theme is lost or obscured. While these observations are not foolproof, they do suggest that a closer look at the condition of the person's home is warranted.

Step 1: Assessing Risk
Clutter Image Rating

The Clutter Image Rating (CIR; Frost et al. 2008) (see Appendix B) is the quickest and most effective way to screen for hoarding problems. It takes less than 5 minutes and can be administered in the office. The CIR is a widely used measure that contains a series of pictures depicting rooms in various states of clutter. There are three rooms depicted (a living room, bed-room, and kitchen), with nine pictures of each room ranging from no clutter to clutter that covers every square foot up to eye level. The clutter pictured consists of objects typically found in hoarded homes (e.g., papers, books, clothes). Observers are asked to pick the picture that best represents the amount of clutter present in their own home in the room being evaluated. This measure was carefully constructed to create differences in clutter that are approximately equal for each interval on the scale from 1 to 9. It offers a shorthand way of evaluating the seriousness of hoarding without having to rely on self-reports of "clutter," which may vary widely based on people's interpretation of the word.

The CIR can be used by an observer visiting the home or by the client in the therapist's office. The psychometric properties of this measure are strong, with high test-retest and interrater reliabilities. Ratings by the cli-ent in the office are highly correlated with ratings by the client and an ob-server in the home (Frost et al. 2008), although in-home CIR ratings appear to be somewhat lower than those CIR ratings obtained in the clinic (Frost et al. 2008). This may reflect an overreporting bias among people seeking help for hoarding. The CIR is highly correlated with other measures of hoarding severity, especially the Clutter Scale from the Saving Inventory—Revised (Dozier and Ayers 2015; Frost et al. 2008) and the Clutter item of the Hoarding Rating Scale interview (Tolin et al. 2010). Correlations with other psychopathologies (e.g., depression, anxiety) are relatively small or nonsignificant and indicate good divergent validity (Dozier and Ayers 2015; Frost et al. 2008). A score of 4 or greater for any room is the suggested cut-off for significant hoarding (Tolin et al. 2010). The CIR appears to be sen-sitive to treatment effects (Frost and Hristova 2011; Frost et al. 2012; Tolin et al. 2007) and may be less susceptible to reporting bias than self-report measures (Frost et al. 2008). CIR means and standard deviations of diagnosed and treatment-seeking samples can be found in Table 3–1.

Activities of Daily Living—Hoarding Scale

The Activities of Daily Living—Hoarding Scale (ADL-H; Frost et al. 2013) (see Appendix E) does not measure the symptoms of hoarding; instead, it measures the effects that hoarding has on normal everyday life. The ADL-H can also be used to screen for level of risk. Fifteen activities of daily living—from everyday behaviors (e.g., eating at a table, sitting on a sofa, preparing food) to behaviors required in special circumstances (e.g., ability to exit the home quickly)—are rated for difficulty of completion using a 5-point scale. Response choices include 1=Can do it easily, 2=Can do it with a little difficulty, 3=Can do it with moderate difficulty, 4=Can do it with great difficulty, and 5=Unable to do it because of the clutter or hoarding problem. A sixteenth item (caring for pets) can be included if relevant. Because some of the items might not be relevant to everyone (e.g., doing laundry), an average score across all answered items is used to calculate the final score. The average score among people with hoarding disorder is 2.2 (SD=0.74) (Frost et al. 2013). Examination of individual item responses on the ADL-H is recommended. Any item rated 3 or above is cause for concern and should be incorporated into the treatment plan. The scale has excellent psychometric properties (Frost et al. 2013) and is sensitive to treatment effects (Frost and Hristova 2011; Frost et al. 2012; Linkovski et al. 2018). The ADL-H is one of the only measures of the impact of hoarding behaviors and has been widely used for that reason. It can be completed by an observer in the home or administered as an interview or a self-report.

Multi-disciplinary Hoarding Risk Assessment or Photographs of Home

Like the CIR, the HOMES Multi-disciplinary Hoarding Risk Assessment (Bratiotis 2009) is a brief screening device used to evaluate the level of risk in a hoarded environment. It is designed to be used in the home and accompanied by conversation with the occupant. The HOMES contains a checklist of problems in five areas of functioning: Health, Obstacles, Mental Health, Endangerment, and Structure & Safety. Checklist items in the Health and Obstacles sections indicate normal activities that are impaired by the clutter (e.g., "Cannot prepare food," "Cannot sleep in bed," "Cannot move freely/safely in home"). Checklist items in the Mental Health section

TABLE 3–1.   Clutter Image Rating means (standard deviations) and ranges for diagnosed or treatment-seeking samples

	Living room	Kitchen	Bedroom
Frost et al. 2012			
Client	3.69 (1.8)	3.36 (1.4)	4.24 (1.8)
	range 1–9	range 1–7	range 1–9
Assessor	3.47 (1.7)	3.24 (1.3)	4.13 (1.6)
	range 1–8	range 1–7	range 1–9
Frost et al. 2008			
Client	3.87 (2.24)	3.79 (2.01)	4.34 (2.16)
	range 1–9	range 1–9	range 1–9
Dozier and Ayers 2015			
Client	4.3 (2.1)	3.6 (1.9)	4.1 (2.2)

cover issues related to insight (e.g., "Does not seem to understand seriousness of problem"). The Endangerment section covers threats to vulnerable individuals (e.g., children, elders, those with disabilities, pets). The Structure & Safety section covers items related to structural damage and safety (e.g., "Flammable items beside heat source," "Leaking roof"). Additional information on household composition, level of imminent harm, and mental and physical capacity is also collected. HOMES is not a quantitative measure, so no psychometric analyses have been reported. It provides a structured approach to evaluating risk associated with hoarding and provides a good starting point for intervention.

If home visits are not feasible, photographs of the home can be a useful aid in screening, assessing risk, and diagnosing hoarding. Fernández de la Cruz et al. (2013) presented pictures of 10 homes of people in three categories: those who had hoarding, those who were "collectors" without hoarding, and those with OCD-based clutter. The professionals easily distinguished the hoarding cases from the collector cases. Sensitivity was high for both individuals with hoarding and collectors (95% and 100%, respectively), but not for those with OCD (32%). Specificity was somewhat lower but still high for both individuals with hoarding and collectors (79% and 88%) and was very high for OCD (97%). Hoarding homes were rated significantly higher than collector or OCD homes on five dimensions: amount of possessions, tidiness, functionality, number of categories, and cleanliness. The implication of these findings is that pictures can be a useful assessment strategy for identification of hoarding problems when a home visit is not feasible.

Step 2: Conducting a Diagnostic Interview

Structured Interview for Hoarding Disorder

The Structured Interview for Hoarding Disorder (SIHD; Nordsletten et al. 2013) (see Appendix A) is a semistructured clinical interview that can be used to establish a formal diagnosis of hoarding disorder. It begins with an examination of the core features (e.g., difficulty discarding), followed by an evaluation of the specifiers, and finally questions to establish a differential diagnosis with OCD. Newer versions also include a risk assessment checklist and differential diagnosis with autism spectrum disorder (Nordsletten et al. 2013). The SIHD has been shown to discriminate hoarding disorder cases with a high degree of sensitivity (correct determination of group status) and specificity (correct determination that the case did not fit the group, e.g., was not a hoarding disorder case) (Nordsletten et al. 2013). The SIHD has been translated into Italian and validated in a clinical sample (Novara et al. 2019).

Administration in the home is recommended for the SIHD. This allows for visual inspection to verify answers about clutter and impairment. If home administration is not feasible, recent photos of the living areas of the home may be a suitable substitute (Fernández de la Cruz et al. 2013). Other sources of verifying information include CIRs (Frost et al. 2008) and pictures (Fernández de la Cruz et al. 2013) provided either by people who have recently visited the home or by the respondent. Some caution is warranted if the reports are from family members who may have a bias to overinflate the severity (Tolin et al. 2010).

Some familiarity with hoarding and experience in the homes of people with hoarding disorder are important for being able to use the SIHD effectively. Many people with hoarding display overinclusive and tangential speech and are easily distracted. Consequently, administration time may be lengthy unless these problems are anticipated. Skip rules throughout the interview help to maximize efficiency.

Step 3: Assessing Symptom Severity

A number of hoarding-dedicated symptom severity measures have been developed to provide a more comprehensive assessment of hoarding severity. Some cover the full range of hoarding symptoms, while others measure a specific symptom (e.g., clutter). These dedicated symptom severity measures vary by the method of administration. Table 3–2 lists these instruments and how they are or can be administered (e.g., interview, self-report, observation).

TABLE 3–2. Methods of administration for hoarding disorder–dedicated symptom severity measures

	Method of administration		
Measure	**Self-report**	**Interview**	**Observation**
Saving Inventory—Revised	X		
Hoarding Rating Scale	X	X	
Activities of Daily Living—Hoarding	X	X	X
Clutter Image Rating	X		X
UCLA Hoarding Severity Scale		X	
Hoarding Assessment Scale	X		
HOMES			X
Children's Saving Inventory			X
Compulsive Acquiring Scale	X		
Pictures			X

Note. HOMES = HOMES Multi-disciplinary Hoarding Risk Assessment.

Saving Inventory—Revised

The most widely used self-report measure of hoarding is the Saving Inventory—Revised (SI-R; Frost et al. 2004) (see Appendix C). The SI-R is a 23-item questionnaire with three subscales: Difficulty Discarding, Excessive Acquisition, and Clutter. At least one study found a four-factor resolution that split the Excessive Acquisition items into two factors: distress-related acquiring and urge-related acquiring (Raines et al. 2015). Items on the SI-R are scored on a scale from 0 to 4, with a potential total score of 92. The number of items making up each of the three subscales varies from seven (Difficulty Discarding and Excessive Acquisition) to nine (Clutter). A considerable amount of research has been done using the SI-R since its introduction. The psychometric properties of the SI-R are good, though the factor structure varies somewhat in different populations. Internal and test-retest reliabilities are excellent (Frost et al. 2004; Kellman-McFarlane et al. 2019), and there is considerable evidence for convergent as well as divergent validity (Frost et al. 2004; Kellman-McFarlane et al. 2019). SI-R total scores are correlated with age, and females appear to score slightly higher than males (Kellman-McFarlane et al. 2019). SI-R scores are also sensitive to the effects of treatment (Ayers et al. 2018; Frost and Hristova 2011; Frost et al. 2012; Steketee et al. 2010; Tolin et al. 2007) The cutoff scores for determining clinically significant hoarding have been developed using receiver operating characteristic (ROC) curves drawn from a large number of cases originating from several major research laboratories across North America and Australia (Kellman-McFarlane et al. 2019). The ability to discriminate diagnosed hoarding cases from community controls and people with anxiety disorders was high for the total score and each of the subscales. The overall optimal cutoff for establishing significant hoarding was a total score of 39, slightly lower than the cutoff found in an earlier study using a smaller sample (Tolin et al. 2011). The sensitivity (correct determination of group status) of the total score cutoff of 39 was high (93%), while the specificity (correct determination that the case did not fit the group, i.e., was not a hoarding case) was slightly lower but still high (81%).

Because hoarding prevalence varies with age (see Chapter 1), a single cutoff does not perform equally well across the life span. Kellman-McFarlane et al. (2019) found three age cohorts with different optimal cutoffs for hoarding caseness. Cutoff scores for determining hoarding disorder decline with age. ROC optimal cutoffs for each of the subscales are shown in Table 3–3. The SI-R has been translated and evaluated for its psychometric properties in several languages, including Chinese/Mandarin, German, Greek, Italian, Portuguese, and Spanish (Fontenelle et al. 2010; Kalogeraki et al. 2020; Melli et al. 2013; Mueller et al. 2009; Novara et al. 2013; Tang et al. 2012; Timpano et al. 2015; Tortella-Feliu et al. 2006).

Hoarding Rating Scale

The Hoarding Rating Scale (HRS; Tolin et al. 2010) (see Appendix D) is a short semistructured interview containing five items that represent the major features of hoarding (difficulty discarding, excessive acquisition, clutter), as well as the problems associated with them (distress, impairment). Responses to each question are ratings on a scale from 0 (no problem) to 8 (extreme problem), with a brief description of what the rating means (e.g., "extreme, nearly all of the living spaces are difficult or impossible to use"). The HRS closely aligns with DSM-5 criteria for hoarding disorder. The interview version of the HRS (HRS-I) has excellent reliability and validity and is widely used as a screener for hoarding. Clients with hoarding problems score higher than community controls or people with OCD, and people with OCD do not differ from community controls on the measure (Tolin et al. 2010). HRS-I scores are highly correlated with the SI-R, and specific items are most highly correlated with corresponding subscales of the SI-R (e.g., Difficulty Discarding, Excessive Acquisition, Clutter). The HRS-I is also sensitive to treatment effects (Frost and Hristova 2011; Steketee et

TABLE 3–3. Receiver operating characteristic (ROC)–established cutoff scores on the Saving Inventory—Revised (SI-R) (Kellman-McFarlane et al. 2019)

Total/Subscale	≤40 years	41–60 years	>60 years
SI-R Total	43	39	33
Difficulty Discarding	15	13	12
Excessive Acquisition	11	8	9
Clutter	17	15	16

al. 2010). ROC analyses indicate that the HRS can reliably distinguish people with hoarding from people who do not hoard, with an optimal cutoff score of 14 (Tolin et al. 2010). As with the SIHD, some familiarity with hoarding disorder is helpful when using the HRS as an interview. Self-report and interview versions of the HRS both possess excellent reliability and validity. Table 3–4 presents typical HRS-I and SI-R scores obtained in diagnosed or treatment-seeking hoarding samples. Ad hoc translations of the HRS have been used in clinical and research settings to assess Spanish-speaking populations (Nordsletten et al. 2018; Rodriguez et al. 2012). The HRS has also been translated and evaluated for its psychometric properties in several languages, including Spanish, Italian, and Japanese (Faraci et al. 2019; Stamatis et al. 2021; Tsuchiyagaito et al. 2017).

Hoarding Disorder—Dimensional Scale

As part of the DSM-5 revision, the Obsessive-Compulsive Spectrum Disorders subworkgroup developed a dimensional self-report measure of hoarding symptoms modeled after the HRS. The Hoarding Disorder—Dimensional Scale (HD-D; LeBeau et al. 2013) contains five items reflecting difficulty discarding, distress, clutter, avoidance, and interference. It does not include a question about acquisition. The psychometric properties of the HD-D have been studied in college student and community samples (Carey et al. 2019; LeBeau et al. 2013), but only in a very small sample of people with hoarding (Mataix-Cols et al. 2013). The scale had a single-factor structure with good internal and test-retest reliability. It discriminated hoarding cases from community controls and showed strong correlations with other measures of hoarding and weaker correlations with nonhoarding ones. More evidence is needed using hoarding samples to validate this measure.

TABLE 3–4. Hoarding Rating Scale—Interview (HRS I) and Saving Inventory—Revised (SI-R) means (standard deviations) for diagnosed or treatment-seeking hoarding disorder samples

	Tolin et al. 2010	Steketee et al. 2010	Frost et al. 2012
HRS-I	24.2 (5.7)	28.2 (5.0)	22.5 (5.5)
SI-R: Total	67.0 (11.1)	61.7 (15.5)	61.4 (11.9)
Difficulty Discarding	22.0 (3.5)	19.8 (4.8)	19.5 (3.8)
Excessive Acquisition	15.9 (5.8)	15.0 (6.7)	15.7 (5.9)
Clutter	29.0 (5.3)	26.9 (6.8)	26.0 (5.9)

UCLA Hoarding Severity Scale

The UCLA Hoarding Severity Scale (UHSS; Saxena et al. 2015) is a 10-item semistructured interview similar to the HRS-I. It includes items reflecting the core features of hoarding (difficulty discarding, excessive acquisition, clutter), functional impairments, and several constructs closely related to hoarding (e.g., perfectionism, indecisiveness, procrastination). Thus, the total score on the UHSS is a somewhat broader measure than the SI-R or other hoarding symptom assessments. Internal consistency of the UHSS total score is good (Cronbach $\alpha=0.70$–0.81) (Ayers et al. 2013; Saxena et al. 2015). The items factor into three subscales: Core Hoarding Symptoms, Clutter and Social Impairment, and Associated Features/Functioning. The subscales were somewhat independent in that the Clutter and Social Impairment subscale did not correlate with either of the other two subscales, and the Core Hoarding Symptoms subscale only modestly correlated with the Associated Features/Functioning subscale. In contrast, the UHSS subscales correlated with all of the SI-R subscales (Saxena et al. 2015). The UHSS total score has been shown to correlate with other measures of hoarding and to distinguish hoarding disorder case individuals from controls (Dozier and Ayers 2015; Saxena et al. 2015). The UHSS has also been shown to be sensitive to treatment effects, including cognitive-behavioral therapy (Ayers et al. 2014) and pharmacotherapy (Saxena and Sumner 2014; Saxena et al. 2007). Saxena and Sumner (2014) describe ongoing efforts to develop a new version of the UHSS (the UHSS-II) that more closely matches the DSM-5 criteria for hoarding disorder.

Hoarding Assessment Scale

The Hoarding Assessment Scale (HAS; Schneider et al. 2008) is a four-item questionnaire with questions on difficulty discarding, clutter, urges to acquire, and functional impairment. A detailed description of each is provided to improve the accuracy of the ratings. Ratings are made on an 11-point scale based on the extent to which this symptom bothered the person during the past week—from "not at all" to "extremely." The HAS has good internal consistency and is significantly correlated with the SI-R and its subscales, but correlations with the Florida Obsessive-Compulsive Inventory hoarding items are small (Schneider et al. 2008). Little else is known about this measure.

Self-report questionnaires and interviews designed to assess hoarding and its severity are no substitute for a visit to the home to observe firsthand the clutter and its effects on the lives of the people in the home. Many people with hoarding problems have difficulty recognizing the nature and extent of their hoarding. Only a walk-through of their home with them can give a full picture of the level of severity. There are several assessment strategies that will help to make the evaluation systematic.

Children's Saving Inventory

Only one instrument has been developed to assess hoarding in children—the Children's Saving Inventory (CSI; Storch et al. 2011). The 21-item scale is designed to be completed by a parent or guardian. It is patterned after the SI-R. The four subscales correspond to those of the SI-R and HRS: Difficulty Discarding, Excessive Acquisition, Clutter, and Distress/Impairment. The total score and subscales have strong internal consistency and test-retest reliability, and they are strongly correlated with other measures of hoarding and less highly correlated with nonhoarding constructs (Storch et al. 2011). A recent attempt to revise the CSI removed the acquisition items to make it more consistent with DSM-5 criteria (Soreni et al. 2018). While the psychometric properties of this revised measure are good, the absence of information about acquisition limits its utility.

Compulsive Acquisition Scale

Excessive acquisition of possessions is a major feature of hoarding disorder (see Chapter 2). Recent findings suggest that 90% or more of people with hoarding disorder acquire in excess, either through compulsive buying or by acquiring free things (Mataix-Cols et al. 2013). Without a careful and thorough assessment of this feature of hoarding, efforts to understand and treat the disorder will be limited. Although there are several existing measures of compulsive buying, only one includes a measure of excessive acquisition of free things. The

Compulsive Acquisition Scale (CAS; Frost et al. 2009) is an 18-item questionnaire measuring both excessive buying and excessive acquisition of free things. The 12-item Buying subscale refers to the effect of buying on financial health, frequency of inappropriate buying (of things never used), and emotional reactions to buying. The 6-item CAS-Free subscale contains items related to feeling compelled to collect free things. These subscales have good internal consistency as well as convergent and divergent validity (Frost et al. 2004). Having separate indices for buying and free acquisition appears to be important. Evidence suggests that the CAS-Free subscale predicts a unique variance related to hoarding and psychiatric impairment (Williams 2012). The factor structure of the CAS appears to vary somewhat in different countries (Faraci et al. 2018; Mueller et al. 2010).

Squalor Measures: Environmental Cleanliness and Clutter Scale and Home Environment Index

A small percentage of people with hoarding live in unsanitary or squalid conditions. Several squalor measures have been developed for use in hoarding cases. The Environmental Cleanliness and Clutter Scale (ECCS; Halliday and Snowdon 2009) is a 10-item scale measuring environmental conditions in the home. The scale includes items depicting hoarding in addition to squalor and precludes a pure assessment of squalor. The 15 items on the Home Environment Index (HEI; Rasmussen et al. 2014) focus on cleanliness in the home, daily cleaning behaviors, and personal hygiene and are rated from 0 (no squalor or symptoms) to 3 (severe symptoms), with specific descriptors for each response choice. The Daily Behaviors section is also scored from 0 to 3 based on the frequency of the behavior (never performed to nearly daily performance). The HEI has demonstrated good reliability and validity. It is highly correlated with hoarding severity and associated to a lesser extent with nonhoarding psychopathology (depression and anxiety symptoms). See Chapter 13 for more information on squalor in hoarding.

Step 4: Assessing Attachments to and Beliefs About Possessions

While difficulty discarding is the core feature of hoarding disorder, it is determined by motives for saving possessions. Strongly held attachments to and beliefs about possessions make discarding them difficult. In general, people with hoarding problems generate more reasons to save possessions than people who do not hoard, but they do not generate fewer reasons to discard

(Frost et al. 1995). Motives to save possessions do not differ in kind from those of people who do not hoard; however, they are more rigidly held and applied to a wider range of possessions (Frost and Gross 1993). A number of measures have been developed to capture these attachments and beliefs.

Saving Cognitions Inventory

The Saving Cognitions Inventory (SCI; Steketee et al. 2003) is a 24-item questionnaire that measures beliefs about possessions. Four types of beliefs have been identified by factor analyses of this scale. The Emotional Attachment subscale reflects the wide variety of emotions that are tied up with possessions. Items in this subscale include feeling that possessions are part of one's identity and discarding them would mean losing a piece of oneself. Also included are feelings of comfort provided by the possession. The Memory subscale reflects concerns about forgetting or losing important information if the item is discarded. Beliefs about control include negative reactions to having one's possessions taken, moved, or even touched by others. Beliefs about responsibility involve concerns over wasting opportunities and not being prepared if items are discarded. Typical scores on the SCI subscales of people with hoarding can be found in Table 3–5.

The SCI has shown good reliability and validity in a variety of studies. Each of the subscales discriminates people with hoarding problems from community controls and people with OCD. The subscales are highly correlated with hoarding symptoms and remain so when depression and OCD symptoms are controlled for (Steketee et al. 2003). The SCI is also sensitive to treatment effects (Frost and Hristova 2011; Frost et al. 2012), and there is evidence that changes in these beliefs mediate changes in symptoms during treatment (Levy et al. 2017). Treatment for hoarding disorder is largely designed to change these beliefs and to loosen attachments to possessions. This should reduce difficulty discarding and lessen excessive acquisition, which in turn should help reduce the level of clutter in the home. Without changes in these attachments and beliefs, lasting change in symptoms is unlikely.

Other Measures

Several other targeted measures of attachments and beliefs have been developed, though few of them have been well validated. One set of beliefs that is not captured by the SCI comprises beliefs that lead to the saving of things that the individual is not attached to and does not want. The rationale behind this motive for saving is moral or ethical, reminiscent of scrupulosity beliefs in OCD (Frost and Steketee 2010). Frost et al. (2018) labeled this phenomenon as "material scrupulosity" and defined it as "a set of rigid beliefs that include an exaggerated sense of duty or moral/ethical responsibility for the

TABLE 3–5. Saving Cognitions Inventory (SCI) means (standard deviations) for diagnosed or treatment-seeking samples

SCI subscale	Frost et al. 2012 N=53	Chou et al. 2018 N=104	Dozier and Ayers 2017 N=84
Emotional Attachment	42.3 (14.4)	37.4 (14.5)	37.0 (13.5)
Responsibility	25.2 (7.9)	23.6 (8.6)	24.6 (7.6)
Memory	22.4 (7.3)	19.1 (6.9)	21.0 (5.5)
Control	16.2 (4.3)	16.4 (3.8)	15.8 (4.2)

care and disposition of possessions to prevent their being harmed or wasted" (p. 20). This is similar to some of the items in the Responsibility subscale of the SCI, but that subscale does not contain the moral or ethical emphasis seen in anecdotal accounts of hoarding (Frost and Steketee 2010).

Measure of Material Scrupulosity

The Measure of Material Scrupulosity (MOMS; Frost et al. 2018) contains nine items, each scored on a 5-point scale. The items emphasize the sense of duty, morality, and guilt related to wasting or harming possessions. The MOMS has shown good internal consistency and was strongly correlated with the SI-R—especially the Difficulty Discarding subscale—in both non-clinical and clinical samples (Frost et al. 2018). MOMS scores predict hoarding severity, especially for difficulty discarding, independent of OCD, OCD-related scrupulosity, and SCI Responsibility scores.

Object Attachment Scale

A similar measure to the SCI is the Object Attachment Scale (OAS; Grisham et al. 2009). The OAS contains 13 items reflecting emotional responses and attitudes toward possessions, including anthropomorphism, identity, and responsibility. In the limited research on this measure, it has shown good reliability and validity and can predict future discarding behavior (Norberg et al. 2015).

Possessions Comfort Scale

The Possessions Comfort Scale (PCS; Hartl et al. 2005) is a 31-item questionnaire assessing the emotional comfort provided by possessions for people with hoarding problems. It contains items related to physical and emotional comfort, vulnerability, and loneliness. Examples are "I feel like my possessions create a protective wall around me" and "Being surrounded by my possessions makes me feel physically comfortable." Response choices range from 1 (strongly disagree) to 7 (strongly agree). The PCS has excellent internal consistency, and people with hoarding problems score significantly higher than community controls (Hartl et al. 2005).

Possessions in View

The Possessions in View (PIV; Hartl et al. 2004) is an 11-item questionnaire designed to assess the extent to which people keep their belongings in sight as visual cues for memory retrieval. Items include "I cannot remember something unless I keep a possession in sight to remind me of it" and "If I put something in storage, I will forget I own it." Items are scored from 1 to 5 (strongly disagree to strongly agree). The scale has good internal consistency, and PIV scores distinguished hoarding from nonhoarding individuals even when differences in confidence in memory were controlled for (Hartl et al. 2004).

Measure of Areas of Overlap to Assess Relationship to Possessions

Dozier et al. (2017) used a series of circles with increasing areas of overlap and asked respondents to indicate which circles best described their relationship to their possessions. Although the measure distinguished a hoarding group from community controls, it was only weakly correlated with existing measures of hoarding and needs further testing to establish adequate validity.

Anthropomorphism Questionnaire

People with hoarding disorder frequently cite the concern of hurting a possession by discarding it as a reason to save things. Although anthropomorphizing objects is normative, people with hoarding disorder appear to experience possessions as having human characteristics more intensely than other people do (Burgess et al. 2018; Neave et al. 2015, 2016). Several measures have been developed to capture this feature in hoarding disorder. Neave et al. (2015) developed the Anthropomorphism Questionnaire (AQ) for use in hoarding cases. The 20-item AQ contains both Current (10 items) and Child (10 items) subscales. Items on the AQ reflect general anthropomorphism, with a few questions about personally owned objects. The Child items focus on toys in early youth, while the Current items focus on attitudes toward technology, nature, and everyday objects. Both subscales show excellent reliability and correlate with other measures of anthropomorphism as well as measures of hoarding.

Graves Anthropomorphism Task Scale

Since people with hoarding disorder develop object-specific attachments to possessions, Burgess et al. set out to develop an anthropomorphism measure that focuses specifically on personally owned objects: the Graves Anthropomorphism Task Scale (GATS; Burgess et al. 2018). Respondents are asked to choose three possessions: their most frustrating technological possession, their favorite comfort object, and a past or present pet. They are then asked 15 questions about each. The questions all pertain to human characteristics of that particular possession (e.g., "I treat X like a human," "X can be lonely without me"). All three subscales showed excellent reliability. The Tech and Comfort subscales were strongly correlated with the AQ and with measures of hoarding symptoms and beliefs. The Pets subscale was only weakly correlated with the AQ and measures of hoarding.

Early Measures of Hoarding

Because hoarding was once thought to be a subtype of OCD, the earliest measures of hoarding are found in omnibus measures of OCD that include a few items about hoarding (e.g., Yale-Brown Obsessive Compulsive Scale [Y-BOCS]). Such measures are not recommended for clinical assessment because they rely on earlier and inaccurate conceptualizations of hoarding and they do not cover the full range of hoarding symptoms. However, there are several comorbid disorders that may need assessing, including obsessive-compulsive disorder, depression, and ADHD. These disorders are highly comorbid with hoarding and may need attention during treatment.

Case Example

John was a 57-year-old man who reported struggling with hoarding and depression for much of his life. He had been in therapy for depression for more than 10 years and was also on medication for it (Effexor). He reported attending a hoarding support group for at least a year, but he still struggled with the problem. John was married and had a high school education. He had worked for a number of years as a custodian but was now on disability with an income of less than $10,000 per year. When he applied for treatment, the initial assessment consisted of the HRS-I, SI-R, SCI, ADL, and CIR. John's HRS-I score was 21, which was well above the hoarding cutoff of 14 and similar to the scores of others in treatment for hoarding (see Table 3–4).

He scored above 4 on each of the core feature items as well as the distress and interference items. His SI-R total score of 67 was also well above the recommended maximum of 39 points for his age group (see Table 3–3). The SI-R subscale scores (Difficulty Discarding=22, Excessive Acquisition=21, Clutter=24) were also well above the established cutoffs (see Table 3–3).

John's therapist-rated CIR from the home visit was 3.67 for the main living areas (living room, kitchen, bedroom). The most significant clutter was in the bedroom, with a CIR score of 6, which matched John's self-reported CIR rating for that room. A CIR rating of 6 reflects clutter that would make any activity in the room extremely difficult. The ratings for the living room (3) and kitchen (2) indicated less severe clutter.

John's ADL-H score was 2.57, well above the severity cutoff. Examination of the individual items indicated that because of the hoarding, only 2 of the 15 activities could be done without difficulty. Five activities were problematic for him. Sitting on a chair or sofa was moderately difficult (rating of 3). Using the refrigerator, eating at a table, and moving freely about the house could only be done with great difficulty (rating of 4). Most importantly, he was unable to find important paper documents in his home (rating of 5) because of the clutter. Knowledge about the difficulty of these activities was used to establish his treatment goals.

John's SCI reflected a mixed pattern of attachments to possessions. His scores on emotional attachments to possessions (34) and his beliefs about the need to keep objects as memory aids (28) were both very high and were comparable to, if not higher than, those seen in studies of people with hoarding disorder (see Table 3–5). His scores on responsibility and control (11 and 10, respectively) were substantially lower than those of most people with hoarding disorder and comparable to values seen in nonclinical samples (Steketee et al. 2003). This mixed pattern of attachments helped to shape the focus of treatment.

Conclusion

Hoarding is a complex disorder and requires a careful assessment of impairments, symptoms, and motives for saving. There now exist a host of well-validated and frequently used assessments for hoarding disorder. They range in content and procedures and can be implemented easily, even for cases in which home visits are not feasible. We recommend a four-step assessment protocol when preparing for hoarding disorder treatment (see Table 3–6 for an outline). The first step should always be an assessment of risk. Three of the instruments reviewed here are useful for this purpose: the CIR, the HOMES, and the ADL-H. All will provide a clear sense of the hoarding symptoms' level of danger to the client, their family members,

TABLE 3–6.   Recommended assessment protocol when preparing for
              hoarding disorder treatment

Step 1: Assess risk

Clutter Image Rating

Multi-disciplinary Hoarding Risk Assessment

Activities of Daily Living—Hoarding Scale

Step 2: Conduct a diagnostic interview

Structured Interview for Hoarding Disorder

Hoarding Rating Scale—Interview

Step 3: Assess symptom severity

Saving Inventory—Revised

UCLA Hoarding Severity Scale

Compulsive Acquisition Scale

Step 4: Assess attachments to and beliefs about possessions and motives

Saving Cognitions Inventory

Object Attachment Scale

Measure of Material Scrupulosity

Possessions Comfort Scale

Possessions in View

and neighbors. The information gained from these instruments will clarify whether immediate action is warranted before starting treatment. The second step is a diagnostic interview. The gold standard for this is the SIHD. One shorter option is to use the HRS-I, supplemented with a clinical interview, to rule out other disorders as the cause of the hoarding behavior. The third step is to assess hoarding severity with several easy-to-administer instruments. The most well-validated is the SI-R, which provides a general quantitative index of severity as well as scores on each of the three main features of hoarding (difficulty discarding, excessive acquisition, clutter). Having an index of severity for each of these features will provide a baseline with which to monitor progress in treatment. The UHSS is an alternative that also provides assessment of several related difficulties. Additional information can be collected with instruments that target specific features of hoarding, such as clutter (CIR) and excessive acquisition (CAS). The fourth step is to obtain information on the motives for hoarding. A number of instruments have been developed for this purpose. These not only can be useful in understanding the nature of the client's difficulties but also can help to frame the focus of therapy and to create strategies to modify beliefs about and attachments to possessions. Decisions about which ones to administer should be guided by the needs of the individual client.

KEY CLINICAL POINTS

- A four-step assessment protocol is recommended for hoarding cases: assessing risk, conducting a diagnostic interview, assessing symptom severity, and assessing attachments to and beliefs about possessions.

- Home visits are strongly recommended for the assessment of hoarding, although when they are not feasible, photographs of the home may be useful.

- The Structured Interview for Hoarding Disorder is the gold standard for diagnosis of the disorder.

- Hoarding subscales of existing measures of OCD are not recommended for more than initial screening purposes.

- Several well-validated symptom severity measures are available to assess hoarding, including the Saving Inventory—Revised and the Hoarding Rating Scale.

- Assessment of the frequency and intensity of excessive acquisition (e.g., buying, free acquisition, stealing) is an important part of preparation for treatment.

- Assessment of the motives for saving, including attachments to and beliefs about possessions, is necessary for treatment planning.

- In some cases, evaluation of sanitation in the home is warranted as part of the assessment of risk.

References

Ayers CR, Wetherell JL, Schiehser D, et al: Executive functioning in older adults with hoarding disorder. Int J Geriatr Psychiatry 28(11):1175–1181, 2013 23440720

Ayers CR, Saxena S, Espejo E, et al: Novel treatment for geriatric hoarding disorder: an open trial of cognitive rehabilitation paired with behavior therapy. Am J Geriatr Psychiatry 22(3):248–252, 2014 23831173

Ayers CR, Dozier ME, Twamley EW, et al: Cognitive rehabilitation and exposure/sorting therapy (CREST) for hoarding disorder in older adults: a randomized clinical trial. J Clin Psychiatry 79(2):16m11072, 2018 28541646

Bratiotis C: HOMES Multi-disciplinary Hoarding Risk Assessment. 2009. Available at: https://vet.tufts.edu/wp-content/uploads/HOMES_SCALE.pdf. Accessed February 27, 2020.

Burgess AM, Graves LM, Frost RO: My possessions need me: anthropomorphism and hoarding. Scand J Psychol 59(3):340–348, 2018

Carey E, Bolger A, Wootton B: Psychometric properties of the Hoarding Disorder—Dimensional Scale. J Obsessive Compuls Relat Disord 21:91–96, 2019

Chou CY, Mackin RS, Delucchi KL, Mathews CA: Detail-oriented visual processing style: its role in the relationships between early life adversity and hoarding-related dysfunctions. Psychiatry Res 267:30–36, 2018 29883858

Dozier ME, Ayers CR: Validation of the Clutter Image Rating in older adults with hoarding disorder. Int Psychogeriatr 27(5):769–776, 2015 25391419

Dozier ME, Ayers CR: The etiology of hoarding disorder: a review. Psychopathology 50(5):291–296, 2017 28810245

Dozier ME, Taylor CT, Castriotta N, et al: A preliminary investigation of the measurement of object interconnectedness in hoarding disorder. Cognit Ther Res 41:799–805, 2017 32669747

Faraci P, Perdighe C, Del Monte C, Saliani AM: Reliability, validity and factor structure of the Compulsive Acquisition Scale (CAS). Clin Neuropsychiatry 15(1):42–49, 2018

Faraci P, Perdighe C, Del Monte CS, Saliani A: Hoarding Rating Scale—Interview (HRS-I): reliability and construct validity in a nonclinical sample. International Journal of Psychology and Psychological Therapy 19:345–352, 2019

Fernández de la Cruz L, Nordsletten AE, Billotti D, Mataix-Cols D: Photograph-aided assessment of clutter in hoarding disorder: is a picture worth a thousand words? Depress Anxiety 30(1):61–66, 2013 22930673

Fontenelle IS, Prazeres AM, Borges MC, et al: The Brazilian Portuguese version of the Saving Inventory—Revised: internal consistency, test-retest reliability, and validity of a questionnaire to assess hoarding. Psychol Rep 106(1):279–296, 2010 20402454

Frost RO, Gross RC: The hoarding of possessions. Behav Res Ther 31(4):367–381, 1993 8512538

Frost RO, Hristova V: Assessment of hoarding. J Clin Psychol 67(5):456–466, 2011 21351103

Frost RO, Steketee G: Stuff: Compulsive Hoarding and the Meaning of Things. Boston, MA, Houghton Mifflin Harcourt, 2010

Frost RO, Hartl TL, Christian R, Williams N: The value of possessions in compulsive hoarding: patterns of use and attachment. Behav Res Ther 33(8):897–902, 1995 7487849

Frost RO, Steketee G, Grisham J: Measurement of compulsive hoarding: saving inventory-revised. Behav Res Ther 42(10):1163–1182, 2004 15350856

Frost R, Steketee G, Tolin D, Renaud S: Development and validation of the Clutter Image Rating. J Psychopathol Behav Assess 30(3):193–203, 2008

Frost RO, Tolin DF, Steketee G, et al: Excessive acquisition in hoarding. J Anxiety Disord 23(5):632–639, 2009 19261435

Frost RO, Steketee G, Tolin DF: Diagnosis and assessment of hoarding disorder. Annu Rev Clin Psychol 8:219–242, 2012 22035242

Frost RO, Hristova V, Steketee G, Tolin DF: Activities of Daily Living Scale in hoarding disorder. J Obsessive Compuls Relat Disord 2(2):85–90, 2013 23482436

Frost RO, Gabrielson I, Deady S, et al: Scrupulosity and hoarding. Compr Psychiatry 86:19–24, 2018 30041077

Grisham JR, Frost RO, Steketee G, et al: Formation of attachment to possessions in compulsive hoarding. J Anxiety Disord 23(3):357–361, 2009 19201154

Halliday G, Snowdon J: The Environmental Cleanliness and Clutter Scale (ECCS). Int Psychogeriatr 21(6):1041–1050, 2009 19589191

Hartl TL, Frost RO, Allen GJ, et al: Actual and perceived memory deficits in individuals with compulsive hoarding. Depress Anxiety 20(2):59–69, 2004 15390215

Hartl TL, Duffany SR, Allen GJ, et al: Relationships among compulsive hoarding, trauma, and attention-deficit/hyperactivity disorder. Behav Res Ther 43(2):269–276, 2005 15629755

Kalogeraki L, Vitoratou S, Tsaltas E, et al: Factor structure and psychometric properties of the Greek version of Saving Inventory-Revised (SI-R) in a non-clinical sample. Psychiatriki 31(2):105–117, 2020 32840215

Kellman-McFarlane K, Stewart B, Woody S, et al: Saving Inventory—Revised: psychometric performance across the lifespan. J Affect Disord 252:358–364, 2019 30999092

LeBeau R, Mischel E, Simpson H, et al: Preliminary assessment of obsessive–compulsive spectrum disorder scales for DSM-5. J Obsessive Compuls Relat Disord 2:114–118, 2013

Levy HC, Worden BL, Gilliam CM, et al: Changes in saving cognitions mediate hoarding symptom change in cognitive-behavioral therapy for hoarding disorder. J Obsessive Compuls Relat Disord 14:112–118, 2017 29170732

Linkovski O, Zwerling J, Cordell E, et al: Augmenting Buried in Treasures with in-home uncluttering practice: pilot study in hoarding disorder. J Psychiatr Res 107:145–150, 2018 30419524

Mataix-Cols D, Billotti D, Fernández de la Cruz L, Nordsletten AE: The London field trial for hoarding disorder. Psychol Med 43(4):837–847, 2013 22883395

Melli G, Chiorri C, Smurra R, Frost R: Psychometric properties of the paper-and-pencil and online versions of the Italian Saving Inventory—Revised in nonclinical samples. Int J Cogn Ther 6:40–56, 2013

Mueller A, Crosby RD, Frost RO, et al: Fragebogen zum zwanghaften Horten (FZH)—Validierung der deutschen Version des Saving Inventory—Revised (German Compulsive Hoarding Inventory [FZH]—Evaluation of the German version of the Saving Inventory—Revised). Verhaltenstherapie 19(4):243–250, 2009

Mueller A, Crosby RD, Linsenbühler S, et al: Evaluation of the German version of the Compulsive Acquisition Scale. Zeitschrift für Klinische Psychologie und Psychotherapie: Forschung und Praxis 39(3):161–169, 2010

Neave N, Jackson R, Saxton T, Hönekopp J: The influence of anthropomorphic tendencies on human hoarding behaviors. Pers Individ Dif 72:214–219, 2015

Neave N, Tyson H, McInnes L, Hamilton C: The role of attachment style and anthropomorphism in predicting hoarding behaviours in a non-clinical sample. Pers Individ Dif 99:33–37, 2016

Norberg MM, Keyan D, Grisham JR: Mood influences the relationship between distress intolerance and discarding. J Obsessive Compuls Relat Disord 6:77–82, 2015

Nordsletten AE, Fernández de la Cruz L, Pertusa A, et al: The Structured Interview for Hoarding Disorder (SIHD): development, usage and further validation. J Obsessive Compuls Relat Disord 2(3):346–350, 2013

Nordsletten AE, Fernández de la Cruz L, Aluco E, et al: A transcultural study of hoarding disorder: insights from the United Kingdom, Spain, Japan, and Brazil. Transcult Psychiatry 55(2):261–285, 2018 29508639

Novara C, Bottesi G, Dorz S, Pastore M: The Saving Inventory—Revised (SI-R): study of the validity of the three-factor structure in Italian community samples. Psicoterapia Cognitiva e Comportamentale 19:309–322, 2013

Novara C, Cavedini P, Dorz S, et al: Structured Interview for Hoarding Disorder (SIHD): an Italian validation with diagnosed clinical patients. Eur J Psychol Assess 35(4):512–520, 2019

Raines AM, Allan NP, Oglesby ME, et al: Specific and general facets of hoarding: a bifactor model. J Anxiety Disord 34:100–106, 2015 26210824

Rasmussen JL, Steketee G, Frost RO, et al: Assessing squalor in hoarding: the Home Environment Index. Community Ment Health J 50(5):591–596, 2014 24292497

Rodriguez CI, Herman D, Alcon J, et al: Prevalence of hoarding disorder in individuals at potential risk of eviction in New York City: a pilot study. J Nerv Ment Dis 200(1):91–94, 2012 22210369

Saxena S, Sumner J: Venlafaxine extended-release treatment of hoarding disorder. Int Clin Psychopharmacol 29(5):266–273, 2014 24722633

Saxena S, Brody AL, Maidment KM, Baxter LR Jr: Paroxetine treatment of compulsive hoarding. J Psychiatr Res 41(6):481–487, 2007 16790250

Saxena S, Ayers CR, Dozier ME, Maidment KM: The UCLA Hoarding Severity Scale: development and validation. J Affect Disord 175:488–493, 2015 25681559

Schneider A, Storch E, Geffken G, et al: Psychometric properties of the Hoarding Assessment Scale in college students. Illness, Crisis & Loss 16:227–236, 2008

Soreni N, Cameron D, Vorstenbosch V, et al: Psychometric evaluation of a revised scoring approach for the Children's Saving Inventory in a Canadian sample of youth with obsessive-compulsive disorder. Child Psychiatry Hum Dev 49(6):966–973, 2018 29797231

Stamatis CA, Muroff J, Bocanegra ES, et al: A Spanish Translation of the Hoarding Rating Scale: differential item functioning and convergent validity. J Psychopathol Behav Assess 43(4):946–959, 2021

Steketee G, Frost RO, Kyrios M: Cognitive aspects of compulsive hoarding. Cognit Ther Res 27:463–479, 2003

Steketee G, Frost RO, Tolin DF, et al: Waitlist-controlled trial of cognitive behavior therapy for hoarding disorder. Depress Anxiety 27(5):476–484, 2010 20336804

Storch EA, Muroff J, Lewin AB, et al: Development and preliminary psychometric evaluation of the Children's Saving Inventory. Child Psychiatry Hum Dev 42(2):166–182, 2011 20886284

Tang T, Wang J, Tang S, Zhao L: Psychometric properties of the Saving Inventory—Revised in Chinese university students sample. Chin J Clin Psychol 20(1):21–24, 2012

Timpano KR, Çek D, Fu ZF, et al: A consideration of hoarding disorder symptoms in China. Compr Psychiatry 57:36–45, 2015 25483851

Tolin DF, Frost RO, Steketee G: An open trial of cognitive-behavioral therapy for compulsive hoarding. Behav Res Ther 45(7):1461–1470, 2007 17306221

Tolin DF, Frost RO, Steketee G: A brief interview for assessing compulsive hoarding: the Hoarding Rating Scale—Interview. Psychiatry Res 178(1):147–152, 2010 20452042

Tolin DF, Meunier SA, Frost RO, Steketee G: Hoarding among patients seeking treatment for anxiety disorders. J Anxiety Disord 25(1):43–48, 2011 20800427

Tortella-Feliu M, Fullana MA, Caseras X, et al: Spanish version of the Savings Inventory—Revised: adaptation, psychometric properties, and relationship to personality variables. Behav Modif 30(5):693–712, 2006 16894237

Tsuchiyagaito A, Horiuchi S, Igarashi T, et al: Factor structure, reliability, and validity of the Japanese version of the Hoarding Rating Scale—Self-Report (HRS-SR-J). Neuropsychiatr Dis Treat 13:1235–1243, 2017 28533685

Williams AD: Quality of life and psychiatric work impairment in compulsive buying: increased symptom severity as a function of acquisition behaviors. Compr Psychiatry 53(6):822–828, 2012 22197214

CHAPTER 4
Insight and Motivation

Gold-standard treatments for obsessive-compulsive disorder (OCD) such as exposure and response prevention and medication have not fared well when used to treat hoarding (Abramowitz et al. 2003; Matsunaga et al. 2010; Rufer et al. 2006). Treatments designed specifically for hoarding have fared better (Bodryzlova et al. 2019; Muroff et al. 2011; Steketee 2014). However, although clients are significantly improved following hoarding-specific treatment, many still display functional impairment because of their hoarding (Tolin et al. 2015). Many authors have speculated that the poorer response to treatment is a result of limited insight and poor motivation to change (Abramowitz et al. 2003; Saxena and Maidment 2004). Poor insight might also explain a delay in seeking treatment (Damecour and Charron 1998) and the relatively high dropout rates in hoarding treatment (Mataix-Cols et al. 2002). Low or fluctuating motivation during treatment that is observed among individuals with hoarding problems might also be related to poor insight (Hartl and Frost 1999; Tolin et al. 2007). This chapter will explore insight and motivation for change in hoarding disorder.

Level of Insight in Hoarding Disorder
Poor Problem Recognition (Anosognosia)

Poor insight can be defined in several ways in the context of hoarding (Frost et al. 2010). Anosognosia is the most basic form of poor insight and refers to a lack of awareness of the severity of a problem. This form of lack of insight is most often used in conjunction with disorders such as schizophrenia, dementia, and other neurocognitive disorders (Amador et al. 1994; Galeone et al. 2011). In hoarding disorder, anosognosia includes lack of recognition of the negative consequences of excessive acquisition, difficulty discarding, and/or excessive clutter. Complicating this picture is that it may be possible to recognize a symptom (e.g., excessive acquisition, excessive clutter) while not recognizing it is a problem (i.e., it is possible to recognize clutter yet not see it as a problem). A similar variant of this is an indifference to symptoms. In other words, the individual may recognize that the behaviors are problematic but be indifferent to the consequences. The DSM-5 insight specifier for hoarding disorder is in line with the anosognosia concept and focuses on the recognition of the extent to which the hoarding beliefs and behaviors are problematic (American Psychiatric Association, 2013, p. 247).

Studies that examine the recognition of a problem—in hoarding samples—have shown a confusing picture. Kim et al. (2001) interviewed elder service caseworkers about their hoarding clients. The majority of the clients were judged by their service provider as having no insight (73%) or little insight (12%). Only 15% of the case clients were judged to acknowledge the irrationality of their hoarding behavior. Frost et al. (2000) surveyed health department personnel about hoarding complaints that led to action by local health departments in Massachusetts. Despite serious levels of squalor, only half of identified individuals acknowledged the lack of sanitation, and fewer than a third willingly cooperated with authorities to remedy the situation.

Research done on family and friend informants also suggests problems with recognition of the negative consequences of hoarding behaviors. Tolin et al. (2010) surveyed a large number ($N > 500$) of family and friends of individuals with hoarding problems about their loved one's level of insight. The measure used conformed closely to the anosognosia definition of insight. Informants were told: "We would like to know just how clearly (your loved one) recognizes the problem he/she has with hoarding." They were first asked to rate their loved one's insight on a question adapted from the Yale-Brown Obsessive Compulsive Scale (Y-BOCS) interview. There were five response choices along with an explanation of each (Table 4–1). The mean scores of family and friend informants' judgments of their hoarding loved ones were between "fair" and "poor" insight. More telling, however, is that

TABLE 4–1. Hoarding Insight (Problem Recognition) Scale

Score	Label	Description
0	Excellent, fully rational	Fully recognizes that hoarding behavior is a problem, even though it may be bad.
1	Good insight	Readily acknowledges that their acquisition, clutter, and/ or difficulty discarding is a problem. However, when at home or out shopping/acquiring, has difficulty seeing the problem with acquiring and discarding.
2	Fair insight	May admit clutter is a problem but only reluctantly admits that their behavior has caused the problem. When at home or out shopping/acquiring, has difficulty seeing that they have a problem with acquiring or discarding.
3	Poor insight	Maintains that acquisition, difficulty discarding, and clutter are under control or not a problem. When discussing the problem, acknowledges that they might have a problem, but still underestimates the severity.
4	Lacks insight, delusional	Convinced that they have no problems with acquisition, clutter, or difficulty discarding. Argues that there is no problem, despite contrary evidence.

Source. Adapted from Tolin et al. 2010.

more than half (55%) of the hoarding loved ones were described as having poor insight (36%) or lacking insight/delusional (19%), suggesting that a large number of hoarding individuals may have some degree of anosognosia. In addition, family and friend informants were asked a series of questions about the severity of hoarding, including the extent to which the living area was cluttered; the extent to which clutter, difficulty discarding, and acquisition were problems; and the extent to which the loved one had difficulty discarding. These questions were followed by their estimation of how their hoarding loved ones would answer these questions for themselves. For each question, there was a significant discrepancy between the informants' judgments and their estimation of their loved one's judgments. Informants rated the hoarding as more severe than their loved ones would rate it to be.

In a comprehensive study of hoarding cases in community agencies, Woody et al. (2020) measured insight as a judgment by service providers of whether the individual understood the "severity or consequences of their hoarding behavior." Across four different communities, between 41% and 55% of identified hoarding clients had poor insight (problem recognition) as judged by their service providers.

Tolin et al. (2012) surveyed health care and service professionals about their experiences with hoarding clients. Participants reported that their hoarding clients showed significantly poorer insight into the nature of their problem compared with nonhoarding clients and failed to acknowledge the severity of it or its impact on others.

Despite these indications of poor insight, research in other contexts suggests that insight may not be as poor as it appears. The London Field Trial for Hoarding Disorder (Mataix-Cols et al. 2013) used the DSM-5 criteria for insight (understanding of the presence of a problem) and found that in only a small percentage of hoarding disorder cases could the individual be considered to lack insight or be delusional. Specifically, 86% of participants in the trial were classified as having "good or fair insight" (recognition of a problem), 10% were considered to have "poor insight" (limited recognition of a problem), and only 3% had "absent insight" (no recognition of a problem). While this was a small trial that sampled from people who self-identified as having hoarding problems, it indicates that a substantial number of individuals with hoarding disorder do possess insight. Consistent with this conclusion, Tolin et al. (2008a) found that 85% of a large sample of people with hoarding problems who volunteered for an internet study on hoarding indicated that they would seek therapy for it if it were available. However, it may be that those without insight were less likely to volunteer for these studies and thus were underrepresented.

Other research also suggests that hoarding participants in research studies are relatively accurate in evaluating their symptoms, and in some cases even overestimate their problems with hoarding. Frost and Steketee (2010) describe a case referred to them by a psychiatrist who indicated that the hoarding was severe. At the home inspection, however, the level of clutter was not close to what would constitute hoarding disorder. This may reflect the fact that for some people, unacceptable clutter may constitute a few small areas with more items than necessary, while for others, areas saturated with large numbers of possessions may not be considered cluttered. To get around this problem, Frost et al. (2008) developed a pictorial representation of three rooms in varying states of clutter (see Chapter 3 and Appendix B). The Clutter Image Rating (CIR) consists of nine pictures of each room (bedroom, living room, kitchen), with clutter ranging from little or none (score of 1) to chest-high with no path (score of 9). Individuals diagnosed with hoarding disorder completed the CIR both in the office and in their homes, while a research assistant completed the CIR in each individual's home. Scores on the CIR completed in the home by the individuals with hoarding were highly correlated with those on the CIR completed by the independent assessor in the home ($r=0.94$). Furthermore, the composite score for individuals with hoarding (mean=3.80, SD=1.77) was not significantly different from the composite rating of the experimenter visiting the participants' homes (mean = 3.70, SD = 1.81). These findings suggest that most people with hoarding disorder can accurately judge the amount of clutter in their home.

While the CIR ratings of participants with hoarding problems were relatively accurate, their responses to questions about clutter on a questionnaire overestimated clutter and its consequences compared with the ratings of the independent evaluator. Questions on the self-report questionnaire concerned functionality (e.g., "To what extent does clutter in the room take up space intended for other purposes?" "To what extent is it difficult to walk through the room because of the clutter?" "To what extent would it be easy to find what one is looking for in the room?"). In this sample, it is clear that when accompanied in the home by an independent assessor, individuals who self-identify as having hoarding problems do not underestimate the amount of clutter and may overestimate the impact clutter has on their functioning. It should be noted, however, that since many of these participants were seeking treatment for hoarding, there may have been an incentive to highlight or overestimate its consequences.

The Frost et al. (2008) study indicates that people who recognize they have a problem with hoarding can accurately assess the extent of the clutter in their homes. However, there is an odd phenomenon that has been noticed in the perception of clutter, in that it depends on when and where the assessment takes place. Frost and Steketee (2010) describe the case of a woman who sought treatment for hoarding. She demonstrated good insight but described an unusual experience each time the therapist arrived and left her home. Whenever she was home alone, she did not notice the clutter. But when the therapist arrived, it became excruciatingly clear to her just how dysfunctional her home had become. At that realization, she became extremely distressed, and her thoughts turned to what a "worthless" person she had become. She later admitted desperately wanting the therapist to leave. When the therapist did leave, she became her old self and did not notice the clutter. Her depressed mood lifted, and she could get on with her life. The cycle repeated itself with each visit. In this context, her blindness to the clutter was a strategy, albeit not a conscious one, to escape feeling overwhelmed and worthless.

This is not the only case of what Frost and Steketee (2010) have come to call "clutter blindness." Many others have told similar stories. For instance, one gentleman left out a whole room when making a drawing of his home at the beginning of treatment. The room was so cluttered that he could not open the door, and the room was lost to him. Clutter blindness also seems to play out when we ask clients to take pictures of their homes. When we look at the pictures with the clients while in the clinic, clients are often horrified by what they see. Many have a hard time believing that their home looks that bad. It appears that these individuals have habituated to living in a cluttered space, but when they see a two-dimensional representation of it, it is like seeing their home through someone else's eyes. This may reflect habituation, indifference to one's home environment, or a form of cognitive avoidance. Gregory et al. (2011) reported similar phenomena among individuals living in squalid conditions. Most participants correctly identified squalor when shown pictures, and even expressed concern for individuals living in those conditions, but did not recognize their own squalor.

While agreement on the amount of clutter in the home between people with hoarding behaviors and independent assessors (Frost et al. 2008) indicates that people with hoarding disorder appear to be insightful about their hoarding, reports from family members and friends suggest that in more than half of hoarding cases individuals have poor insight or are delusional with respect to their hoarding (Tolin et al. 2010). Dimauro et al. (2013) suggest that one explanation for this apparent discrepancy might be that family and friends overestimate hoarding severity because of the long-standing frustration and hostility that characterize their relationship with their hoarding loved ones (Tolin et al. 2008b). To examine this possibility, they compared hoarding severity and functional impairment reported by participants with hoarding behaviors and a close friend or family member. Family and friends' ratings of the severity of their loved one's hoarding were significantly greater than the ratings by the hoarding loved one, especially on the CIR as well as excessive acquisition, squalor, global severity, and level of insight. However, when these comparisons were corrected to control for the level of hostility and rejection expressed by family members, only two comparisons remained significant (excessive acquisition and poor insight). These findings suggest that family and friends may overreport hoarding symptoms, possibly because of their negative relationship with the hoarding loved one. However, the negative relationship did not account for all the differences.

To examine this further, Dimauro et al. (2013) compared responses of people with hoarding disorder with those of an independent evaluator who visited their home on measures of hoarding severity and level of impairment. There were relatively few differences in responses between participants with hoarding behaviors and independent evaluators, and those showing differences presented a mixed picture. On a measure of overall impairment due to hoarding, participants with hoarding problems rated themselves as significantly *more* impaired than did the independent evaluators, although on ratings of clutter based on the CIR, the independent evaluators gave higher clutter ratings than did the hoarding participants. Overall, however, these findings suggest that participants with hoarding behaviors are reasonably accurate when assessing the severity of their hoarding.

In a similar study comparing estimates of hoarding severity and problem recognition of family and friend informants with those of hoarding participants, Drury et al. (2015) found few differences on measures of hoarding severity or insight. Level of insight based on clinical interviews with individuals with hoarding did not differ from levels of insight based on clinical interviews with a friend/family informant.

For the most part, studies using independent evaluators indicate that most individuals with hoarding behaviors who volunteer for studies of hoarding have good insight. However, there are an unknown number of people with hoarding disorder who do not volunteer to be in these studies. People with hoarding behaviors who have poor insight may be unlikely to participate, making these findings unrepresentative of the full population of people with hoarding disorder. There are some indications that those who don't volunteer to be in these studies might have more severe symptoms and less insight than those who do. In the study cited above, Drury et al. (2015) solicited family and friend informants and attempted to get their loved ones who hoarded to volunteer to be in the study. They compared the informant responses for loved ones who volunteered with those for loved ones who did not volunteer. The severity of hoarding was judged to be significantly worse in the individuals who did not volunteer, and more importantly, their level of insight was worse. Among participants with hoarding behaviors who volunteered, only 12.5% were judged to have poor or absent insight (recognition of extent of a problem). Among participants with hoarding behaviors who did not volunteer, 55% were judged by family and friends to have poor or absent insight. This figure is nearly identical to that obtained by Tolin et al. (2010) in their study of family and friend informants.

These findings suggest that the samples used in most studies (i.e., volunteers) may not be representative of the population of individuals with hoarding problems. Woody et al. (2020) examined this hypothesis by comparing insight and accuracy of symptom severity measures in volunteers from research samples with similar measures from samples drawn from individuals coming to the attention of community agencies (i.e., people who did not respond to solicitations to be in research studies of hoarding). Combining data from various sites generated a large number of cases ($N = 824$). The community samples looked quite different from the research samples on a number of important variables. Individuals in community samples were significantly older, were more likely to be male, had lower socioeconomic status, lived with more clutter and more squalor, and had poorer insight into hoarding severity and consequences. Only 15% of the research volunteers were judged by an interviewer to have poor insight, while the community sample participants judged to have poor insight ranged from 41% to 63%. Other research has found that hoarding individuals who use community agency services display more severe hoarding problems (Bratiotis 2013).

It appears that research volunteers may differ from the broader population of people with hoarding disorder. Those who volunteer to be in studies on hoarding appear to have reasonably good insight (i.e., problem recognition), but a substantial portion of people with hoarding disorder who do not volunteer may not recognize the problematic nature of their behavior. People who show up for treatment are likely to have reasonably good insight (problem recognition), but those who don't or who refuse efforts by family members to seek treatment may not.

Defensiveness: Admission vs. Recognition

From the research on insight in hoarding, it appears that some people with hoarding problems recognize it as a problem and are willing to participate in studies on it, whereas others do not, based on judgments of community agency officials who are assigned to work with them. However, this research equates *admission* of a problem with *recognition* of a problem. It is possible that people with hoarding disorder may refuse to admit they have a problem and be quite insistent about it but in reality recognize that they do have difficulties due to the hoarding. There are several reasons to think this might be the case. Investigators have observed that even individuals who appear to lack insight go to great lengths to conceal what is behind their front door. Children of parents who hoard describe a phenomenon called "doorbell dread" (Frost and Steketee 2010). An unexpected visitor produces panic in the family, as they scramble to hide the clutter from the view of the visitor. They know that other people would judge them harshly because of the clutter or, worse, turn them in to authorities who may try to throw their possessions away. This suggests at least some recognition of a problem in their home.

Admission of a hoarding problem is heavily influenced by context. If someone from the local health department were to show up at your door and say they have had complaints about you and want to inspect your home to decide whether to take action against you, how would you respond? Or what about an elder service worker who says that your neighbors do not believe you can take care of yourself properly? Would you let them in? Or would you argue with them about the right to tell you how to live? In such a context, it does not seem likely that the resident would agree with the health department or elder service worker about the condition of the home even if they did recognize it as a problem. The worker is likely to leave that situation with the belief that the resident has no insight (recognition of a problem). In reality, what is observed in these cases is the absence of admission and not the absence of recognition. Hoarding clients may be able to admit to a problem when discussing clutter with a compassionate and supportive helper, but not with someone whom they perceive as threatening. Whether someone with hoarding disorder will admit a problem may be dictated by a perceived threat to their freedom. The motivation to restore personal freedom that is perceived to be lost or threatened (psychological reactance) has a long history of research in psychology (Brehm 1966). When people perceive that their personal freedom is lost or threatened, they are motivated to take steps to restore it. This could involve denial of or avoidance of admitting a problem pointed out by others. Psychological reactance theory has been adapted to therapy contexts in order to understand the behavior of clients in therapy who resist therapists' suggestions or instructions (Dowd and Wallbrown 1993). Therapeutic reactance seems to characterize many interactions between hoarding clients and their therapists (Christensen and Dreist 2001; Hartl and Frost 1999). We have found it difficult to establish homework assignments in therapy with individuals with hoarding behaviors. In fact, a number of our clients have a negative reaction to the word "homework." One of my clients put it simply: "I know myself, and if you tell me what to do, I won't do it." Maintaining control over possessions (i.e., not allowing anyone to touch or move them) is a characteristic of people with hoarding (Steketee et al. 2003). This might be an additional manifestation of their attempts to regain freedom from being controlled by others.

Another motive for responding defensively regarding hoarding symptoms may be a desire to protect oneself from decrements in self-worth and compromised self-identity, as happened with our clutter blindness case. Recent studies have highlighted the role of identity and attachment in hoarding (see Chapter 5). Possessions play a crucial role in the sense of identity for those with hoarding—in terms of both maintaining an idealized past and providing the opportunity for a fantasized future. Both of these motives appear to bolster self-esteem and improve a sense of self-worth.

High levels of perfectionism characterize people with hoarding problems (Frost and Gross 1993). The most putative feature of perfectionism is that self-worth becomes contingent on being perfect and not making mistakes (DiBartolo et al. 2004). In the context of hoarding, these mistakes take the form of violating beliefs about the value of possessions. Other research suggests such a connection as well. Hoarding symptoms in students and OCD patients have been tied to self-ambivalence or the presence of conflicting beliefs about oneself (Frost et al. 2007) and lowered self-worth (García-Soriano and Belloch 2012; García-Soriano et al. 2012). In a sample of patients with hoarding disorder, Chou et al. (2018) examined the relationship between self-criticism, shame, and hoarding. Both self-criticism and shame were associated with more severe hoarding symptoms and hoarding beliefs. The greater the severity of hoarding symptoms, the more the individual responds with self-hatred and shame. In light of this phenomenon, it is not surprising that people with hoarding problems would develop strategies to avoid acknowledging the hoarding (e.g., clutter blindness) or even recognizing the issue (denial of a problem when confronted), as well as keep others from discovering it (doorbell dread). In this context, what appears to be lack of insight (not recognizing the problem) may in reality be an attempt to defend oneself from compromised self-identity and declining self-worth by refusing to admit there is a problem.

Determining why people with hoarding react so defensively to the suggestion that they have a problem comes from research on how other people react to them. Chasson et al. (2018) examined three aspects of stigma related to hoarding: the extent to which people with hoarding are seen as different, bad, and to blame for their condition. In a survey of a large number of adults, people with hoarding were viewed as "different" from the general population to a greater extent than people with OCD, those with substance abuse issues, or those who have spent time incarcerated. They were held in more disdain ("they are bad") than people with OCD, and they were judged to be more to blame for their condition than people with OCD or severe mental illness. Furthermore, family members with a relative with hoarding behaviors viewed individuals with hoarding as more bad and more to blame for their condition than did people who did not have a family member with hoarding.

Tolin et al. (2008b) found similar negative views of people with hoarding among family and friends. Family and friends of individuals with hoarding reported more rejecting attitudes (e.g., criticism, hostility) than did family members of OCD patients (Amir et al. 2000) and schizophrenia patients (Kreisman et al. 1979). These rejecting attitudes were related to the perceived patient's insight (problem recognition) as well as the severity of the hoarding symptoms. In this study, family members' perception of their hoarding loved one's level of insight predicted patient rejection by family and friends beyond the effect of hoarding severity.

Rejecting attitudes toward people with hoarding are not limited to family or the general public. Tolin et al. (2012) surveyed professional organizers and health care and social service professionals about their experiences with and attitudes toward both hoarding and nonhoarding clients. Hoarding clients produced significantly more frustration, irritation, and patient rejecting attitudes than nonhoarding clients. Hoarding clients led their service providers to feel more hopeless and helpless. The service providers reported feeling more relieved when these clients missed or canceled a session compared with their nonhoarding clients and even wished the clients could be transferred to another provider.

Such negative views of people with hoarding problems get conveyed in subtle and not-so-subtle ways. One of the most apparent is the language used in discussions of hoarding. When people refer to someone with a hoarding problem as a "hoarder," it conflates the disorder with the person's identity, suggesting that this is the sum total of who that person is. Such language is usually perceived as stigmatizing by people with the lived experience of hoarding. In a YouTube video, Lee Shuer and Becca Belofsky Shuer (2021) address this issue by describing what this experience is like and the importance of using affirming language that is acceptable to hoarding clients.

Several things are apparent in the research on insight (problem recognition) and defensiveness in hoarding disorder. First, insight (problem recognition) is reasonably good among people who show up for treatment or who volunteer to be research participants. Second, family and friends tend to overestimate the lack of insight in their loved ones who hoard, and this tendency appears to be related to the negative emotional relationship that has developed over the hoarding symptoms. Third, a substantial number of those with hoarding problems (especially those identified by community agencies for their hoarding) appear to community agency professionals and family members to have limited or no insight (problem recognition). Finally, an unknown number of these individuals may deny symptoms and fail to acknowledge the hoarding as a way to protect themselves from criticism and lowered self-esteem. Future research addressing these issues is needed to clarify the true nature of insight in hoarding disorder.

Overvalued Ideation

The literature on OCD has confused problem recognition (the anosognosia definition of insight) with overvalued ideation. OCD research on insight has focused on the extent to which the ideas are overvalued rather than the extent to which the symptoms are problematic (Veale 2007). For instance, the DSM-5 insight specifier for OCD focuses on recognition of the "excessive or unreasonable" nature of the obsessions and compulsions rather than awareness of the severity of the problem or its consequences. The focus is more on the strength and rigidity of the thinking than on problem recognition.

Studies of overvalued ideation in OCD have consistently found that individuals with both OCD and hoarding symptoms have poorer insight (more overvalued ideation) than OCD patients without hoarding symptoms (De Berardis et al. 2005; Jakubovski et al. 2011; Matsunaga et al. 2002; Samuels et al. 2007; Torres et al. 2012). In these studies, however, it is not clear whether the overvalued ideation measured referred to the OCD symptoms or the hoarding symptoms.

In hoarding disorder, the excessive and unreasonable beliefs (overvalued ideas) have to do with the value of possessions, which will be outlined in Chapter 5. These include beliefs about possessions that are related to opportunity and identity, comfort and safety, responsibility, and aesthetic value (see Table 5–1). However, it may not be accurate to define these beliefs as problems with insight because they do not directly pertain to recognition of the consequences of hoarding. Nevertheless, judgments of the value of possessions are at the core of hoarding disorder and drive the excessive acquisition, difficulty discarding, and resultant clutter. Hoarding individuals who have good insight (problem recognition) will more than likely have high levels of overvalued ideas about possessions. These ideas are part of the disorder itself. It is difficult to imagine someone whose behavior meets the criteria for hoarding disorder who would not have overvalued ideas about their possessions. The strength and rigidity of the beliefs can vary from mild to delusional and more than likely affect treatment outcomes. Indeed, much of the treatment for hoarding disorder focuses on changing these beliefs about possessions. Describing people with overvalued ideas about the value of possessions as lacking insight confuses insight with the disorder itself.

Motivation

Each of the characteristics reviewed here (poor problem recognition, defensiveness, overvalued ideation) will have significant effects on motivation for treatment, establishment of a working relationship, and adherence to a treatment protocol. Many individuals with hoarding problems avoid seeking help, even though they may be seeing a therapist for other problems. In a sample of people seeking help for anxiety disorders at a specialty clinic, Tolin et al. (2011) found that 13% had serious hoarding problems despite never mentioning hoarding during their regular intake, and more than a third of them scored above the clinical cutoff on one or more of the subscales of the Saving Inventory—Revised.

Once in therapy, people with hoarding problems appear to have a hard time establishing a good working relationship with their therapist (Tolin et al. 2012). Among professionals working with hoarding clients, scores on the Working Alliance Inventory were significantly lower for hoarding than for nonhoarding clients. Among the specific behaviors that contributed to this were failing to appear at or arriving late for sessions or canceling sessions; arguing or repeatedly questioning the rationale for treatment; failing to complete homework; and getting distracted by other problems. Therapists found themselves getting into debates with their hoarding clients rather than working cooperatively on the problem. Not surprisingly, the hoarding clients were rated as not receiving as much benefit from the work as nonhoarding clients. Some of these difficulties may be due to the therapeutic reactance mentioned earlier. Therapists who are more directive and authoritarian may face more difficulties in motivating hoarding clients.

Other characteristics of hoarding are likely to contribute to motivational problems in treatment. High levels of anxiety sensitivity and intolerance of distress (Grisham et al. 2018)—as well as the tendency to avoid negative emotional experiences (Wheaton et al. 2013)—will increase the likelihood the homework will not be completed and that diverting the focus to other issues will occur during sessions. Attentional deficits will contribute to their problems staying on task (Steketee and Frost 2014) (see Chapter 2). The shame (Chou et al. 2018) and high levels of criticism from family, friends, and authorities (Chasson et al. 2018) will increase their tendency to use avoidance as a coping strategy. The lack of cognitive flexibility will make it difficult for hoarding clients to see alternatives and solve problems easily (Carbonella and Timpano 2016).

The hoarding symptoms themselves can influence motivation to change. Many of our hoarding clients tell us that their acquiring episodes are the only activity that gives them joy. The episodes are intensely pleasurable, and if part of the goal of therapy is to take them away, motivation to cooperate will be limited. In most hoarding cases, the overvalued ideas regarding the value of possessions are strong and rigid. The sense of loss of opportunity or identity that goes along with discarding possessions can be powerful. Without a clear rationale for letting go of treasured possessions, compliance with homework will be limited.

The social world of clients with hoarding will also have a significant impact on motivation to work on the problem. Families characterized by hostility and criticism, which are common in hoarding cases, will make sustained motivation a challenge. If the client has been through a cleanout or had relatives get rid of their stuff without their permission, there will be great sensitivity regarding anyone's efforts to make them throw things away.

Specialized therapist training in how to approach hoarding problems will circumvent some of these issues. Established treatments for hoarding involve a heavy dose of motivational interviewing (Steketee and Frost 2014). Also, efforts at training family members in motivational interviewing techniques have shown some promise (Chasson et al. 2014).

KEY CLINICAL POINTS

- Several processes are at work that lead to the judgment that someone with hoarding has poor insight, including poor problem recognition, defensiveness, and overvalued ideation.

- People with hoarding may recognize that their behavior is problematic but be unwilling to admit it when confronted.

- People with hoarding are often stigmatized by the public and professionals whose job it is to help them, leading to defensiveness and reluctance to admit a problem.

- Overvalued ideas about possessions are part of the disorder itself and not a reflection of poor insight.

- Psychological reactance (perceived threat to freedom) can impair progress in treatment unless it is recognized and addressed.

- Poor problem recognition, defensiveness, and overvalued ideation have significant effects on motivation for treatment.

References

Abramowitz JS, Franklin ME, Schwartz SA, Furr JM: Symptom presentation and outcome of cognitive-behavioral therapy for obsessive-compulsive disorder. J Consult Clin Psychol 71(6):1049–1057, 2003 14622080

Amador XF, Flaum M, Andreasen NC, et al: Awareness of illness in schizophrenia and schizoaffective and mood disorders. Arch Gen Psychiatry 51(10):826–836, 1994 7944872

American Psychiatric Association: Diagnostic and Statistical Manual of Mental Disorders, 5th Edition. Arlington, VA, American Psychiatric Association, 2013

Amir N, Freshman M, Foa EB: Family distress and involvement in relatives of obsessive-compulsive disorder patients. J Anxiety Disord 14(3):209–217, 2000 10868980

Bodryzlova Y, Audet JS, Bergeron K, O'Connor K: Group cognitive-behavioural therapy for hoarding disorder: systematic review and meta-analysis. Health Soc Care Community 27(3):517–530, 2019 30033635

Bratiotis C: Community hoarding task forces: a comparative case study of five task forces in the United States. Health Soc Care Community 21(3):245–253, 2013 23199135

Brehm JW: A Theory of Psychological Reactance. New York, Academic Press, 1966

Carbonella JY, Timpano KR: Examining the link between hoarding symptoms and cognitive flexibility deficits. Behav Ther 47(2):262–273, 2016 26956657

Chasson GS, Carpenter A, Ewing J, et al: Empowering families to help a loved one with hoarding disorder: pilot study of family-as-motivators training. Behav Res Ther 63:9–16, 2014 25237830

Chasson GS, Guy AA, Bates S, Corrigan PW: They aren't like me, they are bad, and they are to blame: a theoretically-informed study of stigma of hoarding disorder and obsessive-compulsive disorder. J Obsessive Compuls Relat Disord 16:56–65, 2018

Chou CY, Tsoh J, Vigil O, et al: Contributions of self-criticism and shame to hoarding. Psychiatry Res 262:488–493, 2018 28939393

Christensen DD, Dreist JH: The challenge of obsessive-compulsive disorder hoarding. Prim Psychiatry 8:79–86, 2001

Damecour CL, Charron M: Hoarding: a symptom, not a syndrome. J Clin Psychiatry 59(5):267–272, quiz 273, 1998 9632043

De Berardis D, Campanella D, Gambi F, et al: Insight and alexithymia in adult outpatients with obsessive-compulsive disorder. Eur Arch Psychiatry Clin Neurosci 255(5):350–358, 2005 15711867

DiBartolo P, Frost R, Chang P, et al: Shedding light on the relationship between personal standards and psychopathology: the case for contingent self-worth. J Ration-Emot Cogn-Behav Ther 22:237–250, 2004

Dimauro J, Tolin DF, Frost RO, Steketee G: Do people with hoarding disorder under-report their symptoms? J Obsessive Compuls Relat Disord 2(2):130–136, 2013 23524977

Dowd ET, Wallbrown F: Motivational components of client reactance. J Couns Dev 71(5):533–538, 1993

Drury H, Nordsletten A, Ajmi S, et al: Accuracy of self and informant reports of symptom severity and insight in hoarding disorder. J Obsessive Compuls Relat Disord 5:37–42, 2015

Frost RO, Gross RC: The hoarding of possessions. Behav Res Ther 31(4):367–381, 1993 8512538

Frost RO, Steketee G: Stuff: Compulsive Hoarding and the Meaning of Things. Boston, MA, Houghton Mifflin Harcourt, 2010

Frost RO, Steketee G, Williams L: Hoarding: a community health problem. Health Soc Care Community 8(4):229–234, 2000 11560692

Frost R, Kyrios M, McCarthy K, Matthews Y: Self-Ambivalence and Attachment to Possessions. J Cogn Psychother 21:232–242, 2007

Frost R, Steketee G, Tolin D, Renaud S: Development and validation of the Clutter Image Rating. J Psychopathol Behav Assess 30(3):193–203, 2008

Frost R, Tolin D, Maltby N: Insight-related challenges in the treatment of hoarding. Cognit Behav Pract 17:404–413, 2010

Galeone F, Pappalardo S, Chieffi S, et al: Anosognosia for memory deficit in amnestic mild cognitive impairment and Alzheimer's disease. Int J Geriatr Psychiatry 26(7):695–701, 2011 21495076

García-Soriano G, Belloch A: Exploring the role of obsessive-compulsive relevant self-worth contingencies in obsessive-compulsive disorder patients. Psychiatry Res 198(1):94–99, 2012 22386566

García-Soriano G, Clark DA, Belloch A, et al: Self-worth contingencies and obsessionality: a promising approach to vulnerability? J Obsessive Compuls Relat Disord 1(3):196–202, 2012

Gregory C, Halliday G, Hodges J, Snowdon J: Living in squalor: neuropsychological function, emotional processing and squalor perception in patients found living in squalor. Int Psychogeriatr 23(5):724–731, 2011 21108862

Grisham JR, Roberts L, Cerea S, et al: The role of distress tolerance, anxiety sensitivity, and intolerance of uncertainty in predicting hoarding symptoms in a clinical sample. Psychiatry Res 267:94–101, 2018 29880277

Hartl TL, Frost RO: Cognitive-behavioral treatment of compulsive hoarding: a multiple baseline experimental case study. Behav Res Ther 37(5):451–461, 1999 10228316

Jakubovski E, Pittenger C, Torres AR, et al: Dimensional correlates of poor insight in obsessive-compulsive disorder. Prog Neuropsychopharmacol Biol Psychiatry 35(7):1677–1681, 2011 21640153

Kim HJ, Steketee G, Frost RO: Hoarding by elderly people. Health Soc Work 26(3):176–184, 2001 11531193

Kreisman DE, Simmens SJ, Joy VD: Rejecting the patient: preliminary validation of a self-report scale. Schizophr Bull 5(2):220–222, 1979 462140

Mataix-Cols D, Marks IM, Greist JH, et al: Obsessive-compulsive symptom dimensions as predictors of compliance with and response to behaviour therapy: results from a controlled trial. Psychother Psychosom 71(5):255–262, 2002 12207105

Mataix-Cols D, Billotti D, Fernández de la Cruz L, Nordsletten AE: The London Field Trial for Hoarding Disorder. Psychol Med 43(4):837–847, 2013 22883395

Matsunaga H, Kiriike N, Matsui T, et al: Obsessive-compulsive disorder with poor insight. Compr Psychiatry 43(2):150–157, 2002 11893994

Matsunaga H, Hayashida K, Kiriike N, et al: Clinical features and treatment characteristics of compulsive hoarding in Japanese patients with obsessive-compulsive disorder. CNS Spectr 15(4):258–265, 2010 20414175

Muroff J, Bratiotis C, Steketee G: Treatment for hoarding behaviors: a review of the evidence. Clin Soc Work J 39:406–423, 2011

Rufer M, Fricke S, Moritz S, et al: Symptom dimensions in obsessive-compulsive disorder: prediction of cognitive-behavior therapy outcome. Acta Psychiatr Scand 113(5):440–446, 2006 16603035

Samuels JF, Bienvenu OJ III, Pinto A, et al: Hoarding in obsessive-compulsive disorder: results from the OCD Collaborative Genetics Study. Behav Res Ther 45(4):673–686, 2007 16824483

Saxena S, Maidment KM: Treatment of compulsive hoarding. J Clin Psychol 60(11):1143–1154, 2004 15389621

Shuer L, Belofsky Shuer B: Lee and Becca talk Buried in Treasures, language, clutter stigma, and HOPE. Available at: www.youtube.com/watch?v=cJ7NvM-Ka6UU. Accessed September 15, 2021.

Steketee G: Individual cognitive and behavioral treatment for hoarding, in The Oxford Handbook of Hoarding and Acquiring. Edited by Frost RO, Steketee G. Oxford, UK, Oxford University Press, 2014, pp 260–273

Steketee G, Frost RO: Phenomenology of hoarding, in The Oxford Handbook of Hoarding and Acquiring. Edited by Frost RO, Steketee G. Oxford, UK, Oxford University Press, 2014, pp 19–32

Steketee G, Frost RO, Kyrios M: Cognitive aspects of compulsive hoarding. Cognit Ther Res 27:463–479, 2003

Tolin DF, Frost RO, Steketee G: An open trial of cognitive-behavioral therapy for compulsive hoarding. Behav Res Ther 45(7):1461–1470, 2007 17306221

Tolin DF, Frost RO, Steketee G, et al: The economic and social burden of compulsive hoarding. Psychiatry Res 160(2):200–211, 2008a 18597855

Tolin DF, Frost RO, Steketee G, Fitch KE: Family burden of compulsive hoarding: results of an internet survey. Behav Res Ther 46(3):334–344, 2008b 18275935

Tolin D, Fitch K, Frost R, Steketee G: Family informants' perceptions of insight in compulsive hoarding. Cognit Ther Res 34:69–81, 2010

Tolin DF, Meunier SA, Frost RO, Steketee G: Hoarding among patients seeking treatment for anxiety disorders. J Anxiety Disord 25(1):43–48, 2011 20800427

Tolin D, Frost R, Steketee G: Working with hoarding vs. non-hoarding clients: a survey of professionals' attitudes and experiences. J Obsessive Compuls Relat Disord 1:48–53, 2012

Tolin DF, Frost RO, Steketee G, Muroff J: Cognitive behavioral therapy for hoarding disorder: a meta-analysis. Depress Anxiety 32(3):158–166, 2015 25639467

Torres AR, Fontenelle LF, Ferrão YA, et al: Clinical features of obsessive-compulsive disorder with hoarding symptoms: a multicenter study. J Psychiatr Res 46(6):724–732, 2012 22464941

Veale D: Treating obsessive-compulsive disorder in people with poor insight and overvalued ideation, in Psychological Treatment of Obsessive-Compulsive Disorder: Fundamentals and Beyond. Washington, DC, American Psychological Association, 2007, pp 267–280

Wheaton MG, Berman NC, Fabricant LE, Abramowitz JS: Differences in obsessive-compulsive symptoms and obsessive beliefs: a comparison between African Americans, Asian Americans, Latino Americans, and European Americans. Cogn Behav Ther 42(1):9–20, 2013 23134374

Woody SR, Lenkic P, Bratiotis C, et al: How well do hoarding research samples represent cases that rise to community attention? Behav Res Ther 126:103555, 2020 32044474

PART II
Etiology

CHAPTER 5
Cognitive-Behavioral Model

Much of the research on the etiology of hoarding disorder has been driven by a cognitive-behavioral model of hoarding (Figure 5–1) (Frost and Hartl 1996; Steketee and Frost 2003). The model posits a number of factors that interact to produce excessive acquisition, saving behavior, difficulty discarding, and disorganization of living spaces (Table 5–1). Foremost among the factors are vulnerabilities that may predispose people to develop hoarding disorder. A second factor is deficits in information processing or executive function that characterize people with the disorder and play a role in symptom severity. A third factor is the nature of the emotional attachments that form the meanings people give to their possessions. Finally, all of these factors operate together to reinforce acquiring and saving behavior and underlie the inability to manage possessions. Each of these factors has been subject to scrutiny and elaboration. This chapter will detail the essential features of each factor.

Vulnerabilities

A number of potential factors may make people vulnerable to the development of hoarding disorder. Since the earliest studies, it has been clear that

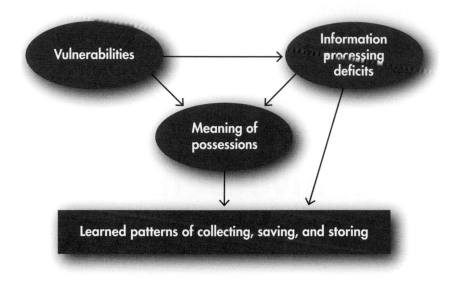

FIGURE 5–1.   Cognitive-behavioral model of hoarding.

hoarding runs in families (Frost and Gross 1993). It is estimated that up to 30%–50% of the variance in hoarding is genetic (see Chapter 6 for more details). Comorbidity with other mental disorders is common in hoarding, with the most frequent comorbid disorder being depression (see Chapter 2). Trauma history may also be a vulnerability factor; up to half of people with hoarding problems have experienced a significant trauma (Frost et al. 2011a). A fourth potential vulnerability factor has shown up in several studies but has not been studied extensively: a large percentage of people with hoarding disorder are significantly disabled or in poor physical health—more than would be expected for their age (Raines et al. 2015; Tolin et al. 2008). The medical conditions are serious and chronic and include severe arthritis and other joint problems, severe asthma and other lung problems, hypertension, diabetes, heart trouble, kidney and liver diseases, stroke, ulcers, cancer, and several more. In addition, people with hoarding problems have a higher-than-average BMI and a higher degree of obesity than would be expected for their age (Timpano et al. 2011; Tolin et al. 2008). Whether these medical conditions are true vulnerability factors, disease correlates, or consequences of the disorder is unknown.

Dysfunctions in emotion regulation have been hypothesized to be vulnerability factors for the development of hoarding as well. The forms of emotion regulation that have been studied in hoarding include anxiety sensitivity, distress tolerance, negative urgency, and experiential avoidance.

TABLE 5–1. Summary of specific features of the cognitive-behavioral model

Vulnerabilities	Genetics
	Comorbidity
	Trauma history
	Poor physical health or disability
	Emotion dysregulation
	Perfectionism
	Attachment deficits
Information processing deficits	Attention
	Memory
	Cognitive flexibility
	Categorization
	Perception
	Association
	Decision-making
Meaning of possessions	Opportunity and identity-related meanings
	Comfort and safety-related meanings
	Responsibility-related meanings
	Aesthetic-related meanings
Reinforcement patterns	Negative reinforcement
	Positive reinforcement
	Absence of learning

Anxiety sensitivity or the fear of anxiety-related sensations is associated with catastrophic interpretations of anxiety-related symptoms, which lead to heightened distress and increased avoidance (Medley et al. 2013). A growing body of studies link anxiety sensitivity with hoarding severity, particularly difficulty discarding (Coles et al. 2003; Grisham et al. 2018; Medley et al. 2013). A related construct—intolerance of distress or the inability to tolerate negative emotional states—is also found in people suffering from hoarding disorder (Grisham et al. 2018). For individuals low in distress tolerance, negative emotional states are seen as unbearable and unmanageable, leading to increased avoidance behaviors. High levels of anxiety sensitivity and low levels of distress tolerance are hallmarks of anxiety disorders; both also characterize people with hoarding problems (Phung et al. 2015; Shaw et al. 2015; Timpano et al. 2009).

Another related vulnerability factor for hoarding is negative urgency or the tendency to act impulsively when experiencing negative affect (Shaw and Timpano 2016). One hoarding disorder client expressed it in the following way: "If I don't get [purchase] this, I feel like I could just die." In a study incorporating all three of these vulnerability constructs, Grisham et al. (2018) found that although all three were related to hoarding, intolerance of distress was the strongest and most unique predictor. Moreover, Grisham et al. found that beliefs about responsibility for possessions partially mediated the relationship between distress tolerance and hoarding behavior. This is consistent with the hypothesis that distress intolerance leads to heightened beliefs about responsibility for the well-being of possessions (e.g., not wasting them). These beliefs then lead to hoarding behaviors.

Finally, a potential vulnerability factor that relates to each of these is experiential avoidance. Experiential avoidance involves the unwillingness to have unpleasant or negative experiences—including emotions, thoughts, and memories—resulting in behaviors designed to avoid or escape them. People with hoarding disorder appear to have higher levels of experiential avoidance, though perhaps not as high as those displayed by people with other anxiety disorders (Wheaton et al. 2013). Both experiential and behavioral avoidance predict hoarding severity and each of the features of hoarding (difficulty discarding, excessive acquisition, clutter) (Ayers et al. 2013).

Both evaluative concerns and striving dimensions of perfectionism correlate strongly with hoarding, as predicted by the cognitive-behavioral model of hoarding (Burgess et al. 2018b; Frost and Gross 1993; Frost et al. 2013; Grisham et al. 2018). It is hypothesized that perfectionism leads to avoidance of discarding as well as excessive acquiring in order to bypass mistakes that will be later regretted (Frost and Hartl 1996). Perfectionism may be an especially important vulnerability factor since Muroff et al. (2014) found that high levels of perfectionism interfere with treatment outcomes for people with hoarding disorder. Closely related to perfectionism is the intolerance of uncertainty, which has also been found in people with hoarding disorder and which interferes with their treatment outcomes (Castriotta et al. 2019).

Recent literature has begun to investigate the role of attachment deficits as a vulnerability factor for the development of hoarding disorder. Kyrios et al. (2018) postulate that negative early developmental experiences produce insecure attachments to people and may facilitate the development of hoarding to compensate. Reports have compiled data on those with early life experiences of poor maternal care, maternal overprotection and overcontrol (Chen et al. 2017), and lower levels of early family warmth (Kyrios et al. 2018). These experiences are thought to lead to ambivalence and uncertainty about one's self (Danet and Secouet 2018; Frost et al. 2007) as well as poor self-concept (Kings et al. 2017), which may result in overattachment to possessions as a form of compensation (Kyrios et al. 2018). Several studies have shown a link between attachment problems and the tendency to anthropomorphize possessions, which has been found to be related to hoarding (Burgess et al. 2018b; Neave et al. 2015, 2016). Norberg et al. (2018) found that anxious attachment was linked to excessive acquisition through distress tolerance and anthropomorphism. Kwok et al. (2018) found that stronger anthropomorphism was linked to the likeability of objects through perceived sentimental and instrumental value. A recent review and theoretical analysis suggested that dysfunctional attachments to both people and possessions may facilitate the development of hoarding behaviors (Mathes et al. 2020). It should be noted, however, that people with hoarding disorder typically suffer decades of criticism and rejection from friends, family, and authorities and experience considerable shame as a result (Chou et al. 2018). These experiences could easily explain the dysfunctional attachments observed in this population. Rather than being the cause, dysfunctional attachments may be a consequence of hoarding behaviors.

Information Processing Deficits

From the earliest descriptions of the phenomena, a number of information processing deficits have been associated with hoarding behaviors. In a review of subsequent research on performance-based measures of cognitive processing in hoarding disorder, Woody et al. (2014) concluded that the evidence supports problems with planning, problem-solving, visuospatial learning and memory, sustained attention, working memory, and organization among people with hoarding disorder. One of the most highly replicated of these is problems with attention. Anecdotal accounts of having difficulty staying on task when discarding—as well as "churning" through possessions without making effective decisions—are legendary, along with descriptions of distracted and tangential speech (Frost and Steketee 2010; Hartl et al. 2005).

A number of studies have highlighted the association between hoarding and symptoms of ADHD—particularly inattention (for a review, see Woody et al. 2014). Approximately 30% of patients with hoarding problems suffer from ADHD, and substantially more have struggles that do not quite meet diagnostic criteria for that disorder (Frost and Hristova 2011; Hartl et al. 2005). People with both hoarding and ADHD experience greater impairments in daily living (Hall et al. 2013). The association of hoarding with ADHD appears to be stronger than the association between hoarding and OCD. Tolin and Villavicencio (2011) reported that ADHD symptoms of inattention predicted hoarding symptoms after negative affect was controlled for, whereas OCD symptoms did not. This effect was apparent only for inattention, not for hyperactivity. In a large sample drawn from the World Health Organization's World Mental Health Survey Initiative, Fullana et al. (2013) found that symptoms of inattention in childhood were associated with greater hoarding symptoms later in life, even after OCD symptoms were controlled for. The association did not hold for symptoms of hyperactivity. Lynch et al. (2015), in a review of ADHD studies of hoarding, concluded that ADHD and hoarding disorder share executive function deficits in spatial working memory, planning, and inhibition. These findings suggest neuropsychological deficits in hoarding that may not be specific to ADHD but instead represent broader neurocognitive impairment with symptoms that resemble ADHD (Tolin and Villavicencio 2011).

Closely related to attentional problems are reported difficulties with memory. Hoarding disorder patients report more difficulties with their memory (Tolin et al. 2018), but differences in actual memory dysfunction are mixed. Some studies have found differences between hoarding and non-hoarding groups in visual memory and delayed recall, whereas other studies have failed to find memory-related differences (Hartl et al. 2004; Sumner et al. 2016). More robust findings have been in regard to confidence in memory. People with hoarding disorder doubt their ability to recall important information related to possessions, and describe the need to keep objects in sight in order to facilitate their memory (Hartl et al. 2005; Kyrios et al. 2018).

Drawing from research on neurocognitive performance in hoarding disorder, Carbonella and Timpano (2016) hypothesized that cognitive flexibility deficits are an additional information processing problem in hoarding disorder (i.e., "the ability to inhibit material and attend flexibly between different mental sets" [p. 262]). These investigators found evidence for a general deficit in cognitive flexibility, but not a specific one. People with hoarding tendencies had more trouble attending to things in their environment in a flexible way when there were distracting stimuli. Hoarding-related distracting stimuli did not exacerbate this effect. Cognitive flexibility deficits may be related to the inattention displayed by people with hoarding problems and the often-observed "churning" behavior and ineffective attempts to organize possessions.

People with hoarding disorder are also hypothesized to have difficulties with categorization and concept formation (Frost and Hartl 1996; McMillan et al. 2013). Studies have found that people with hoarding difficulties form underinclusive category boundaries, leading to problems with organizing (Luchian et al. 2007; Wincze et al. 2007). Each object is perceived to be so unique and complex that it belongs in its own category, making the organizing of possessions by category problematic. Consequently, the normal organizing strategy of grouping "like with like" does not work. Rather than having no organizational strategy, however, people with hoarding disorder appear to organize their possessions visually and spatially. Objects go into a pile somewhere in the room and a mental note is made of the location. Over time a mental map is created with the spatial location of each item registered (e.g., on the left side of the pile about a foot down). This system may work for a small number of items, such as on a desk or worktable, but when applied to all possessions, it becomes unmanageable.

Some perceptual abnormalities have been observed among people who hoard, though there is relatively little research on the topic. Specifically, anecdotal reports of a phenomenon called "clutter blindness" have appeared in the literature (Frost and Steketee 2010) (see Chapter 4). One woman told her therapist that when home alone, she does not notice the clutter. Yet when her therapist visits, she notices it, and it makes her feel embarrassed and depressed. This may reflect a sort of habituation to the clutter or a more perception-based problem.

Another hypothesized information processing deficit that has received little attention is that people with hoarding disorder experience a richer set of associations with possessions or potential possessions. One gentleman with hoarding disorder complained that his mind was too hard to navigate: "It's like a tree with too many branches. Everything is connected. Every branch leads somewhere, and there are so many branches that I get lost. They are too thick to see through" (Frost and Steketee 2010, p. 201).

Impaired decision-making, which has been widely observed among hoarding disorder patients, may link each of the information processing deficits to hoarding. Frost and Hartl (1996) suggested that hoarding symptoms stem in large part from impaired decision-making capacity. Individuals with hoarding disorder report more problems with decision-making than do people with OCD as well as nonclinical control groups (Cougle et al. 2013; Frost and Gross 1993; Hayward and Coles 2009). Furthermore, relatives of hoarding probands are rated as having more problems with decisions than are relatives of nonhoarding probands, suggesting that indecisiveness may be part of a hoarding phenotype (Frost et al. 2011b; Samuels et al. 2007). A problem with decision-making also predicts hoarding severity, along with each of the core features of hoarding independent of other vulnerability factors such as depression and anxiety (Frost et al. 2011b; Kyrios et al. 2018). Decision-making fears have been linked to poor memory confidence (Nedeljkovic et al. 2009).

Connecting vulnerabilities to information processing deficits, the cognitive-behavioral model suggests that the evaluative concern dimension of perfectionism influences hoarding symptoms by increasing indecisiveness (Frost and Hartl 1996). Burgess et al. (2018a) found support for this hy-

pothesis, particularly for the avoidance of decision-making (decisional procrastination). The relationship between evaluative concerns perfectionism
and hoarding symptoms (difficulty discarding, excessive acquisition, clutter) is through its effects on decisional procrastination. The implication of
these findings is that people who are highly perfectionistic procrastinate in
making decisions, and their procrastination, in turn, is associated with an
increase in the severity of hoarding symptoms.

Meaning of Possessions

The meaning that possessions have for people gives rise to decisions to save
or let go of them. Meaning is variously described in the research literature
as motives, beliefs, attachments, cognitions, or reasons for saving. The meanings are wide-ranging and generally reflect the reasons most people give for
saving things. In fact, in the earliest study on this topic, the reasons for saving that were given by people who were struggling with hoarding were virtually identical to the reasons for saving given by people who did not hoard
(Frost and Gross 1993). The difference between these groups was not in what
reasons they gave, but in how strongly they endorsed those reasons and how
rigidly and extensively they applied them. These meanings can be organized
into four categories: opportunity and identity-related meanings, comfort- and
safety-related meanings, responsibility-related meanings, and aesthetically
related meanings. The categories overlap, and most people with hoarding
problems report meanings in several and often all of these categories. However, some research has suggested that certain of these categories are stronger predictors of hoarding severity than others.

Opportunity and Identity

A frequent theme reported by people with hoarding disorder is that their
belongings provide opportunities that cannot or should not be passed up.
Frost and Steketee (2010, p. 134) quote a woman with a serious hoarding
problem on the topic: "Life is a river of opportunities. If I don't grab everything interesting, I'll lose out. Things will pass me by. The stuff I have is
like a river. It flows into my house, and I try to keep it from flowing out. I
want to stop it long enough to take advantage of it." The reasoning reflected in this quote is often repeated by people with hoarding disorder. As
most people in society age and mature, they learn that in order to move forward and take advantage of what life has to offer, they must give up some
opportunities that present themselves in order to pursue others. People with
hoarding disorder appear to be unwilling to do so, especially with respect
to the opportunities that possessions provide. One such opportunity relates

to a sense of identity or self-concept. A common refrain among people with hoarding disorder is "I see my belongings as extensions of myself; they are part of who I am" (Frost and Gross 1993). This is not an unusual belief. As far back as 1890, the noted philosopher and psychologist William James (1890) commented, "A man's self is the sum-total of all that he can call his" (p. 353), and "between what a man calls me and what he simply calls mine, the line is difficult to draw" (p. 319). For most, the identification with possessions is normal and adaptive. A growing body of literature suggests that in hoarding disorder, possessions become integrated into self-concept in a pathological way because the self-concept in people with hoarding problems is fragile. As a result, possessions become crucial to them for defining who they are. For example, Irene, one of the main characters in the book *Stuff: Compulsive Hoarding and the Meaning of Things* (Frost and Steketee 2010), had more than 300 cookbooks, and she saved the cooking section of each newspaper as well as recipes from magazines. But she never cooked. When she looked at these items, she fantasized about being a good cook and the dinner parties she would put on for her friends. These books and recipes allowed her to dream about the person she wanted to be—a sort of fictionalized or ideal future identity. These thoughts were also reflected in the thousands of newspapers that she saved with the intention of someday reading them. These possessions were not really a part of her real self; instead, they were part of a fictionalized future one. They became integrated into her self-concept, but in a pathological way. Markus and Nurius (1986) describe this as a "possible self," reflecting how people think about their potential and future.

The research literature is consistent with this idea. Hoarding severity is associated with higher levels of ambivalence about the self and self-worth (Frost et al. 2007), and people who hoard show confusion about who they are and what they believe in (Claes et al. 2016). Kings et al. (2017) suggest that people with hoarding disorder save possessions to address this self-ambivalence, and consequently they extend what James thought was a normal process of integrating identity with possessions to a much wider array of objects, making getting rid of any one of them difficult. These investigators propose that people with hoarding disorder search for certainty regarding their identity in possessions and that their possessions serve as identity substitutes. This work has led investigators to explore attachment-related problems in hoarding disorder (Claes et al. 2016; Kyrios et al. 2018; Mathes et al. 2020).

While many possessions are saved to create a fantasized future self, many possessions are also saved to preserve an idealized past self. Possessions serve as cues to past experiences (Cherrier and Ponnor 2010). Most people with hoarding disorder describe this feeling as needing the possession to preserve memories. In reality, this is a form of extreme sentimental saving. Almost everyone saves things of sentimental value. They preserve an association with a person, place, or event, like a ticket stub from a favorite concert. Developmental psychologists call this form of thinking "essentialism" (Bloom 2010). The ticket stub has an essence—a meaning that goes beyond the physical characteristics of the stub itself. The essence is applied to it by the holder of the ticket. The billion-dollar memorabilia industry is built on the phenomenon of essentialism. Whether the item is shoes worn by a legendary basketball player or chunks of concrete from the Berlin Wall, the object connects the owner to that piece of the object's history. In its more extreme form, it is what James Frazer called "superstitious magic," a belief that objects that were once close to someone or something (contiguity) can transfer something to the new owner (Frazer 1940). This belief is the basis for voodoo religious and magical spells, but it is held to some degree by all of us.

The ticket stub is also a trigger for memories associated with an event. Without the trigger, would the memories still be there? This is the question many people with hoarding disorder ask when considering whether to get rid of a possession. One of our recent cases described her experience in deciding whether to get rid of a tricycle that her daughter used to ride: "It feels like I'm letting go of the little girl. I feel like I'm destroying the past, like it never happened. I'm erasing that time period. If I throw this out, then it never happened."

Little is known about the nature of these memories. However, some recent interest has come from the cognitive psychology area of study on the "Proust effect." Marcel Proust's novel *Remembrance of Things Past* contains a famous example of memories of things lost to time. In the first volume of the novel, the narrator describes eating a madeleine cookie and being transported back to a time in his childhood when a favorite relative fed him cookies and tea. All of the sensory experiences came back to him as he ate the cookie—the sights, sounds, and smells—with a vividness that did not occur when simply recalling early childhood. This is much like the experience of hearing a song from childhood or adolescence. The music prompts more than a sterile memory. It brings back the visceral feelings of actually being there.

As with most human traits, there is probably great variability in the extent to which this phenomenon is experienced. Is it possible that people with hoarding disorder experience this Proust effect through the visual system? Does the sight of a possession transport them back to the time that the possession was used, with all of the thoughts and feelings attached? Preliminary data suggest that it does (Frost et al. 2019). This might explain why it seems much easier for people with hoarding disorder to let go of things if those things are out of sight. The sight of the possession carries with it an unusually heavy memory that includes much more of the past experience than is the case for people who do not hoard.

Comfort and Safety

Frost and Steketee (2010) report that in one of their hoarding cases, the client declared after a particularly difficult day: "I just wanted to go home and gather my treasures around me." Frost and Hartl (1996) suggest that for people who hoard, their possessions become safety signals in a world seen as dangerous. Even the thought of getting rid of a possession seems to violate this sense of safety and create feelings of vulnerability. Kellett (2007) echoes this idea in his "site-security" model of hoarding and suggests that for people with hoarding disorder, objects form the only source of comfort, safety, and security. This idea is not entirely new. Nearly 50 years ago, a little-known Spanish psychiatrist, Juan Antonio Vallejo-Nágera, described a condition he called "soteric neurosis" (Fontenelle 2016). He named it after the Greek goddess of safety, Soteria. He claimed the condition was the opposite of a phobia—instead of a physical stimulus becoming associated with fear, the stimulus (a possession) becomes imbued with "an absurd and unjustified sense of safety and protection" (Fontenelle 2016, p. 86). Perhaps he was onto something.

Reports by people with significant hoarding of the extent to which their possessions provide comfort and safety are highly correlated with hoarding symptoms (Frost et al. 1995). Themes of safety in possessions may be especially relevant for people with hoarding disorder who have experienced significant trauma. While half of people with hoarding disorder have experienced significant trauma, only a small percentage of them develop PTSD (Frost et al. 2011a). Perhaps the safety signal value of their possessions masks their PTSD symptoms. For example, Frost and Steketee (2010) describe the case of a woman with hoarding disorder whose PTSD symptoms emerged only when her progress in hoarding treatment led to focusing on possessions in the bedroom where she had experienced a violent sexual assault. Although this sense of safety is spoken of often by people with hoarding problems, it is as yet unexamined by the research community.

Responsibility

Although many motives for saving possessions among people with hoarding disorder reflect intentional saving, most people with hoarding disorder also save possessions they do not want. In such cases, the motivation for saving is rooted in a sense of responsibility. People with hoarding disorder report feeling responsible for finding a use for all of their possessions, for not wasting valuable opportunities provided by them, for the well-being of their possessions, and for saving things that might be useful to others, and they feel ashamed when they don't have something when they need it (Steketee et al. 2003). The sense of responsibility reflected in these statements has been shown to correlate with hoarding severity in a variety of studies (Steketee et al. 2003; Timpano et al. 2015).

A more intense form of responsibility concerns the moral implications of ownership. For example, Frost and Steketee (2010) describe the case of a woman struggling to get rid of a wool glove with a hole in it, despite the fact that she knew she would never wear or use it for anything. She alternated between weeping with the guilt she felt over wasting over 90% of the wool and raging at the store for "tricking" her into buying such inferior merchandise. Her moral dilemma over waste extended to most things in her life, which is what brought her into treatment. Even the word "waste" made her cringe. Frost and colleagues call this form of responsibility "material scrupulosity" to reflect the extent to which not discarding (not wasting) is a moral or ethical imperative. They define material scrupulosity as an "exaggerated sense of duty or moral/ethical responsibility for the care and disposition of possessions to prevent them from being harmed or wasted" (Frost et al. 2018, p. 20).

There are a variety of ways that material scrupulosity can be expressed in hoarding disorder. The avoidance of waste is a hallmark of this motive. People with hoarding disorder will go to great lengths to avoid waste. Failure to do so leaves them feeling guilty and morally corrupt. We have had cases where the individual could not let go of a trash bag that was only three quarters full. One man tore the labels off of food cans to use them for stationary and writing paper. Perhaps the most dysfunctional waste avoidance is the saving and consuming of food that is well past its use date and sometimes already rotting. The operating principle seems to be that possessions can't be discarded until they are maximally used up.

A behavioral consequence of waste avoidance and beliefs about maximum usage is the intense work required before hoarding clients can let go of an object. Many people with hoarding disorder insist that they do not have a problem getting rid of things, but rather that they just do not have enough time to do it and are exhausted by the effort. Close observation of their attempts to discard reveals enormous effort and time spent in trying to find a responsible way to dispose of objects. The individual becomes exhausted by the effort that yields too little discarding to keep up with the ongoing acquisition. An outsider looking in may assume a lack of insight and motivation, but in reality, the person is working tirelessly on their problem, but in a way that ensures failure.

Closely related is the "good home syndrome," in which people with hoarding disorder cannot consider letting something go unless they have found a good enough home for it. They need extensive reassurance that wherever the item goes, it will be used to its full potential and not wasted. Often this concern is so rigid that no home qualifies, and the object must be kept even though the person does not want it. This insistence is, in a sense, an attempt to maintain ownership (i.e., control over the object) without possession of it.

Concerns about and avoidance of waste appear to be major motives for both excessive acquisition and saving behavior (Dozier and Ayers 2014; Frost et al. 2015; Haws et al. 2012). They are among the most frequent rationales given by people with hoarding disorder for their difficulty discarding (Bratiotis et al. 2019). The avoidance-of-waste motive was the strongest and most consistent predictor of both excessive acquisition and difficulty discarding in several large studies of hoarding disorder (Dozier and Ayers 2014; Frost et al. 2015). Consistent with this, at least one study reported higher levels of environmental conscientiousness among people who hoard (Frost and Gross 1993). While environmental conscientiousness has a prosocial quality, its rigid expression here can be pathological. Fear of waste as a motivator for saving possessions may vary across cultures. Timpano et al. (2015) reported that concerns over usefulness and waste were the only beliefs related to hoarding symptoms among Chinese students, while American students showed a wider array of beliefs (e.g., opportunity and identity, safety and security, aesthetics).

Another expression of material scrupulosity is the need to make sure that possessions are not harmed. This concern appears to be rooted in the tendency to attribute humanlike characteristics (e.g., motives, emotions, feelings) to inanimate objects. Although some degree of anthropomorphism is normative, it can become problematic when the objects are atypical or the attributions of humanlike traits are extreme. Anecdotal accounts of anthropomorphism in hoarding are common. For example, Frost and Steketee (2010) describe the account of a woman with hoarding disorder who was trying to discard an empty yogurt container: "The thought crossed my mind: maybe the container would rather be dry instead of sitting there for a long time, humid." She continued, "I also had to resist apologizing to the container. . . . I felt responsible for giving it as comfortable a ride as possible" (p. 272). Several studies have confirmed the link between anthropomorphism and hoarding disorder and hoarding beliefs (Burgess et al. 2018b; Neave et al. 2015, 2016; Timpano and Shaw 2013).

Aesthetics

Saving for aesthetic reasons in hoarding is an understudied area, yet the frequency of attachments to beautiful things is very common in individuals with hoarding compared with nonclinical controls and people with other anxiety disorders (Dozier and Ayers 2014; Frost et al. 2015). The appreciation for the beauty in physical objects has led to speculation that this aspect of hoarding disorder may reflect a form of giftedness (Frost and Steketee 2010). Anecdotal observations indicate that recognition of the aesthetic qualities of objects often leads people with hoarding to acquire them with the intention of creating some kind of art or display. However, while materials necessary for completing such a project are collected, little or no effort goes into actually creating the product, possibly because of difficulties with sustained attention and organization. This also may be an example of the creating of a future self that does not correspond to the current one.

Reinforcement Patterns

In a study of patterns of use of possessions, Frost et al. (1995) discovered that greater hoarding severity was associated with less frequent use of possessions. In other words, once a possession enters the home, it is seldom used or interacted with. Interaction with a possession in a home that is in disarray is likely to focus on whether and where to keep it. Both of these questions are related to problem areas for people with hoarding disorder. Struggles with organization and decision-making are likely to make such consideration unpleasant, leading individuals to abandon the effort. Consideration of getting rid of a possession will be difficult due to the emotion dysregulation difficulties outlined above (e.g., anxiety sensitivity, distress tolerance, negative urgency). The preference for avoiding negative affect (experiential avoidance) suggests that the lack of interaction with possessions in the home is due to avoidance of the extreme emotional arousal during the act of discarding (e.g., anxiety, grief, guilt, anger, sadness). Saving behavior is therefore negatively reinforced because it allows for escape from or avoidance of negative emotional states. For example, in one of our earliest cases, the client began weeping at the thought of selling a book she had not looked at in 30 years. "I just feel like I could die," was her comment. She put the book down and went into the other room, busying herself with straightening up the kitchen table. In this sequence, she avoided the experience of negative emotions by stopping her consideration of discarding. She prevented the experience of negative emotions by not even raising the question of whether to save the things she had collected. Therefore, there was virtually no processing of any possession in her home in regard to the importance of it to her current self. This prevents the processing of feedback that would correct the dysfunctional meanings and attachments.

When avoidance behaviors lead to little or no discarding, there is no opportunity to learn the true consequences (or benefits) of letting go of possessions and no opportunity to develop a different way of interacting with possessions. Many people with hoarding disorder fear catastrophic emotional reactions to discarding that will be with them for the rest of their lives. Clients frequently report not only a fear of the distress they will experience if they let go of a cherished possession but also the fear that the horrible feeling will never go away. Only discarding (or not acquiring) and living with the actual consequences can disabuse them of those fears.

In addition to this negative reinforcement pattern, acquiring and saving are also positively reinforced. Buying or collecting free things is often reported as the most fun activity people with hoarding disorder enjoy. Many describe it as a "high" or like a drug. Acquiring behavior is clearly positively reinforced by such experiences. Occasionally the high occurs when people find a valued treasure amid the piles in a room, but for the most part, positive reinforcement for saving the stuff already in the home comes in the form of its contribution to the "fantasized future self" mentioned earlier. For Irene (the woman who saved cookbooks), whenever she looked at a cookbook amid the piles of things in her home, she began to fantasize about the dinner parties she would hold. That fantasy was reinforcing enough to lead her to keep the cookbook, even though she knew she would never have a dinner party unless she could deal with the clutter. This pattern is the opposite of that of people who do not hoard. For the most part, people keep things they use. Their use positively reinforces the saving behavior. For Irene, it is not the use of the possessions that is reinforcing, but the dreams of who she could be when she looks at them. By keeping all the cookbooks, she can preserve the dream.

Conclusion

The cognitive-behavioral model of hoarding outlined in this chapter represents an attempt to organize the rapidly expanding understanding of this difficult disorder. This model was designed to provide a template for studying hoarding problems and to aid in future research by guiding the generation of testable hypotheses. The model incorporates four general features: vulnerabilities, information processing deficits, exaggerated attachments to and beliefs about possessions, and reinforcement patterns that tie these features together. When the model was first proposed (Frost and Hartl 1996), our knowledge of hoarding was limited. Since that time, research findings have been generally consistent with the model and have elaborated on what we know about each of these features. During cognitive-behavioral treatment for hoarding, this model forms much of the patient education regarding hoarding disorder. Each of these features are examined to create a profile of the client's hoarding problem (see Chapter 7).

KEY CLINICAL POINTS

- Much of the research on hoarding to date has been driven by a cognitive-behavioral model that posits four contributing factors: vulnerabilities, information processing deficits, perceived meanings of possessions, and patterns of reinforcement for acquiring and saving.

- Existing research suggests a number of vulnerabilities for hoarding, including genetics, emotional dysregulation, comorbidities, perfectionism, and—potentially—attachment deficits.

- Information processing deficits in hoarding include attention, memory, categorization, cognitive flexibility, and decision-making.

- For people with hoarding behaviors, the exaggerated meanings of possessions are related to four overlapping categories: opportunity and identity, comfort and safety, responsibility, and aesthetics.

- Excessive acquisition and saving behaviors in hoarding disorder are both positively and negatively reinforced, leading to the avoidance of discarding.

- The tendency to avoid discarding leads to the absence of learning the true importance of possessions.

References

Ayers CR, Wetherell JL, Schiehser D, et al: Executive functioning in older adults with hoarding disorder. Int J Geriatr Psychiatry 28(11):1175–1181, 2013 23440720

Bloom P: How Pleasure Works: The New Science of Why We Like What We Like. New York, WW Norton, 2010

Bratiotis C, Steketee G, Dohn J, et al: Should I keep it? Thoughts verbalized during a discarding task. Cognit Ther Res (43):1075–1085, 2019

Burgess A, Frost RO, Marani C, Gabrielson I: Imperfection, indecision, and hoarding. Curr Psychol 37(2):445–453, 2018a

Burgess AM, Graves LM, Frost RO: My possessions need me: anthropomorphism and hoarding. Scand J Psychol 59(3):340–348, 2018b 29608213

Carbonella JY, Timpano KR: Examining the link between hoarding symptoms and cognitive flexibility deficits. Behav Ther 47(2):262–273, 2016 26956657

Castriotta N, Dozier ME, Taylor CT, et al: Intolerance of uncertainty in hoarding disorder. J Obsessive Compuls Relat Disord 21:97–101, 2019 32670782

Chen D, Bienvenu OJ, Krasnow J, et al: Parental bonding and hoarding in obsessive-compulsive disorder. Compr Psychiatry 73:43–52, 2017 27915218

Cherrier H, Ponnor T: A study of hoarding behavior and attachment to material possessions. Qualitative Market Research 13(1):8–23, 2010

Chou CY, Mackin RS, Delucchi KL, Mathews CA: Detail-oriented visual processing style: its role in the relationships between early life adversity and hoarding-related dysfunctions. Psychiatry Res 267:30–36, 2018 29883858

Claes L, Müller A, Luyckx K: Compulsive buying and hoarding as identity substitutes: the role of materialistic value endorsement and depression. Compr Psychiatry 68:65–71, 2016 27234185

Coles ME, Frost RO, Heimberg RG, Steketee G: Hoarding behaviors in a large college sample. Behav Res Ther 41(2):179–194, 2003 12547379

Cougle JR, Fitch KE, Jacobson S, Lee HJ: A multi-method examination of the role of incompleteness in compulsive checking. J Anxiety Disord 27(2):231–239, 2013 23511304

Danet M, Secouet D: Insecure attachment as a factor in hoarding behaviors in a non-clinical sample of women. Psychiatry Res 270:286–292, 2018 30278410

Dozier ME, Ayers CR: The predictive value of different reasons for saving and acquiring on hoarding disorder symptoms. J Obsessive Compuls Relat Disord 3(3):220–227, 2014 32670784

Fontenelle LF: Vallejo-Nágera (1926-1990) and the concept of "soteric neurosis": a forgotten sketch of hoarding disorder in the obsessive-compulsive spectrum literature. J Med Biogr 24(1):85–89, 2016 24658218

Frazer JG: The Golden Bough, Abridged Edition. New York, Macmillan, 1940

Frost RO, Gross RC: The hoarding of possessions. Behav Res Ther 31(4):367–381, 1993 8512538

Frost RO, Hartl TL: A cognitive-behavioral model of compulsive hoarding. Behav Res Ther 34(4):341–350, 1996 8871366

Frost RO, Hristova V: Assessment of hoarding. J Clin Psychol 67(5):456–466, 2011 21351103

Frost RO, Steketee G: Stuff: Compulsive Hoarding and the Meaning of Things. Boston, MA, Houghton Mifflin Harcourt, 2010

Frost RO, Hartl TL, Christian R, Williams N: The value of possessions in compulsive hoarding: patterns of use and attachment. Behav Res Ther 33(8):897–902, 1995 7487849

Frost RO, Kyrios M, McCarthy K, Matthews Y: Self-ambivalence and attachment to possessions. J Cogn Psychother 21:232–242, 2007

Frost RO, Steketee G, Tolin DF: Comorbidity in hoarding disorder. Depress Anxiety 28(10):876–884, 2011a 21770000

Frost RO, Tolin D, Steketee G, Oh M: Indecisiveness and hoarding. Int J Cogn Ther 4:253–262, 2011b

Frost RO, Hristova V, Steketee G, Tolin DF: Activities of Daily Living Scale in hoarding disorder. J Obsessive Compuls Relat Disord 2(2):85–90, 2013 23482436

Frost RO, Steketee G, Tolin DF, et al: Motives for acquiring and saving in hoarding disorder, OCD, and community controls. J Obsessive Compuls Relat Disord 4:54–59, 2015 25729641

Frost RO, Gabrielson I, Deady S, et al: Scrupulosity and hoarding. Compr Psychiatry 86:19–21, 2018 30041077

Frost RO, Wraga MJ, Eldevik MM, et al. The Proust phenomenon may be interfering with your ability to discard. Paper presented at annual meeting of the International OCD Foundation. Austin, TX, July 2019

Fullana MA, Vilagut G, Mataix-Cols D, et al: Is ADHD in childhood associated with lifetime hoarding symptoms? An epidemiological study. Depress Anxiety 30(8):741–748, 2013 23606213

Grisham JR, Roberts L, Cerea S, et al: The role of distress tolerance, anxiety sensitivity, and intolerance of uncertainty in predicting hoarding symptoms in a clinical sample. Psychiatry Res 267:94–101, 2018 29886277

Hall BJ, Tolin DF, Frost RO, Steketee G: An exploration of comorbid symptoms and clinical correlates of clinically significant hoarding symptoms. Depress Anxiety 30(1):67–76, 2013 23213052

Hartl TL, Frost RO, Allen GJ, et al: Actual and perceived memory deficits in individuals with compulsive hoarding. Depress Anxiety 20(2):59–69, 2004 15390215

Hartl TL, Duffany SR, Allen GJ, et al: Relationships among compulsive hoarding, trauma, and attention-deficit/hyperactivity disorder. Behav Res Ther 43(2):269–276, 2005 15629755

Haws K, Naylor R, Coulter R, Bearden W: Keeping it all without being buried alive: understanding product retention tendency. J Consum Psychol 22(2):224–236, 2012

Hayward L, Coles M: Elucidating the relation of hoarding to obsessive compulsive disorder and impulse control disorders. J Psychopathol Behav Assess 31:220–227, 2009

James W: The Principles of Psychology. New York, Henry Holt, 1890

Kellett S: Compulsive hoarding: a site-security model and associated psychological treatment strategies. Clin Psychol Psychother 14:413–427, 2007

Kings CA, Moulding R, Knight T: You are what you own: reviewing the link between possessions, emotional attachment, and the self-concept in hoarding disorder. J Obsessive Compuls Relat Disord 14:51–58, 2017

Kwok C, Grisham JR, Norberg MM: Object attachment: humanness increases sentimental and instrumental values. J Behav Addict 7(4):1132–1142, 2018 30311771

Kyrios M, Mogan C, Moulding R, et al: The cognitive-behavioural model of hoarding disorder: evidence from clinical and non-clinical cohorts. Clin Psychol Psychother 25(2):311–321, 2018 29266639

Luchian SA, McNally RJ, Hooley JM: Cognitive aspects of nonclinical obsessive-compulsive hoarding. Behav Res Ther 45(7):1657–1662, 2007 17014824

Lynch F, McGillivray J, Moulding R, Byrne L: Hoarding in attention deficit hyperactivity disorder: understanding the comorbidity. J Obsessive Compuls Relat Disord 4:37–46, 2015

Markus H, Nurius P: Possible selves. Am Psychol 41:954–969, 1986

Mathes BM, Timpano KR, Raines AM, Schmidt NB: Attachment theory and hoarding disorder: a review and theoretical integration. Behav Res Ther 125:103549, 2020 31923776

McMillan SG, Rees CS, Pestell C: An investigation of executive functioning, attention and working memory in compulsive hoarding. Behav Cogn Psychother 41(5):610–625, 2013 23116570

Medley AN, Capron DW, Korte KJ, Schmidt NB: Anxiety sensitivity: a potential vulnerability factor for compulsive hoarding. Cogn Behav Ther 42(1):45–55, 2013 23505992

Muroff J, Steketee G, Frost RO, Tolin DF: Cognitive behavior therapy for hoarding disorder: follow-up findings and predictors of outcome. Depress Anxiety 31(12):964–971, 2014 24277161

Neave N, Jackson R, Saxton T, Hönekopp J: The influence of anthropomorphic tendencies on human hoarding behaviors. Pers Individ Dif 72:214–219, 2015

Neave N, Tyson H, McInnes L, Hamilton C: The role of attachment style and anthropomorphism in predicting hoarding behaviours in a non-clinical sample. Pers Individ Dif 99:33–37, 2016

Nedeljkovic M, Moulding R, Kyrios M, Doron G: The relationship of cognitive confidence to OCD symptoms. J Anxiety Disord 23(4):463–468, 2009 19022617

Norberg MM, Crone C, Kwok C, Grisham JR: Anxious attachment and excessive acquisition: the mediating roles of anthropomorphism and distress intolerance. J Behav Addict 7(1):171–180, 2018 29444605

Phung PJ, Moulding R, Taylor JK, Nedeljkovic M: Emotional regulation, attachment to possessions and hoarding symptoms. Scand J Psychol 56(5):573–581, 2015 26183596

Raines AM, Allan NP, Oglesby ME, et al: Specific and general facets of hoarding: a bifactor model. J Anxiety Disord 34:100–106, 2015 26210824

Samuels JF, Bienvenu OJ III, Pinto A, et al: Hoarding in obsessive-compulsive disorder: results from the OCD Collaborative Genetics Study. Behav Res Ther 45(4):673–686, 2007 16824483

Shaw AM, Timpano KR: An experimental investigation of the effect of stress on saving and acquiring behavioral tendencies: the role of distress tolerance and negative urgency. Behav Ther 47(1):116–129, 2016 26763502

Shaw AM, Timpano KR, Steketee G, et al: Hoarding and emotional reactivity: the link between negative emotional reactions and hoarding symptomatology. J Psychiatr Res 63:84–90, 2015 25732668

Steketee G, Frost R: Compulsive hoarding: current status of the research. Clin Psychol Rev 23(7):905–927, 2003 14624821

Steketee G, Frost RO, Kyrios M: Cognitive aspects of compulsive hoarding. Cognit Ther Res 27:463–479, 2003

Sumner JM, Noack CG, Filoteo JV, et al: Neurocognitive performance in unmedicated patients with hoarding disorder. Neuropsychology 30(2):157–168, 2016 26301774

Timpano K, Shaw A: Conferring humanness: the role of anthropomorphism in hoarding. Pers Individ Dif 54:383–388, 2013

Timpano KR, Buckner JD, Richey JA, et al: Exploration of anxiety sensitivity and distress tolerance as vulnerability factors for hoarding behaviors. Depress Anxiety 26(4):343–353, 2009 19123454

Timpano KR, Exner C, Glaesmer H, et al: The epidemiology of the proposed DSM-5 hoarding disorder: exploration of the acquisition specifier, associated features, and distress. J Clin Psychiatry 72(6):780–786, quiz 878–879, 2011 21733479

Timpano KR, Çek D, Fu ZF, et al: A consideration of hoarding disorder symptoms in China. Compr Psychiatry 57:36–45, 2015 25483851

Tolin DF, Villavicencio A: Inattention, but not OCD, predicts the core features of hoarding disorder. Behav Res Ther 49(2):120–125, 2011 21193171

Tolin DF, Frost RO, Steketee G, et al: The economic and social burden of compulsive hoarding. Psychiatry Res 160(2):200–211, 2008 18597855

Tolin DF, Hallion LS, Wootton BM, et al: Subjective cognitive function in hoarding disorder. Psychiatry Res 265:215–220, 2018 29751168

Wheaton MG, Berman NC, Fabricant LE, Abramowitz JS: Differences in obsessive-compulsive symptoms and obsessive beliefs: a comparison between African Americans, Asian Americans, Latino Americans, and European Americans. Cogn Behav Ther 42(1):9–20, 2013 23134374

Wincze JP, Steketee G, Frost RO: Categorization in compulsive hoarding. Behav Res Ther 45(1):63–72, 2007 16530724

Woody SR, Kellman-McFarlane K, Welsted A: Review of cognitive performance in hoarding disorder. Clin Psychol Rev 34(4):324–336, 2014 24794835

CHAPTER 6
Neurobiology

Phenomenological differences between hoarding disorder and other mental disorders support its inclusion in DSM-5 (American Psychiatric Association 2013) as a diagnostic entity separate from obsessive-compulsive disorder (OCD). A complication in interpreting the findings of studies of etiology and pathology is that they vary in how hoarding symptoms were assessed. At the same time, because it has only recently been introduced into the classification, the neurobiology of hoarding disorder in humans is a newly burgeoning field, making it somewhat premature to draw firm conclusions. In this chapter, we focus on the genetics, neural correlates, and neuropsychological correlates of hoarding disorder. The assessment strategies for the reviewed studies are described. In addition, we discuss translational animal models of hoarding behaviors and highlight questions for further study.

Genetics
The earliest studies of hoarding suggested that between 50% and 85% of individuals with hoarding symptoms (based on hoarding-specific assessments) described a first-degree relative as a "pack rat" or as having hoarding problems (Frost and Gross 1993; Pertusa et al. 2008). Since then, a number of studies have supported the hypothesis that hoarding behavior is at least partly genetic. Steketee et al. (2012) compared the family histories of hoarding among a sample of individuals diagnosed with hoarding (*n*=217), individuals with

OCD (*n*=96), and a community control (*n*=130). Of those with diagnosed hoarding, 36% grew up in a cluttered home, compared with 16% of those with OCD and 10% of community controls. In subsamples matched for age and gender, more individuals with hoarding behaviors reported a parent with significant clutter and difficulty discarding (53%) than did individuals with OCD (24%) or community controls (18%). For any first-degree relative, the findings were similar (57%, 30%, and 26%, respectively). The effects were also similar for excessive acquisition. Across all three groups, mothers and sisters were more likely to be described as having hoarding symptoms (i.e, difficulty discarding, excessive acquisition, clutter) than fathers or brothers.

Several studies have reported on the genetics of hoarding in families of patients with OCD or Gilles de la Tourette syndrome (GTS). Samuels et al. (2007) examined 219 families with OCD-affected siblings to determine chromosomal regions that might be linked to hoarding behavior. Among the 624 participants, 38% reported hoarding obsessions or compulsions on the Yale-Brown Obsessive Compulsive Scale (Y-BOCS). Strong linkage was discovered to a marker on chromosome 14. Lochner et al. (2005) also used the Y-BOCS hoarding items to examine genetic correlates of hoarding in 315 adult OCD patients. Eighteen percent of the OCD patients had hoarding symptoms. Few differences in genotype frequencies were found between OCD patients with hoarding symptoms and those without. Some differences were found in a subset of patients (Afrikaners), but the small sample involved prevented firm conclusions. In a linkage study, Mathews et al. (2007) assessed 11 mutigenerational families that had at least two or more OCD-affected members. Hoarding status was assessed using the Y-BOCS and clinical interviews. Over 30% of the interviewed participants had significant hoarding symptoms. The findings suggested that hoarding was highly heritable. Zhang et al. (2002) conducted a genome scan of hoarding on 77 sibling pairs concordant for a GTS diagnosis. Twenty-six of the pairs were concordant for hoarding and 28 were discordant, and for 23 pairs neither sibling had hoarding symptoms. Hoarding status was determined using the Y-BOCS. The findings suggested linkage of hoarding symptoms to specific regions on three chromosomes (4q, 5q, and 17q).

Although the findings from these studies are suggestive, there are several reasons for caution in interpreting them. Each of these samples was drawn from populations with other disorders (OCD or GTS), and therefore the findings may not be generalizable to a broader population. In fact, except for the Lochner et al. (2005) study, the high frequency of hoarding observed in these studies does not reflect the levels of comorbidity seen in studies using more accurate hoarding measures. This raises questions about the accuracy of their assessment of hoarding symptoms. Relatedly, each of these studies relied on the two hoarding questions included in the Y-BOCS (presence or absence of hoarding/saving obsessions and of hoarding/collecting compulsions). The literature strongly suggests that such assessments are highly inaccurate and do not capture the full nature of the hoarding phenomenon (see Chapter 3 for more information on assessment of hoarding).

Taylor et al. (2010) corrected for some of these problems by examining hoarding in a sample of 307 twin pairs. They also used the Hoarding subscale from the short version of the Obsessive-Compulsive Inventory—Revised (OCI-R; Foa et al. 2002) to assess hoarding severity. In this study, genetic factors accounted for 42% of the variance in hoarding symptoms, with the remainder attributable to environmental factors. Though the assessment in this study was an improvement over the use of the Y-BOCS measure, the OCI-R still does not adequately assess the full scope of hoarding symptoms.

Other studies have corrected for the sampling and measurement problems by studying large samples derived from twin registries and relying on well-validated measures of hoarding severity. Iervolino et al. (2009) used U.K. Twin Registry data to investigate hoarding among more than 4,000 individuals. Cutoffs for hoarding caseness were based on the receiver operating characteristic (ROC) analysis with established cutoff scores on the Hoarding Rating Scale—Self Report (HRS-SR), a measure used as a template for the development of the DSM-5 criteria (see Chapter 3). Because of the small number of male participants, their heritability analyses were based only on female participants. The polychoric correlation showed greater similarity among monozygotic twins (0.52) than among dizygotic twins (0.27). Genetic factors were estimated to account for approximately 50% of the variance in hoarding symptoms.

Using adult twin pairs and their family members from the Netherlands Twin Register (total sample $N=15,914$), Mathews et al. (2014) found that genetic factors accounted for approximately 36% of the variance in hoarding using the HRS-SR. Similarly, López-Solà et al. (2014) used the HRS-SR to indicate caseness among 3,475 twin pairs from the Australian Twin Registry in examining genetic sex differences. Greater heritability was observed among females (38%) than among males (25%).

In a series of studies, Ivanov and colleagues (2013, 2017) examined heritability in adolescents and young adults from the Swedish Twin Registry using the HRS-SR. The first examined the heritability of hoarding in a population-based study of 15-year-olds (Ivanov et al. 2013). Heritability was found to vary by gender. For boys, the interclass correlation for monozygotic twins (0.44) was significantly higher than for dizygotic boys (0.17). For girls, there was no difference in the interclass correlation between monozygotic (0.35) and dizygotic (0.41) twins. The model suggested that for boys, genes accounted for 32% of the variance in hoarding symptoms, while shared environmental factors contributed very little (4%). For girls, genes accounted for very little variance in hoarding symptoms (2%), while shared environment accounted for 32%. The clutter item of the HRS-SR was slightly modified in this study to account for the fact that youth often do not have control over all of the rooms in their home.

In a follow-up study, Ivanov et al. (2017) estimated the relative contributions of genetic and environmental factors to hoarding symptoms using three cohorts of twins from the Swedish Twin Registry, 15-year-olds (N=7,905), 18-year-olds (N=2,495), and 20- to 28-year-olds (N=6,218). A slightly modified version of the HRS-SR was used to determine hoarding caseness. The overall heritability estimates varied by age and were 41% for 15-year-olds, 31% for 18-year-olds, and 29% for 20- to 28-year-olds. As in the Ivanov et al. (2013) study, heritability estimates for 15-year-olds also varied by sex (33% for boys, 17% for girls). Also, shared environmental effects accounted for significant variance in hoarding symptoms for 15-year-old girls. While heritability of hoarding symptoms decreased with the ascending age cohorts, the fact that there was stability of hoarding symptoms over time appeared to be due to genetic factors.

Hoarding Behaviors Attributable to Another Medical Condition vs. Hoarding Disorder

In Chapter 2, we noted that hoarding behaviors due to physical, perceptual, or cognitive deficits (e.g., brain damage, dementia) are not considered when one is determining whether the DSM-5 criteria for hoarding disorder are met. Although several case reports and a lesion overlap study reported hoarding symptoms after brain lesions in the orbitofrontal cortex, medial prefrontal cortex, and anterior cingulate cortex (Anderson et al. 2005; Cohen et al. 1999; Hahm et al. 2001; Mendez and Shapira 2008; Nakaaki et al. 2007; Volle et al. 2002), caution should be taken when extrapolating these findings to hoarding disorder because of phenomenological differences between such acquired hoarding behaviors and hoarding disorder. In hoarding behaviors attributable to another medical condition, there is typically a sudden onset of the hoarding behaviors, whereas hoarding disorder typically starts in childhood/adolescence and increases in each decade. Further, acquisition behaviors displayed by those with hoarding behaviors attributable to another medical condition (e.g., purposeless, stereotypic, with seemingly no interest in the items themselves [Anderson et al. 2005; Volle et al. 2002]) are different in nature from those observed in hoarding disorder. Additionally, some individuals with hoarding behaviors attributable to another medical condition do not exhibit distress when discarding possessions (Anderson et al. 2005), whereas difficulty parting with possessions is a diagnostic criterion for DSM-5 hoarding disorder.

Structural Abnormalities

Using structural MRI and positron emission tomography (PET), studies have investigated the presence of brain abnormalities associated with hoarding behaviors in patients with co-occurring OCD, dementia, and other neurological disorders and in patients with DSM-5 hoarding disorder.

MRI Studies in Patients With Co-occurring OCD, Dementia, and Other Neurological Disorders

Valente et al. (2005) examined gray matter abnormalities in 19 OCD patients (33% of whom endorsed hoarding obsessions and 28% of whom endorsed hoarding compulsions on the Y-BOCS) compared with 15 healthy controls using voxel-based morphometry. They found dysfunction of the orbitofrontal, cingulate, thalamic, and temporolimbic regions in OCD consistent with what has been found in other studies. Specifically, they reported in OCD participants—relative to control subjects—both increased gray matter in posterior orbitofrontal and parahippocampal regions and decreased gray matter in the left anterior cingulate cortex. Additionally, they found inverse correlations between gray matter in the medial thalamus and obsessive-compulsive symptom severity (Valente et al. 2005). Fouche and colleagues (2017) conducted a multisite mega-analysis of 412 OCD patients (20% of whom endorsed hoarding symptoms currently or in their lifetime) compared with 368 healthy controls. They found decreased cortical thickness in OCD patients compared with healthy controls in the superior and inferior frontal, precentral, posterior cingulate, middle temporal, inferior parietal, and precuneus gyri—consistent with earlier work showing that differences in cortical thickness and gray matter volume are associated with OCD and further adding support to a frontostriatal model of OCD (Fouche et. al 2017). The hoarding dimension was associated with increased cortical thickness in the bilateral inferior frontal gyri; left lateral orbitofrontal, superior parietal, middle temporal, and lateral occipital gyri; right superior frontal and medial orbitofrontal gyri; and cuneus (Fouche et. al 2017). On the other hand, studies of patients with neurological impairments like focal brain lesions resulting in collecting behavior (Anderson et al. 2005) suggest that damage to the mesial frontal region (including the right polar sector and the anterior cingulate) is associated with these behaviors. A study of 49 patients with frontotemporal dementia and either hoarding behaviors (29% endorsing new-onset hoarding) or obsessive-compulsive behaviors reported that hoarding behaviors were associated with decreased thickness in the left temporal, insular, and anterior cingulate cortices (Mitchell et al. 2019). Taken together, these studies involve reductions in cortical volumes in the frontal cortex and other regions spanning the orbitofrontal cortex, prefrontal cortex, anterior cingulate, parahippocampus, caudate, insula, and parietal, temporal, and occipital regions. The wide range of assessment tools used in these studies for determining hoarding behaviors limits the conclusions that can be drawn from this work.

MRI Studies in Patients With Hoarding Disorder

To date, there appears to be only one study on structural brain abnormality in hoarding disorder (Yamada et al. 2018). The team examined gray matter abnormalities in 17 patients with presentations that met DSM-5 criteria for hoarding disorder, 17 OCD patients without hoarding disorder (OCD patients who showed any hoarding symptoms on the dimensional Y-BOCS were excluded), and 17 healthy controls using voxel-based morphometry. In stark contrast to prior structural studies, they found a significantly increased prefrontal gray matter volume in the hoarding disorder group compared with the OCD and healthy control groups, specifically in Brodmann areas 10 and 11. This finding must be interpreted with caution because of the small sample size. Nevertheless, this study highlights how prefrontal abnormalities may be important in hoarding disorder pathology.

Functional Neuroanatomy

Early studies of functional abnormalities compared individuals with OCD who had hoarding symptoms and individuals with OCD without hoarding symptoms, while later studies involved individuals with presentations that met criteria for hoarding disorder. Studies can be further distinguished based on whether they were conducted in a resting state (e.g., typically performed with subjects lying down with eyes closed) or during symptom provocation (e.g., while subjects perform a task that is meant to elicit hoarding symptoms).

PET and MRI Studies in OCD Patients With and Without Hoarding Symptoms

One resting-state fluorodeoxyglucose-PET study found that 12 OCD patients with hoarding symptoms had less activity at rest in the dorsal anterior cingulate and cuneus compared with healthy controls and OCD patients without hoarding symptoms (Saxena and Maldment 2004). In a subsequent resting-state study of 20 unmedicated patients with hoarding symptoms (10 of whom had comorbid OCD), the authors found significantly lower glucose metabolism in the bilateral dorsal and ventral anterior cingulate cortex than was seen in controls (Saxena 2008); these regions were different from those typically associated with OCD. Both studies suggest that patterns of brain activity differ between hoarding disorder and OCD.

In contrast, symptom provocation studies (An et al. 2009; Mataix-Cols et al. 2004; Tolin et al. 2009, 2012) implicate abnormalities in the ventromedial prefrontal/anterior cingulate cortices and subcortical limbic structures (e.g., amygdala/hippocampus). One study compared patients with OCD—some of whom self-reported hoarding symptoms—with healthy control participants while they were presented with pictures of items (e.g., old newspapers, empty food containers) and asked to imagine discarding these possessions. The authors found that OCD patients had higher activation during the hoarding-related blocks in the orbitofrontal cortex, fusiform gyrus, and precentral gyrus than did the healthy controls (Mataix-Cols et al. 2004). Another study compared individuals with OCD who had hoarding symptoms and those who did not have hoarding symptoms with healthy controls during provocation of hoarding-related anxiety (e.g., while being presented with pictures of commonly saved items and with the audio instructions: "Imagine that these objects belong to you, and you must throw them away forever"). Provocation of symptoms unrelated to anxiety was included as a control. The authors found greater activation in the bilateral anterior ventromedial prefrontal cortex for OCD patients with hoarding symptoms than for OCD patients without hoarding symptoms and healthy controls during hoarding-related (but not symptom-unrelated) anxiety provocation (An et al. 2009). Tolin and colleagues (2009) compared 12 individuals with severe hoarding symptoms (two had comorbid OCD) and 12 healthy controls. Participants made decisions while in the functional MRI (fMRI) scanner about whether to keep or discard items that were personal or did not belong to them. Once the decision was made, the item was saved or destroyed. The authors found that during the decision process, individuals with hoarding disorder had increased activation of the lateral orbitofrontal cortex and parahippocampal gyrus compared with healthy controls. The decision to keep (as opposed to the decision to discard) their possessions was associated with greater activity in the anterior cingulate cortex, superior and middle temporal gyri, medial frontal gyrus, precentral gyrus, and cerebellum (Tolin et al. 2009). These results—in individuals primarily without OCD—were similar to the findings described in OCD patients with hoarding symptoms (An et al. 2009).

Functional MRI Studies Using DSM-5 Hoarding Criteria

One of the first studies using DSM-5 criteria compared brain activation patterns during executive function tasks (Stroop and Go/No-Go) in 15 individuals with hoarding disorder, 17 individuals with OCD, and 25 healthy controls (Hough et al. 2016). The findings suggest that individuals with hoarding disorder had significantly greater activity than controls in the anterior cingulate cortex and right dorsolateral prefrontal cortex during the conflict monitoring and response inhibition condition in the Go/No-Go task. In addition, there were activity differences between the hoarding disorder group and the other two groups in the anterior cingulate cortex, anterior insula, orbitofrontal cortex, and striatum, suggesting that brain regions involved in conflict and error processing are abnormally hyperactive in hoarding disorder (Hough et al. 2016).

Another set of studies in individuals with symptoms that met DSM-5 criteria for hoarding disorder were conducted while these patients made decisions about discarding personal possessions (Stevens et al. 2020; Tolin et al. 2009, 2012). Tolin and colleagues (2012) compared 43 patients with DSM-5 hoarding disorder, 31 patients with OCD (without comorbid hoarding disorder), and 33 healthy controls. When deciding about items that did not belong to them, patients with hoarding disorder (compared with participants with OCD and healthy controls) showed lower activity in the anterior cingulate cortex and insula. In contrast, when deciding about items that did belong to them, patients with hoarding disorder had increased activity in the anterior cingulate cortex and insula compared with the other two groups (Tolin et al 2012). These regions—part of the cingulo-opercular network—are associated with cognitive control and decision-making and are functionally connected structures that may be used to identify the emotional significance of an item and generate and regulate the affective state. A second study by the same group (Stevens et al. 2020) recruited 79 adults diagnosed with DSM-5 hoarding disorder and 44 nonhoarding controls and compared these two groups using a fMRI task of decision-making and a control task. Compared with controls, the hoarding disorder group had greater activity in the anterior cingulate cortex and insula during decisions about their own possessions that also correlated with their clutter level and difficulty discarding symptoms. This study replicated the cingulo-opercular abnormalities found in their earlier work (Tolin et al 2012) and further highlights abnormality in the inferior frontal cortex, a region that is important in executive control over semantic processing (Stevens et al. 2020).

In a study assessing cognitive control (using stop- and switch-signal tasks), Suñol and colleagues (2020) compared 17 patients with hoarding disorder, 18 patients with OCD, and 19 healthy controls and found that individuals with hoarding disorder had hyperactivation of the right lateral orbitofrontal cortex during successful response switching. They also reported that hoarding disorder patients had deactivation of frontal regions during error processing in both tasks.

To date, only one known resting-state functional connectivity study has been conducted in hoarding disorder patients (Levy et al. 2019). In this study, 17 patients with hoarding disorder, 8 with major depression, and 10 with co-occurring hoarding disorder and major depression were scanned. Levy and colleagues reported distinct connectivity patterns in hoarding disorder patients, including decreased connectivity in several cingulo-opercular network regions (e.g., orbitofrontal, middle, and superior frontal gyri; caudate nucleus; cuneus) and increased connectivity in the default mode (e.g., precuneus, fusiform gyrus) network. The authors noted that the networks highlighted are associated with information processing, error monitoring, and salience detection and have also been implicated in task-based studies of hoarding disorder (Hough et al. 2016; Stevens et al. 2020; Suñol et al. 2020; Tolin et al 2012).

Taken together, fMRI studies suggest that hoarding disorder is associated with abnormalities in cognitive control, cingulo-opercular, and salience networks. Evidence is limited—because of sample size—and more work is needed, as the abnormal neurophysiology underlying hoarding symptoms may involve structures yet to be detected.

Neuropsychological Studies

From the earliest descriptions of the phenomena, a number of information processing deficits have been associated with hoarding. In a review of subsequent research on performance-based measures of cognitive processing in individuals with hoarding, Woody et al. (2014) concluded that the evidence suggests those with hoarding have problems with planning, problem-solving, visuospatial learning and memory, sustained attention, working memory, and organization. Lynch et al. (2015), in a review of ADHD studies of hoarding, concluded that ADHD and hoarding share executive function deficits in spatial working memory, planning, and inhibition. The authors also suggest that there are greater neuropsychological deficits in hoarding that may not be specific to ADHD. These findings may represent broader neurocognitive impairment with symptoms that resemble ADHD (Tolin and Villavicencio 2011). Part of the broader impairment may include cognitive flexibility. Carbonella and Timpano (2016) hypothesized that cognitive flexibility deficits are an additional information processing problem in hoarding (i.e., "the ability to inhibit irrelevant material and attend flexibly between different mental sets"; p. 262). These investigators found evidence for a general deficit in cognitive flexibility, but not a specific one. For instance, people with hoarding tendencies had more trouble attending to things in their environment in a flexible way when there were distracting stimuli. However, hoarding-related distracting stimuli did not exacerbate this effect (Carbonella and Timpano 2016). Cognitive flexibility deficits may be related to the inattention displayed by people with hoarding problems and the often-observed "churning" behavior and ineffective attempts to organize possessions. People with hoarding are also hypothesized to have difficulties with categorization and concept formation and impaired decision-making (Frost and Hartl 1996; McMillan et al. 2013).

Features of Animal and Human Hoarding Behaviors

Hoarding behaviors across animal species (e.g., "food storing") have been examined and reviewed comprehensively (Vander Wall 1990). These behaviors can include "scatter hoarding," in which food is dispersed in small caches across a wide area, and "larger hoarding," in which food is amassed in a single location. The most recognized food-storing animals are squirrels, but other species with these qualities include Merriam's kangaroo rats, Clark's nutcracker birds, and hamsters. Rats are not considered natural hoarders, since they store food in underground dwellings and typically carry food from one patch to another to secure more food (Keen-Rhinehart et al. 2010). Humans also employ food hoarding—both larger hoarding (e.g., packed refrigerator) and scatter hoarding (e.g., snacks in the car, office, and purse/backpack). These behaviors are adaptive and can be deemed as important in order to have resources on hand in case they are critical for survival.

At the same time, animals can employ different hoarding strategies based on their assessment of risk, also known as the "cache strategy" (Preston 2001; Preston and Jacobs 2001, 2005). For example, it is easier for an animal with a low number of predators to employ a larger hoarding strategy. In times of uncertainty, humans may employ scatter hoarding by withdrawing money from a central location (e.g., the bank) and distributing it among smaller stashes that are in several different locations to mitigate risk. One question to answer is to what extent the animal hoarding behaviors and human hoarding behaviors evolved from a common ancestor as opposed to emerging separately due to environmental needs (e.g., homologous vs. analogous animal hoarding behaviors) (Preston 2014). A behavior that may be analogous is "nesting"—an innate instinct that may be associated with individuals with hoarding disorder, who report they feel safer with their items and more vulnerable without them (Frost and Steketee 2010). These resource allocation behaviors are complex and may reflect neurobiological mechanisms that are wired to cope with the perceived safety of the environment and are important to study further.

The mesolimbocortical system has been implicated in hoarding disorder as well as hoarding behavior in both nonhuman animals and humans regarding decisions to acquire rewarding items (Preston 2011). This mesolimbocortical system employs the neurotransmitter dopamine, which has been linked with animal food hoarding in the nucleus accumbens and ventral tegmentum. Lesions in these regions impair food hoarding and increase activity levels without impacting eating or transporting behaviors.

Translational Animal Models

Preclinical rodent models may contribute to treatment discovery in hoarding disorder. To cover an object, rodents will use their snout and forepaws to lift the bedding material over the object. This behavior was originally linked with anxiety, but in the last decade of research, the task has been seen as a model of compulsive behaviors (Albelda and Joel 2012a, 2012b). Several groups have tested the reliability of marble burying in mice after drug administration (Gawali et al. 2016; Kalariya et al. 2015). The marble-burying test was employed to study atomoxetine—a psychostimulant used to treat ADHD—in a translational study of hoarding behaviors in rodents and humans (Grassi et al. 2016). The test results suggest that attention and inhibitory control are robust target mechanisms for study in translational models.

Conclusion

While there is substantial evidence of the heritability of hoarding, there are questions about gender and age effects that are raised by this research. More definitive work on the genetics of hoarding is needed to answer these questions. Translation of hoarding behaviors across animal species is a fertile ground for psychopharmacology innovation. Advances in neuroimaging technology allow an unprecedented view of the neurobiology of mental illness and have the potential to detect abnormalities with an increasing level of precision. Understanding the neural circuits underlying hoarding behaviors opens up new avenues for intervention, including neuromodulation.

KEY CLINICAL POINTS

- Because of its recent classification, the neurobiology of hoarding disorder in humans is a newly burgeoning field, making it somewhat premature to draw firm conclusions.

- A complication in interpreting the findings of studies of etiology and pathology is that they vary in how hoarding symptoms are assessed.

- Early studies of functional abnormalities compared individuals with OCD who had hoarding symptoms and individuals with OCD without hoarding symptoms, while later studies involved individuals with presentations that met criteria for hoarding disorder.

- Hoarding behaviors attributable to another medical condition may have a sudden onset, whereas hoarding disorder typically starts in childhood/adolescence and increases in severity in each decade.

- Taken together, structural and functional MRI studies and PET studies suggest that hoarding disorder is associated with abnormalities in cognitive control, cingulo-opercular, and salience networks; however, evidence is limited because of sample size.

- A number of information processing deficits have been associated with hoarding, including deficits in planning, problem-solving, visuospatial learning and memory, sustained attention, working memory, and organization.

- Hoarding behaviors have been examined across animal species.

- Preclinical rodent models may contribute to treatment discovery in hoarding disorder.

References

Albelda N, Joel D: Animal models of obsessive-compulsive disorder: exploring pharmacology and neural substrates. Neurosci Biobehav Rev 36(1):47–63, 2012a 21527287

Albelda N, Joel D: Current animal models of obsessive compulsive disorder: an update. Neuroscience 211:83–106, 2012b 21925243

American Psychiatric Association: Diagnostic and Statistical Manual of Mental Disorders, 5th Edition. Arlington, VA, American Psychiatric Association, 2013

An SK, Mataix-Cols D, Lawrence NS, et al: To discard or not to discard: the neural basis of hoarding symptoms in obsessive-compulsive disorder. Mol Psychiatry 14(3):318–331, 2009 18180763

Anderson SW, Damasio H, Damasio AR: A neural basis for collecting behaviour in humans. Brain 128 (Pt 1):201–212, 2005 15548551

Carbonella JY, Timpano KR: Examining the link between hoarding symptoms and cognitive flexibility deficits. Behav Ther 47(2):262–273, 2016 26956657

Cohen L, Angladette L, Benoit N, Pierrot-Deseilligny C: A man who borrowed cars. Lancet 353(9146):34, 1999 10023949

Foa EB, Huppert JD, Leiberg S, et al: The Obsessive-Compulsive Inventory: development and validation of a short version. Psychol Assess 14(4):485–496, 2002 12501574

Fouche JP, du Plessis S, Hattingh C, et al; OCD Brain Imaging Consortium: Cortical thickness in obsessive-compulsive disorder: multisite mega-analysis of 780 brain scans from six centres. Br J Psychiatry 210(1):67–74, 2017 27198485

Frost RO, Gross RC: The hoarding of possessions. Behav Res Ther 31(4):367–381, 1993 8512538

Frost RO, Hartl TL: A cognitive-behavioral model of compulsive hoarding. Behav Res Ther 34(4):341–350, 1996 8871366

Frost RO, Steketee G: Stuff: Compulsive Hoarding and the Meaning of Things. Boston, MA, Houghton Mifflin Harcourt, 2010

Gawali NB, Chowdhury AA, Kothavade PS, et al: Involvement of nitric oxide in anticompulsive-like effect of agmatine on marble-burying behaviour in mice. Eur J Pharmacol 770:165–171, 2016 26593708

Grassi G, Micheli L, Di Cesare Mannelli L, et al: Atomoxetine for hoarding disorder: a pre-clinical and clinical investigation. J Psychiatr Res 83:240–248, 2016 27665536

Hahm DS, Kang Y, Cheong SS, Na DL: A compulsive collecting behavior following an A-com aneurysmal rupture. Neurology 56(3):398–400, 2001 11171910

Hough CM, Luks TL, Lai K, et al: Comparison of brain activation patterns during executive function tasks in hoarding disorder and non-hoarding OCD. Psychiatry Res Neuroimaging 255:50–59, 2016 27522332

Iervolino AC, Perroud N, Fullana MA, et al: Prevalence and heritability of compulsive hoarding: a twin study. Am J Psychiatry 166(10):1156–1161, 2009 19687130

Ivanov VZ, Mataix-Cols D, Serlachius E, et al: Prevalence, comorbidity and heritability of hoarding symptoms in adolescence: a population based twin study in 15-year olds. PLoS One 8(7):e69140, 2013 23874893

Ivanov VZ, Nordsletten A, Mataix-Cols D, et al: Heritability of hoarding symptoms across adolescence and young adulthood: a longitudinal twin study. PLoS One 12(6):e0179541, 2017 28658283

Kalariya M, Prajapati R, Parmar SK, Sheth N: Effect of hydroalcoholic extract of leaves of Colocasia esculenta on marble-burying behavior in mice: implications for obsessive-compulsive disorder. Pharm Biol 53(8):1239–1242, 2015 25885941

Keen-Rhinehart E, Dailey MJ, Bartness T: Physiological mechanisms for food-hoarding motivation in animals. Philos Trans R Soc Lond B Biol Sci 365(1542):961–975, 2010 20156819

Levy HC, Stevens MC, Glahn DC, et al: Distinct resting state functional connectivity abnormalities in hoarding disorder and major depressive disorder. J Psychiatr Res 113:108–116, 2019 30928618

Lochner C, Kinnear CJ, Hemmings SM, et al: Hoarding in obsessive-compulsive disorder: clinical and genetic correlates. J Clin Psychiatry 66(9):1155–1160, 2005 16187774

López-Solà C, Fontenelle LF, Alonso P, et al: Prevalence and heritability of obsessive-compulsive spectrum and anxiety disorder symptoms: a survey of the Australian Twin Registry. Am J Med Genet B Neuropsychiatr Genet 165B(4):314–325, 2014 24756981

Lynch F, McGillivray J, Moulding R, Byrne L: Hoarding in attention deficit hyperactivity disorder: Understanding the comorbidity. J Obsessive Compuls Relat Disord 4:37–46, 2015

Mataix-Cols D, Wooderson S, Lawrence N, et al: Distinct neural correlates of washing, checking, and hoarding symptom dimensions in obsessive-compulsive disorder. Arch Gen Psychiatry 61(6):564–576, 2004 15184236

Mathews CA, Nievergelt CM, Azzam A, et al: Heritability and clinical features of multigenerational families with obsessive-compulsive disorder and hoarding. Am J Med Genet B Neuropsychiatr Genet 144B(2):174–182, 2007 17290446

Mathews CA, Delucchi K, Cath DC, et al: Partitioning the etiology of hoarding and obsessive-compulsive symptoms. Psychol Med 44(13):2867–2876, 2014 25066062

McMillan SG, Rees CS, Pestell C: An investigation of executive functioning, attention and working memory in compulsive hoarding. Behav Cogn Psychother 41(5):610–625, 2013 23116570

Mendez MF, Shapira JS: The spectrum of recurrent thoughts and behaviors in frontotemporal dementia. CNS Spectr 13(3):202–208, 2008 18323753

Mitchell E, Tavares TP, Palaniyappan L, Finger EC: Hoarding and obsessive-compulsive behaviours in frontotemporal dementia: clinical and neuroanatomic associations. Cortex 121:443–453, 2019 31715541

Nakaaki S, Murata Y, Sato J, et al: Impairment of decision-making cognition in a case of frontotemporal lobar degeneration (FTLD) presenting with pathologic gambling and hoarding as the initial symptoms. Cogn Behav Neurol 20(2):121–125, 2007 17558256

Pertusa A, Fullana MA, Singh S, et al: Compulsive hoarding: OCD symptom, distinct clinical syndrome, or both? Am J Psychiatry 165(10):1289–1298, 2008 18483134

Preston SD: Effects of stress on decision making in the Merriam's kangaroo rat (Dipodomys merriami). Doctoral dissertation, University of California, Berkeley, 2001 DAI 63-02B:1082

Preston SD: Toward an interdisciplinary science of consumption. Ann N Y Acad Sci 1236:1–16, 2011 21883274

Preston SD: Hoarding in animals: the argument for a homology, in The Oxford Handbook of Hoarding and Aquiring. Edited by Frost RO, Steketee G. Oxford, UK, Oxford University Press, 2014, pp 187–205

Preston SD, Jacobs LF: Conspecific pilferage but not presence affects Merriam's kangaroo rat cache strategy. Behav Ecol 12(5):517–523, 2001

Preston SD, Jacobs LF: Cache decision making: the effects of competition on cache decisions in Merriam's kangaroo rat (Dipodomys merriami). J Comp Psychol 119(2):187–196, 2005 15982162

Samuels JF, Bienvenu OJ III, Pinto A, et al: Hoarding in obsessive-compulsive disorder: results from the OCD Collaborative Genetics Study. Behav Res Ther 45(4):673–686, 2007 16824483

Saxena S: Neurobiology and treatment of compulsive hoarding. CNS Spectr 13 (9, suppl 14):29–36, 2008 18849909

Saxena S, Maidment KM: Treatment of compulsive hoarding. J Clin Psychol 60(11):1143–1154, 2004 15389621

Steketee G, Schmalisch C, Dierberger A, et al: Symptoms and history of hoarding in older adults. J Obsessive Compuls Relat Disord 1:1–7, 2012

Stevens MC, Levy HC, Hallion LS, et al: Functional neuroimaging test of an emerging neurobiological model of hoarding disorder. Biol Psychiatry Cogn Neurosci Neuroimaging 5(1):68–75, 2020 31676206

Suñol M, Martínez Zalacaín I, Picó-Pérez M, et al: Differential patterns of brain activation between hoarding disorder and obsessive-compulsive disorder during executive performance. Psychol Med 50(4):666–673, 2020 30907337

Taylor S, Jang KL, Asmundson GJ: Etiology of obsessions and compulsions: a behavioral-genetic analysis. J Abnorm Psychol 119(4):672–682, 2010 21090873

Tolin DF, Villavicencio A: Inattention, but not OCD, predicts the core features of hoarding disorder. Behav Res Ther 49(2):120–125, 2011 21193171

Tolin DF, Kiehl KA, Worhunsky P, et al: An exploratory study of the neural mechanisms of decision making in compulsive hoarding. Psychol Med 39(2):325–336, 2009 18485263

Tolin DF, Stevens MC, Villavicencio AL, et al: Neural mechanisms of decision making in hoarding disorder. Arch Gen Psychiatry 69(8):832–841, 2012 22868937

Valente AA Jr, Miguel EC, Castro CC, et al: Regional gray matter abnormalities in obsessive-compulsive disorder: a voxel-based morphometry study. Biol Psychiatry 58(6):479–487, 2005 15978549

Vander Wall SB: Food Hoarding in Animals. Chicago, IL, University of Chicago Press, 1990

Volle E, Beato R, Levy R, Dubois B: Forced collectionism after orbitofrontal damage. Neurology 58(3):488–490, 2002 11839860

Woody SR, Kellman-McFarlane K, Welsted A: Review of cognitive performance in hoarding disorder. Clin Psychol Rev 34(4):324–336, 2014 24794835

Yamada S, Nakao T, Ikari K, et al: A unique increase in prefrontal gray matter volume in hoarding disorder compared to obsessive-compulsive disorder. PLoS One 13(7):e0200814, 2018 30011337

Zhang H, Leckman JF, Pauls DL, et al; Tourette Syndrome Association International Consortium for Genetics: Genomewide scan of hoarding in sib pairs in which both sibs have Gilles de la Tourette syndrome. Am J Hum Genet 70(4):896–904, 2002 11840360

PART III
Interventions

CHAPTER 7

Cognitive-Behavioral Therapy

Early attempts to treat hoarding problems were done using cognitive-behavioral therapy (CBT) designed for treating obsessive-compulsive disorder (OCD). Bloch et al. (2014) reviewed 21 studies of standard treatment for OCD patients with and without hoarding (more than 3,000 cases). OCD patients with hoarding symptoms were less likely to respond to treatments that work for OCD than were OCD patients without hoarding problems. With developing information about the fundamental features of hoarding and the cognitive-behavioral model of hoarding (Frost and Hartl 1996; Steketee and Frost 2003), efforts to develop a treatment specifically designed for hoarding disorder have made some progress (Ayers et al. 2014; Steketee and Frost 2013; Tolin et al. 2017). Targeting hoarding symptoms with CBT conducted by a therapist (via individual or group treatment) has shown therapeutic promise (Bodryzlova et al. 2019; Mathews et al. 2016, 2018; Tolin et al. 2015). Regardless of modality, however, clinically relevant symptoms remain after treatment. In this chapter, we describe the basic features of the treatment, review evidence for its efficacy, and survey suggested variations and additions to the treatment that reveal areas for improvement as well as new approaches to augment existing treatments.

Cognitive-Behavioral Therapy for Hoarding: Overview

CBT for hoarding is still in its infancy and evolving with each new study. This chapter will provide a brief overview of the basic features of this therapy, followed by a review of research on efficacy, adaptations, and related topics. A number of therapy guides that go into more detail are available (Muroff et al. 2014b; Steketee and Frost 2013; Tolin et al. 2014, 2017). The therapies in some of these guides have been subject to rigorous testing (Steketee and Frost 2013; Tolin et al. 2017). While they vary somewhat in form and style, they share core features. Each of these therapies is collaborative. The first step in each involves psychoeducation about the cognitive, emotional, and motivational underpinnings of the disorder. Success in treatment requires the client to understand how these features contribute to their difficulties with acquiring, discarding, and organizing possessions. These features are articulated by the cognitive-behavioral model of hoarding, discussed in Chapter 5 (Frost and Hartl 1996; Steketee and Frost 2003).

Hoarding disorder is a complex disorder that derives from a combination of factors. During the assessment phase of treatment, it is critical to start building a personal model that explains how the client's problems with organizing, discarding, saving, and excessive acquisition are tied together and maintained. The framework for this model is provided in the general conceptual model of hoarding disorder (see Chapter 5). The specific details vary by individual, but the general elements are present for most cases. The exercise of building a personal model in collaboration with the client fosters a perspective that distances them from their symptoms. It encourages a rational rather than emotional response to possessions. Model building begins with a review of the assessment materials and continues throughout the therapy as new insights are gained with each discarding/nonacquiring exercise.

CBT for hoarding emphasizes the use of motivational interviewing (Miller and Rollnick 2013) to understand the ambivalence experienced by people with this problem. The ambivalence in hoarding disorder is the conflict between wanting an uncluttered home and, at the same time, not wanting to part with cherished possessions. One of the first objectives of CBT for hoarding is to explore and resolve this ambivalence. Resolving the ambivalence is accomplished by focusing on the importance of change and instilling confidence that change is possible. In motivational interviewing terms, the importance of change is the discrepancy between the current life experience and the life experience that is desired. The importance of change in CBT for hoarding is fostered by several exercises related to life values. By exploring and articulating what the client would like their life to be like, the therapist can identify the discrepancy between that state and the current situation. For instance, Ellen, a 72-year-old client with hoarding disorder, complained bitterly about her daughter's refusal to allow Ellen's grandchildren to visit her in her home. By juxtaposing these complaints with elaborations of what she would like those visits to be like, a discrepancy was created between the current state of affairs and her life goals. Juxtaposing this life goal against her current situation created dissonance. The dissonance that this produced was an uncomfortable emotional state that led her to look for ways to reduce or change it. There are two types of change that are possible in this scenario. One is to reduce the discrepancy by changing the goal (i.e., "I can see my grandchildren at their parents' home instead."), and the other is to change the current situation (i.e., "I can clear up the clutter in my living room enough so that they will visit."). Without some degree of confidence that change is possible, most people with hoarding problems choose the first course to reduce the discrepancy. The task of the hoarding therapist is twofold: to heighten the discrepancy between what the client wants their life to be and what it is now, and to create exercises that will give the client confidence that change is possible. Exercises designed to clarify life goals and values are the means to do the first of these. Other means include visualization exercises to clarify clients' images of what they want their home to look like and what activities they want to happen there. Once the discrepancy has been created, the therapist's task is to structure some exercises designed to give the client confidence that they can achieve the change that will allow their goals to be achieved. These can be targeted sessions with a discrete goal, such as clearing a small section of the home or engaging in a discarding or a nonacquiring event. They need to be carefully orchestrated to maximize the degree of success.

Chasson and colleagues (2020) have developed a variation of the visualization exercise that involves a brief virtual reality immersion task in which participants view images of their home without the existing clutter. Following 10 minutes of immersion, participants showed an increase in treatment readiness and a greater confidence that hoarding treatment would be successful.

The values and goals elucidated at the beginning of treatment must be re-explored throughout treatment since clients frequently get overwhelmed with the enormity of the task they face and lose the confidence that change is possible.

Once sufficient motivation has been established, gaining control over excessive acquisition must happen as soon as possible. Although not a diagnostic criterion for hoarding disorder, excessive acquisition characterizes the vast majority of people with hoarding (Frost et al. 2009, 2013). Regardless of the volume of possessions discarded or let go, little progress will be made unless new acquisitions stop coming into the home. Excessive acquiring in hoarding is largely impulsive and driven by intense urges and the inability to resist the urge when a target object is encountered. When the individual is faced with a potential acquisition, their attentional focus narrows so that the decision of whether to acquire is driven by the positive features of the object and not by the myriad of reasons why it should not be acquired (e.g., not enough money, space). Thus, acquiring decisions are based on biased information and not a careful consideration of both the pros and cons of acquiring. One simple exercise to counteract this tendency is to have clients generate a set of questions they should ask themselves before making a decision to acquire. This effectively slows the process, blunts the urge, and allows them to consider the context of their life in making a decision. Clients are asked to create a list of such questions to carry with them and to consult before deciding to acquire.

The strength of the urge to acquire is often so powerful that the individual feels out of control. The goal of CBT for hoarding is to teach the client to tolerate the urge to acquire. This can be accomplished by exposing them to increasingly more powerful urges while they resist acquiring. Creating a hierarchy of situations with various levels of urge intensity, much like a hierarchy used in treating OCD, can be useful in teaching urge tolerance.

For some clients, avoiding acquiring triggers (e.g., favorite store) may be helpful in the beginning of treatment. Many people with hoarding use this strategy in an attempt to control the urge. While such a strategy can be useful at the outset of therapy, it is not a good long-term solution because our culture is not one that allows avoidance of the cues to acquiring.

A complicating factor in treating excessive acquisition is that for many people with hoarding, acquiring is one of their few pleasures in life. Taking this away from them can have negative consequences for their mood. Along with teaching urge tolerance and better decision-making strategies, it is important to help them find alternative and more adaptive sources of pleasure.

Tackling difficulty discarding is perhaps the hardest part of treatment for hoarding. The intense attachments to and beliefs about possessions are often rigidly held and difficult to counteract. When work on discarding is just getting started, it is important for the therapist and client to understand the nature of the client's attachments to possessions (see Chapter 5). The goal of this phase of treatment is to help clients change the nature of their attachments to and beliefs about the things they own. Once these change, discarding and decluttering will become easier. The basic format is to set up behavioral experiments to allow clients to challenge the necessity and importance of each possession. The process is slow, so progress in clearing clutter is not apparent at first. The goal of this part of treatment is to get clients to be able to think more flexibly about their possessions and the importance they hold. This can only be done in the context of attempts to discard. Behavioral experiments should be designed to test specific beliefs (i.e., "I would not be able to stop thinking about this item if I threw it away"). There are a number of ways to set up these experiments. In early versions of the treatment (Steketee and Frost 2013), part of this process involved asking targeted questions about each possession. Subsequent research has suggested, however, that it can be more effective to simply ask the client to describe the possession (Frost et al. 2016). In doing so, clients appear to process information about a possession in ways they had not done before. What has been observed about people with hoarding is that once a possession enters the home, it gets put in a pile somewhere and is virtually never looked at again (Frost et al. 1995). Clients may have a memory of where it is, but no real evaluation of the importance of keeping the possession takes place. Simply asking clients to tell the story of the possession gives them the opportunity to process information about its importance. If this exercise is preceded by a discussion of life goals and values, the decision is usually to discard.

Using a similar approach, David et al. (2019) adapted the cognitive bias modification of interpretation (CBM-I) protocol for application to hoarding-related beliefs. CBM-I is an experimental training procedure designed to alter maladaptive interpretations that lead to symptoms of anxiety and depression (MacLeod and Mathews 2012). Among a sample of college students who scored above the clinical cutoff for difficulty discarding on the Saving Inventory—Revised (SI-R), David et al. (2019) reported significant improvement in hoarding-related beliefs as well as self-reported hoarding symptoms 1 week after a single training session.

With homes that are packed with possessions, this strategy will seem to be too little to effectively clear the clutter. However, the purpose here is to loosen the grip of dysfunctional beliefs about possessions. Later in treatment, clients will be able to move more quickly with decisions about discarding.

Besides addressing acquiring and difficulty discarding, the third major focus of treatment for hoarding is on the organizational skills needed to accomplish decluttering. As outlined in the cognitive-behavioral model of hoarding (see Chapter 5), people with hoarding have a number of information processing and executive function deficits that influence their ability to manage possessions. Strategies for working on these deficits are detailed in various treatment manuals (Steketee and Frost 2013; Tolin et al. 2017). Only a brief overview will be provided here. Many people with hoarding report spending a great deal of time trying, but failing, to get organized. These failures may have much to do with deficits in information processing and organizational skills that have been observed in this population (Woody et al. 2014). This includes difficulties in solving problems, managing attention and distraction, categorizing and organizing, and using and sticking to schedules. Problem-solving difficulties consist of an inability to clearly define the problem (often due to overinclusive thinking), generate possible solutions, and carry through with planned efforts to resolve the problem. Specific training in problem-solving steps is a part of most treatment packages for hoarding disorder.

Hoarding disorder is often comorbid with ADHD (Frost et al. 2011b). Distractibility is frequently a major impediment to adherence to treatment and homework assignments. ADHD symptoms have been shown to be negatively correlated with homework compliance in several treatment trials (Fabricant et al. 2007; Tolin et al. 2007). Attaching attentional training to hoarding treatment is recommended. DiMauro et al. (2014) found that a cognitive remediation program focusing on attention resulted in significant improvement in attention compared with a relaxation-only control among hoarding patients. Likewise, a lack of categorizing and organizing skills frequently impairs attempts to manage clutter. Specific training in how to categorize and organize possessions, create filing systems for paper items, and plan the steps necessary for reorganizing space is part of the treatment regimen. Other major impediments for people with hoarding are arriving late, missing sessions, and not carrying out homework assignments (Christensen and Greist 2001). Much of this can be traced to difficulties with time management. Specific training in establishing and sticking to a schedule is part of the treatment as well. Many—if not most—people with hoarding problems organize the possessions in their world visually and spatially rather than categorically. They rely on visual memory to find objects in their home. For instance, Irene, one of our early clients, could recall with some degree of accuracy where she placed an electricity bill ("It's on the left side of the pile, about a foot down"). For her, it was possible to find possessions by recalling where she had seen them last. When we helped her create a filing system for her papers, she felt lost—like she had no idea where things were—even though she was clearly more efficient in locating them. Several studies have reported improvements in these neuropsychological deficits through CBT (Zakrzewski et al. 2020) or cognitive rehabilitation (Ayers et al. 2020).

Ayers et al. (2014) adapted a cognitive rehabilitation program used for psychotic patients (compensatory cognitive training [Twamley et al. 2012]) to address the well-known executive function and information processing deficits among people with hoarding (e.g., problem-solving, categorization, planning). The protocol was designed for treatment of older adults, although it may be equally useful for younger hoarding populations. The authors called the treatment "Cognitive Rehabilitation and Exposure/Sorting Therapy (CREST) for hoarding." The CREST protocol modified treatment by devoting six sessions to cognitive rehabilitation, and adding further work as needed (vs. two to three sessions in the Steketee and Frost [2013] protocol). In addition, following the findings of an earlier study (Ayers et al. 2011), the protocol also deemphasized the cognitive restructuring aspects of CBT for hoarding and focused more on exposure to discarding.

Evidence Base for Cognitive-Behavioral Therapy for Hoarding

A number of case studies and open trials have examined the efficacy of CBT for hoarding and its variants. Findings from these studies indicate that the treatment is effective, with large pre-post effect sizes—especially for changes in difficulty discarding (Tolin et al. 2015). The frequency of clinically significant change across symptoms ranges from 20% to 40%; however, most individuals continue to experience significant hoarding symptoms posttreatment (Tolin et al. 2015). Both individual and group treatment appear to produce comparable improvement in hoarding severity.

Only six randomized controlled trials (RCTs) have compared CBT for hoarding with a wait list or alternative control. Steketee et al. (2010) randomly assigned hoarding participants to weekly CBT or a 12-week wait list. At the end of the 12 weeks, CBT clients showed significant declines on all hoarding measures, while the wait-list group did not. Analyses of the primary hoarding measures—Hoarding Rating Scale (HRS) and SI-R—demonstrated large effect sizes (Cohen's $d = 1.007$ and 0.896, respectively), indicating that the CBT group improved significantly more than the wait-list group after only 12 weeks. Pre-post analyses of all subjects completing the full 26 sessions of CBT indicated continued improvement from session 12 to session 26. Pre-post effect sizes (d) for the SI-R, its subscales, and the HRS were large—ranging from 1.2 to 2.3. Decline in hoarding symptoms ranged from 27% (SI-R) to 39% (HRS). More than 80% of clients rated themselves as improved, while clinicians rated 71% of clients as improved. Despite the significant effects over time and when compared with a wait-list control in this study, the mean posttest SI-R (44.8) and posttest HRS (17.2) scores were both still above the established cutoffs for clinically significant hoarding severity (Kellman-McFarlane et al. 2019).

Frost et al. (2012) created a peer-facilitated group version of CBT for hoarding called the Buried in Treasures (BIT) Workshop using the Tolin et al. (2014) self-help book *Buried in Treasures*. The workshop involved 13 sessions organized around the chapters in *Buried in Treasures* and was highly structured to enable facilitation by nonclinicians. The chapters in the BIT book roughly followed the order of CBT for hoarding (Steketee and Frost 2013). The first four sessions focused on psychoeducation and motivational enhancement, the next two addressed excessive acquisition, and the four sessions after that included cognitive restructuring exercises and practice in nonacquiring and discarding The final three sessions addressed difficulties encountered in discarding and nonacquiring and preparation for continued work after the end of the workshop.

In a RCT, 38 individuals seeking help with hoarding problems were assigned to the BIT Workshop or a wait-list control. For each of the outcome measures (HRS, SI-R, Clutter Image Rating [CIR], and Activities of Daily Living—Hoarding Scale [ADL-H]), there were significant improvements among the BIT group participants, but not for the wait-list controls. Pre-post effect sizes (*d*) for the SI-R and HRS for the full sample of participants were large, ranging from 1.41 to 2.69, and comparable to those observed by Steketee et al. (2010). Pre-post percentage change was 24% for the SI-R and 27% for the HRS. For the SI-R clutter scale, the change was somewhat lower (19%) than for difficulty discarding (25%) or excessive acquisition (31%). A lower percentage change was noted for the CIR (13%) and ADL-H (14%) as well. After completion of the workshop, 84% of all treated participants rated themselves as "much" or "very much" improved. In addition to these outcome measures, Frost et al. (2012) also included a measure of attachments to possessions (Saving Cognitions Inventory [SCI]). Findings from the SCI indicated that BIT Workshop participants improved significantly more on three of the four subscales than did waitlist participants. Pre-post effect sizes (*d*) were large for three of the subscales (Responsibility: 1.59; Memory: 1.85; Emotional Attachment: 1.24). Only the Control subscale did not show significant improvement. This study replicates findings from an earlier open trial (Frost et al. 2011a) and indicates that a highly structured peer-led workshop run for half the number of sessions of the CBT protocol (Steketee and Frost 2013) can produce similar outcomes. Furthermore, it suggests that change occurs not only in hoarding symptoms but also in the attachments to possessions, which are believed to underlie the behavior. However, as in other studies on the efficacy of CBT for hoarding, posttest scores on the primary symptom measures still average above the clinically significant level (SI-R=46.3; HRS=16.7).

Muroff et al. (2012) randomly assigned individuals seeking help for hoarding to one of three hoarding treatment conditions: group CBT with in-home assistance, group CBT without in-home assistance, and a bibliotherapy-only condition. At the end of 20 sessions (20 weeks), for those in both CBT groups, conditions improved significantly more compared with the bibliotherapy group, with large effect sizes. Improvement conditions from the group CBT (24% to 35%) were comparable to improvement reported in other hoarding treatment outcome studies. There was some indication that in-home assistance facilitated treatment. Mean scores on most measures at posttest for the in-home assistance group were lower than those for the group CBT without in-home assistance. Twenty-one percent of individuals in the group CBT without in-home assistance achieved clinically significant change, while 36% of the group CBT with in-home assistance did so. Effect size (*d*) for the group CBT without in-home assistance was large at 2.0, while the effect size for the group CBT with in-home assistance was 3.3. However, none of these differences between conditions with or without in-home assistance reached statistical significance. The small sample size in this study (*N*=38) may have resulted in inadequate power to detect differences between the two group treatment conditions. As with the other studies, the end state symptom measures still indicated significant hoarding problems in the treated groups (SI-Rs with=43.5 and without = 48.8; HRSs with=22.8 and without=22.1).

In the largest treatment study to date, Mathews et al. (2018) conducted a non-inferiority trial comparing clinician-led group CBT with a peer-led CBT group (BIT Workshop). The 323 individuals with hoarding disorder were randomly assigned to 16 sessions of either clinician-led group CBT or a BIT Workshop. SI-R scores at posttest were reduced by 27.7% for clinician-led group CBT and 25.6% for the peer-led group. The test of non-inferiority indicated that the outcomes were equivalent. The hypothesis that peer-led treatment would be inferior was not supported. Outcomes on the SI-R in this study were comparable to those observed in other hoarding treatment studies (25%–30% reduction in hoarding severity), with roughly 30% achieving remission status. There was somewhat less improvement on functional impairment (AHL-H).

Tolin et al. (2017) developed a version of group CBT for hoarding disorder that emphasized more skill-based exercises than the Steketee and Frost (2013) protocol. In a RCT, the CBT group achieved significantly better outcomes than a wait-list control (Tolin et al. 2019). The treated group had significantly more members who achieved clinically significant change (42%) than the wait-list group (8%) on the SI-R, although the difference was not as large using the HRS-Interview (17% vs. 0%). Similar to other RCTs, the reduction in SI-R scores was approximately 30%, and the end state scores on both the SI-R and the HRS (43 and 17, respectively) indicate that many treated individuals still have clinically significant hoarding symptoms.

Some success has been achieved in adapting CBT for hoarding disorder by providing a stronger emphasis on cognitive rehabilitation. Using a sample of older adults with hoarding disorder (ages >60), Ayers et al. (2018a) compared 26 weeks of CREST with case management, which consisted of support and advocacy delivered by geriatric nurses. CREST participants achieved significantly greater reductions on several hoarding severity measures, including the SI-R total score (38% vs. 25%), the ADL-H (32% vs. 13%), and the Clinical Global Impression (CGI)—Severity of Illness (27%

vs. 12%). In addition, significantly more CREST participants were classified as treatment responders (78%) compared with case management participants (28%) using the CGI-Improvement score. For the SI-R subscales,
only the Clutter subscale showed significantly more improvement for
CREST participants. There were no significant group differences on the
other SI-R subscales, the UCLA Hoarding Severity Scale (UHSS), or the
CIR, although the change percentages for each group were in the predicted
direction. One potential problem with these findings was that despite the
random assignment, there were some preexisting differences that might
have influenced these results. Specifically, the CREST group was older and
more highly educated, while the case management group had more participants who were comorbid for OCD (41% vs. 13%).

Follow-Up Findings

A number of studies have included follow-up data ranging from 1 month
to 1 year. These studies have consistently found that improvements during
therapy remained stable after treatment. Muroff et al. (2012) reported that
up to 1 year after treatment, improvements on primary measures (SI-R and
HRS) were maintained. In addition, at follow-up, 62% of clients were judged
by therapists to be "much" or "very much" improved compared with pretreatment, while 79% of clients rated themselves as "much" or "very much"
improved. Similarly, Ivanov et al. (2018) reported that treatment gains from
internet-assisted CBT for hoarding disorder were maintained for all measures (SI-R, SCI) at 3-month follow-up, with 65% or participants being
classified as "much" or "very much" improved, compared with 50% at posttest. Ayers et al. (2018a) found treatment gains to be maintained (SI-R,
ADL-H) from posttreatment to 9- and 12-month follow-up in a trial of
cognitive rehabilitation–enhanced CBT for hoarding disorder. Other studies
with smaller sample sizes have also found that treatment gains are largely
maintained at follow-up (Ayers et al. 2011; Frost et al. 2011a). In their large
sample, Mathews et al. (2018) reported that treatment gains—as measured
by the SI-R—were sustained at 3 months and at longer follow-up. However, longer time from posttreatment to follow-up was associated with worsening symptoms. Also, functional deficits (AHL-H) rose significantly from
posttreatment to follow-up but remained well below pretreatment levels.
Similarly, Ayers et al. (2018a) found treatment gains were maintained for
the SI-R at 3 and 6 months following treatment using the CREST protocol.
However, there was some increase in functional disability (ADL-H), especially 9–12 months posttreatment. These findings indicate that treatment
effects for CBT for hoarding disorder are generally stable after treatment.
However, it should be noted that posttreatment end points still reflect clin-

ical levels of hoarding severity. Since the absence of further improvement after treatment is observed across these studies, treatments may need to be extended in order to achieve remission.

Predictors of Treatment Outcome

Preliminary evidence suggests that several demographic factors might be related to outcome of CBT for hoarding. A meta-analysis including 10 published treatment studies (Tolin et al. 2015) found that studies with a higher proportion of women had significantly better outcomes on SI-R Difficulty Discarding, Excessive Acquisition, and Clutter, as well as general hoarding severity. In addition, younger individuals fared better than older ones. However, in a subsequent study involving a large sample, Mathews et al. (2018) failed to find a relationship between gender or age and remission following CBT. Also, in a smaller meta-analysis, Bodryzlova et al. (2019) failed to find a gender effect, but they did find a small effect for age.

Few personality variables have been examined in relation to treatment outcome in hoarding disorder. However, Muroff et al. (2011) found higher baseline levels of perfectionism to be associated with poorer outcomes in CBT, which is consistent with anecdotal accounts (Frost and Steketee 2010). Castriotta et al. (2019) found that intolerance of uncertainty—a characteristic closely associated with perfectionism (see Obsessive Compulsive Cognitions Working Group 2005)—increased the odds of treatment nonresponse. Ayers et al. (2018b) found that higher levels of avoidant coping (self-distraction and behavioral disengagement) and denial—as well as greater degree of clutter—predicted poorer outcome.

Some evidence suggests that therapy engagement indices are associated with better outcomes. Ayers et al. (2018b) reported that several motivational variables (maintenance stage and composite readiness for change from the University of Rhode Island Change Assessment questionnaire) (McConnaughy et al. 1983) predicted a better outcome in treating hoarding disorder. In the Tolin et al. (2015) meta-analysis, more sessions attended and more home visits during therapy were associated with treatment success. Mathews et al. (2018) also found that increased attendance at group therapy sessions was associated with better outcomes. However, Bodryzlova et al. (2019) failed to find the number of sessions or home visits to predict outcome in a smaller meta-analysis. Homework completion has also been found to be associated with a better response to treatment (Mathews et al. 2018; Muroff et al. 2011; Tolin et al. 2007).

Attempts to develop sources of motivation from family members have shown promise. Chasson et al. (2014) developed a program that teaches family members to serve as "motivators" for loved ones with hoarding disorder.

In a small pilot investigation, the program resulted in more hopefulness among family members, reduced negative impact of the hoarding symptoms on the family, fewer accommodations for hoarding behaviors, and increased knowledge of motivational interviewing principles by family members.

Mediators of Treatment Response

The cognitive-behavioral model of hoarding (Chapter 5) posits that underlying hoarding symptoms are beliefs about possessions (i.e., saving cognitions) that include emotional attachments, beliefs about the role of possessions in maintaining memory and control over possessions, and a sense of responsibility for the care and preservation of possessions. If these beliefs serve to develop and maintain hoarding behavior, as is posited by the model, then changing them may produce changes in the behavior. Two studies have examined this question by testing whether changes in saving cognitions in therapy mediate changes in hoarding symptoms. Levy et al. (2017) found that changes in saving cognitions during treatment mediated changes in all three dimensions of hoarding symptoms (i.e., excessive acquiring, difficulty discarding, clutter). The SCI total score and each of the subscales (Emotional Attachment, Memory, Responsibility, and Control) mediated change in hoarding symptoms. Consistent with these findings, Tolin et al. (2019) also found that changes in saving cognitions mediated changes in symptoms accounting for approximately 16% of treatment effects.

Variations in and Additions to CBT for Hoarding

High levels of perfectionism characterize many people with hoarding disorder (Frost and Gross 1993), and some evidence suggests that perfectionism interferes with treatment (Muroff et al. 2014a). Consistent with this are anecdotal accounts of clients who are so crippled by perfectionism, self-criticism, and shame that they cannot tolerate anyone knowing about their problem, much less talking with a therapist about it (Chou et al. 2018). Frost and Steketee (2010) describe a case in which the client was so critical of herself for being unable to do the homework "perfectly" that she terminated treatment. Clients with such high levels of self-criticism may have difficulty benefiting from cognitive or behavioral therapies. Compassion-focused therapy (CFT; Gilbert 2010) was developed to help such clients approach their problems from a compassionate perspective rather than a self-critical one. CFT has been reported to improve distress tolerance, self-perception, and disordered cognitions in other disorders (Beaumont et al. 2012). Chou et al. (2020) adapted CFT for use as an adjunct to CBT in the treatment of hoarding disorder.

CFT for hoarding disorder exercises focus on recognition of the universal human tendency to become emotionally attached to possessions. The goal is to reduce the shame associated with disordered behavior and allow more flexible thinking with regard to possessions. Exercises also target emotion regulation and distress tolerance surrounding discarding. In the only trial of CFT for hoarding disorder, Chou et al. (2020) provided CFT to 13 individuals who had recently completed a course of CBT for hoarding disorder but still experienced significant hoarding symptoms. Following a 16-week trial of CFT, SI-R scores decreased by 33%, with a strong effect size ($d=1.45$). Seventy-seven percent of participants had SI-R posttreatment scores below 41 (the then-acknowledged cutoff for clinically significant hoarding symptoms). For 62% of participants, the SI-R posttreatment scores declined by 14 or more points (one of the criteria for clinically significant change). Acceptability ratings for CFT as a treatment for hoarding disorder were high, with 95%–100% of participants rating each dimension of acceptability as "good" or "excellent" (e.g., overall treatment quality, easy to understand, helpful for hoarding, gain new tools, knowledge, likely to apply learned information). While this is only a small open trial, given that these treatment gains occurred for people who had been through CBT for hoarding disorder—and for whom the treatment with CFT was highly acceptable—this therapy may offer considerable power to our ability to successfully treat hoarding disorder. In a similar vein, Moulding et al. (2017) adapted the Steketee and Frost protocol to address self-blame and hopelessness in hoarding. Their 12-week protocol produced clinically significant change in 34% of participants—a result similar to those reported for other CBT for hoarding protocols. Further research is needed to determine whether tailoring a treatment protocol to counteract the effects of stigma and self-blame is an important factor in the treatment of hoarding.

Inference-based therapy (IBT), an alternative treatment for OCD, focuses on the reasoning process underlying obsessional doubt (O'Connor et al. 1999). Specifically, obsessional doubt is hypothesized to develop out of a process termed "inferential confusion"—the confusing of remote possibility with reality. St-Pierre-Delorme et al. (2011) argue that this processing error also characterizes hoarding. According to St-Pierre-Delorme and colleagues, inferential confusion in hoarding includes two levels of inference. The primary inference ("I might need this someday") is followed by a secondary one related to the anticipated consequence ("I will suffer in some way for not having this item"). Symptoms are thought to develop out of interior narratives that come from the primary inference, which may be specific for each client. IBT has been successful in treating OCD—especially patients with high levels of overvalued ideas. St-Pierre-Delorme et al. (2011) argue that IBT may be applied to hoarding since high levels of overvalued ideas are characteristic of people with hoarding (Neziroglu et al. 2012). In a case study, St-Pierre-Delorme et al. (2011) treated a woman suffering from hoarding symptoms with IBT. The therapy involved 10 steps aimed at decreasing the conviction about the primary inference. The client showed substantial progress after the 20-week treatment, although there was some regression at follow-up. Blais et al. (2016) followed with an open trial of IBT for hoarding disorder. Among the participants who completed treatment and completed the primary outcome measure ($n=14$), there was significant improvement from pretest to posttest—with levels of improvement similar to those seen in other studies of CBT. Treatment gains were retained at 6-month follow-up, and as in other studies on hoarding treatment, there was no difference between posttest hoarding severity and follow-up assessment. Participants with depressive personality disorder did not improve with this treatment.

Recent research has emphasized the role of self-identity as a significant etiological factor in hoarding disorder (Kings et al. 2017). Koszegi et al. (2017) have suggested that the discrepancy between the person's real or "authentic" self and what they think they should be ("ought self") is key in the development of hoarding. Possessions help to create a picture of a "possible future self" that can be realized by possessions. Possessions are deemed necessary for them to become the person they want to be. For example, as recounted in Chapter 5, Frost and Steketee (2010) described a woman who saved hundreds of cookbooks and recipes but never cooked. When she looked at her cookbooks, she fantasized about the dinner parties she could have. When she considered letting go of some of them, the dream of her future as a great cook was threatened, and her "future possible self" was destroyed. Koszegi et al. (2017) suggest that hoarding represents a discrepancy between an "authentic self" and an "ought self." They suggest that people's sense of self comes from the role possessions play in who they "ought" to be. Several investigators have attempted to incorporate these ideas into treatment. O'Connor et al. (2018) conducted an open trial of group treatment for hoarding disorder using IBT and emphasizing self-identity for a small number of participants. Pre-post improvement on the SI-R was modest (15%), but by 6-month follow-up it was comparable to that found with other CBT for hoarding disorder outcomes (25%). Pre-post improvement on the HRS was more substantial (28%) and improved further at 6-month follow-up (41%). Overall, participants found the treatment to be acceptable, especially in understanding how hoarding relates to their sense of self. Participants all felt the self-identity component of treatment facilitated their decluttering. However, combining these features (inference-based approach and self-identity focus) prevents drawing conclusions about either one. Nonetheless, the focus on self-identity may prove to play a significant role in treatment efficacy.

Home visits between therapy sessions are a recommended part of CBT for hoarding disorder. A meta-analysis of hoarding treatment outcomes found more home visits to be associated with better treatment outcomes (Tolin et al. 2015), and adding in-home decluttering help to treatments that do not automatically include it is both feasible and effective (Linkovski et al. 2018). However, some studies have failed to find a relationship between home work and outcome (Bodryzlova et al. 2019).

Attempts to provide in-home assistance via the internet have shown promise. Ivanov et al. (2018) provided internet support between group treatment sessions for hoarding disorder. In this open trial, clients had access to an online support system adapted from one used in the treatment of anxiety and depression (COMMIT; Månsson et al. 2017). The protocol included homework assessment and monitoring, uploading of pictures, communication with the therapist through messaging, personalized feedback, and guidance on homework. The treatment produced large effect sizes and symptom reduction comparable to that in other treatment outcome studies, with progress maintained at 3-month follow-up. All participants used the COMMIT system an average of 4 hours each week, which increased homework time. Patients reported high levels of satisfaction and especially noted the importance of support from the therapist.

Muroff and Otte (2019) pilot-tested webcam sessions with three clients who did not respond to regular CBT for hoarding disorder. Two of the three improved substantially, and all three reported a strong therapeutic alliance. The clients reported appreciation for the in-home nature of the work and that the webcam contact made them feel that the clinician was with them in the home. Consistent with reports from group therapy participants, clients reported that having the clinician view them in the home made them more accountable.

Muroff et al. (2010) evaluated outcomes of an online peer-moderated support group. New members to the support group showed significant improvement over the 15 months of the study, with large effect sizes. Long-standing members of the group showed less powerful effects.

St-Pierre-Delorme and O'Connor (2016) provided five sessions of virtual reality (VR) decluttering to hoarding disorder clients who had just completed a course of IBT for hoarding disorder (O'Connor et al. 2005). CIR scores for the bedroom declined modestly, but significantly more than those of a non-VR control; however, there were no significant effects observed on the Kitchen or Living Room CIR. Participants reported feeling immersed in the technology, suggesting some promise for VR in treating hoarding disorder. This study supports the feasibility of using VR to treat hoarding disorder, but the outcomes were small, suggesting more work is needed to demonstrate the usefulness of VR for hoarding disorder.

Other attempts to borrow protocols from treatments of other disorders have shown some promise in treating hoarding. Contingency management strategies produce some of the largest effect sizes in the treatment of substance use disorders (Petry 2010). Difficulties in the treatment of hoarding (insight, ambivalence regarding change, motivation, comorbidity) represent barriers that have been addressed with contingency management in other disorders. In light of these considerations, Worden et al. (2017) conducted an open trial of 16 sessions of group CBT for hoarding disorder augmented by contingency management. Independent evaluators conducted six home visits to assess progress and determine rewards for decluttering. Participants received $30 for each one-point reduction in CIR scores, and $10 for each one-point reduction that was maintained at the following assessment. Treatment completers averaged $139 in rewards during the treatment.

Changes in SI-R scores were significant, with very large effect sizes and a 32%–43% reduction in symptom severity. Seventy percent were judged to be "much" or "very much" improved by clinicians, while 90% rated themselves as "much" or "very much" improved. Comparison of the contingency management group with data from other groups using the same CBT protocol at the same clinic (i.e., benchmarked sample) suggested that contingency management adds considerable power. The pre-post effect size on the SI-R total score was 2.59 for the participants receiving contingency management augmentation and 1.97 for the benchmarked sample. Participants reported high levels of satisfaction with treatment, although 2 of the 14 who began treatment dropped out of the contingency management portion because of increased anxiety and pressure they experienced from the contingency management protocol. Sixty-seven percent of the treatment completers achieved clinically significant change.

The authors suggest that contingency management may incentivize taking risks with discarding, and this results in expanded self-efficacy regarding change. More research is needed to determine whether contingency management was the active factor in this study rather than the extra accountability generated by six home visits to evaluate the level of clutter. Other questions need answering as well, including the best ways to evaluate change and the optimal amount of reward. Nevertheless, these findings, although derived from a small sample, represent the best outcomes to date in the treatment research literature.

Conclusion

RCTs of CBT for hoarding indicate that it is an effective treatment across a range of outcome measures, including hoarding symptoms, functional impairment, and hoarding-related beliefs. Nevertheless, posttreatment symptoms and impairment remain problematic for many sufferers. Research on impediments to treatment efficacy has revealed potential areas for improvement. Problems with treatment engagement and motivation are well-known in hoarding cases, and attempts to address them have shown promise. Other impediments, such as perfectionism, intolerance of uncertainty, and avoidant coping, can be addressed by existing protocols, although this is as of yet unexplored. New emphases and modifications of CBT have shown promise, including improved home visit protocols, increased focus on cognitive remediation, compassion- and identity-focused approaches, and the use of virtual reality and contingency management. The next generation of CBT for hoarding disorder will undoubtedly include some combination of these features.

KEY CLINICAL POINTS

- Randomized controlled trials have established cognitive-behavioral therapy (CBT) for hoarding disorder as an effective treatment.

- Improvements seen in CBT for hoarding are largely maintained for up to 1 year.

- A highly structured, peer-led workshop (Buried in Treasures Workshop) following a CBT protocol has been found to produce outcomes similar to those seen with CBT for hoarding disorder.

- Perfectionism and intolerance of uncertainty are associated with poor response to CBT for hoarding disorder.

- Indices of poor motivation (e.g., missing sessions, low homework compliance) predict poorer outcomes in CBT for hoarding disorder.

- Changes in hoarding symptoms during treatment have been found to be mediated by decreases in the strength of attachments to and beliefs about possessions.

- Despite the effectiveness of CBT for hoarding disorder, a substantial number of individuals with hoarding disorder remain clinically impaired by their hoarding symptoms after treatment.

References

Ayers CR, Wetherell JL, Golshan S, Saxena S: Cognitive-behavioral therapy for geriatric compulsive hoarding. Behav Res Ther 49(10):689–694, 2011 21784412

Ayers CR, Saxena S, Espejo E, et al: Novel treatment for geriatric hoarding disorder: an open trial of cognitive rehabilitation paired with behavior therapy. Am J Geriatr Psychiatry 22(3):248–252, 2014 23831173

Ayers CR, Dozier ME, Twamley EW, et al: Cognitive Rehabilitation and Exposure/Sorting Therapy (CREST) for hoarding disorder in older adults: a randomized clinical trial. J Clin Psychiatry 79(2):16m11072, 2018a 28541646

Ayers CR, Pittman JOE, Davidson EJ, et al: Predictors of treatment outcome and attrition in adults with hoarding disorder. J Obsessive Compuls Relat Disord 23:100465, 2018b 32670783

Ayers CR, Davidson EJ, Dozier ME, Twamley EW: Cognitive rehabilitation and exposure/sorting therapy for late-life hoarding: effects on neuropsychological performance. J Gerontol B Psychol Sci Soc Sci 75(6):1193–1198, 2020 31246258

Beaumont E, Galpin A, Jenkins P: "Being kinder to myself": a prospective comparative study, exploring post-trauma therapy outcome measures, for two groups of clients, receiving either Cognitive Behaviour Therapy or Cognitive Behaviour Therapy and Compassionate Mind Training. Couns Psychol Rev 23:31–43, 2012

Blais M, Bodryzlova Y, Aardema F, O'Connor K: Open trial of inference-based therapy in the treatment of compulsive hoarding. Journal of Psychology and Clinical Psychiatry 6:00403, 2016

Bloch MH, Bartley CA, Zipperer L, et al: Meta-analysis: hoarding symptoms associated with poor treatment outcome in obsessive-compulsive disorder. Mol Psychiatry 19(9):1025–1030, 2014 24912494

Bodryzlova Y, Audet JS, Bergeron K, O'Connor K: Group cognitive-behavioural therapy for hoarding disorder: systematic review and meta-analysis. Health Soc Care Community 27(3):517–530, 2019 30033635

Castriotta N, Dozier ME, Taylor CT, et al: Intolerance of uncertainty in hoarding disorder. J Obsessive Compuls Relat Disord 21:97–101, 2019 32670782

Chasson GS, Carpenter A, Ewing J, et al: Empowering families to help a loved one with hoarding disorder: pilot study of Family-As-Motivators training. Behav Res Ther 63:9–16, 2014 25237830

Chasson G, Hamilton E, Luxon A, et al: Rendering promise: enhancing motivation for change in hoarding disorder using virtual reality. J Obsessive Compuls Relat Disord 25:100519, 2020

Chou CY, Tsoh J, Vigil O, et al: Contributions of self-criticism and shame to hoarding. Psychiatry Res 262:488–493, 2018 28939393

Chou CY, Tsoh JY, Shumway M, et al: Treating hoarding disorder with compassion-focused therapy: a pilot study examining treatment feasibility, acceptability, and exploring treatment effects. Br J Clin Psychol 59(1):1–21, 2020 31271462

Christensen DD, Greist JH: The challenge of obsessive-compulsive disorder hoarding. Prim Psychiatry 8:79–86, 2001

David J, Baldwin P, Grisham J: To save or not to save: the use of cognitive bias modification in a high-hoarding sample. J Obsessive Compuls Relat Disord 23:100457, 2019

DiMauro J, Genova M, Tolin DF, Kurtz MM: Cognitive remediation for neuropsychological impairment in hoarding disorder: a pilot study. J Obsessive Compuls Relat Disord 3(2):132–138, 2014

Fabricant L, Frost RO, Tolin DF, Steketee G: The role of homework in the treatment of compulsive hoarding. Paper presented at the annual meeting of the Association of Behavioral and Cognitive Therapies, Philadelphia, PA, November 2007

Frost RO, Gross RC: The hoarding of possessions. Behav Res Ther 31(4):367–381, 1993 8512538

Frost RO, Hartl TL: A cognitive-behavioral model of compulsive hoarding. Behav Res Ther 34(4):341–350, 1996 8871366

Frost RO, Steketee G: Stuff: Compulsive Hoarding and the Meaning of Things. Boston, MA, Houghton Mifflin Harcourt, 2010

Frost RO, Hartl TL, Christian R, Williams N: The value of possessions in compulsive hoarding: patterns of use and attachment. Behav Res Ther 33(8):897–902, 1995 7487849

Frost RO, Tolin DF, Steketee G, et al: Excessive acquisition in hoarding. J Anxiety Disord 23(5):632–639, 2009 19261435

Frost RO, Pekareva-Kochergina A, Maxner S: The effectiveness of a biblio-based support group for hoarding disorder. Behav Res Ther 49(10):628–634, 2011a 21831357

Frost RO, Steketee G, Tolin DF: Comorbidity in hoarding disorder. Depress Anxiety 28(10):876–884, 2011b 21770000

Frost RO, Ruby D, Shuer LJ: The Buried in Treasures Workshop: waitlist control trial of facilitated support groups for hoarding. Behav Res Ther 50(11):661–667, 2012 22982080

Frost RO, Rosenfield E, Steketee G, Tolin D: An examination of excessive acquisition in hoarding disorder. J Obsessive Compuls Relat Disord 2:338–345, 2013

Frost RO, Ong C, Steketee G, Tolin DF: Behavioral and emotional consequences of thought listing versus cognitive restructuring during discarding decisions in hoarding disorder. Behav Res Ther 85:13–22, 2016 27537707

Gilbert P: Compassion Focused Therapy: Distinctive Features. London, Routledge, 2010

Ivanov VZ, Enander J, Mataix-Cols D, et al: Enhancing group cognitive-behavioral therapy for hoarding disorder with between-session Internet-based clinician support: a feasibility study. J Clin Psychol 74(7):1092–1105, 2018 29411356

Kellman-McFarlane K, Stewart B, Woody S, et al: Saving Inventory—Revised: psychometric performance across the lifespan. J Affect Disord 252:358–364, 2019 30999092

Kings C, Moulding R, Knight T: You are what you own: reviewing the link between possessions, emotional attachment, and the self-concept in hoarding disorder. J Obsessive Compuls Relat Disord 14:51–58, 2017

Koszegi N, O'Connor K, Bodryzlova Y: Etiological models of hoarding disorder. Journal of Psychology and Clinical Psychiatry 7(5):00453, 2017

Levy HC, Worden BL, Gilliam CM, et al: Changes in saving cognitions mediate hoarding symptom change in cognitive-behavioral therapy for hoarding disorder. J Obsessive Compuls Relat Disord 14:112–118, 2017 29170732

Linkovski O, Zwerling J, Cordell E, et al: Augmenting Buried in Treasures with in-home uncluttering practice: pilot study in hoarding disorder. J Psychiatr Res 107:145–150, 2018 30419524

MacLeod C, Mathews A: Cognitive bias modification approaches to anxiety. Annu Rev Clin Psychol 8:189–217, 2012 22035241

Månsson KN, Klintmalm H, Nordqvist R, Andersson G: Conventional cognitive behavioral therapy facilitated by an Internet-based support system: feasibility study at a psychiatric outpatient clinic. JMIR Res Protoc 6(8):e158, 2017 28838884

Mathews CA, Uhm S, Chan J, et al: Treating Hoarding Disorder in a real-world setting: results from the Mental Health Association of San Francisco. Psychiatry Res 237:331–338, 2016 26805562

Mathews CA, Mackin RS, Chou CY, et al: Randomised clinical trial of community-based peer-led and psychologist-led group treatment for hoarding disorder. BJPsych Open 4(4):285–293, 2018 30083381

McConnaughy EA, Prochaska J, Velicer W: Stages of change in psychotherapy: measurement and sample profiles. Psychotherapy 20:368–375, 1983

Miller WR, Rollnick S: Motivational Interviewing: Helping People Change, 3rd Edition. New York, Guilford, 2013

Moulding R, Nedeljkovic M, Kyrios M, et al: Short-term cognitive-behavioural group treatment for hoarding disorder: a naturalistic treatment outcome study. Clin Psychol Psychother 24(1):235–244, 2017 26750388

Muroff J, Otte S: Innovations in CBT treatment for hoarding: transcending office walls. J Obsessive Compuls Relat Disord 23:100471, 2019

Muroff J, Steketee G, Himle J, Frost R: Delivery of internet treatment for compulsive hoarding (D.I.T.C.H.). Behav Res Ther 48(1):79–85, 2010 19800051

Muroff J, Bratiotis C, Steketee G: Treatment for hoarding behaviors: a review of the evidence. Clin Soc Work J 39:406–423, 2011

Muroff J, Steketee G, Bratiotis C, Ross A: Group cognitive and behavioral therapy and bibliotherapy for hoarding: a pilot trial. Depress Anxiety 29(7):597–604, 2012 22447579

Muroff J, Steketee G, Frost RO, Tolin DF: Cognitive behavior therapy for hoarding disorder: follow-up findings and predictors of outcome. Depress Anxiety 31(12):964–971, 2014a 24277161

Muroff J, Underwood P, Steketee G: Group Treatment for Hoarding Disorder: Therapist Guide. Oxford, UK, Oxford University Press, 2014b

Neziroglu F, Weissman S, Allen J, McKay D: Compulsive hoarders: how do they differ from individuals with obsessive compulsive disorder? Psychiatry Res 200(1):35–40, 2012 22748189

Obsessive Compulsive Cognitions Working Group: Psychometric validation of the obsessive belief questionnaire and interpretation of intrusions inventory—Part 2: Factor analyses and testing of a brief version. Behav Res Ther 43(11):1527–1542, 2005 16299894

O'Connor K, Todorov C, Robillard S, et al: Cognitive-behaviour therapy and medication in the treatment of obsessive-compulsive disorder: a controlled study. Can J Psychiatry 44(1):64–71, 1999 10076743

O'Connor KP, Aardema F, Pélissier M-C: Beyond Reasonable Doubt: Reasoning Processes in Obsessive-Compulsive Disorder and Related Disorders. Chichester, UK, Wiley, 2005

O'Connor K, Bodryzlova Y, Audet J-S, et al: Group cognitive-behavioural treatment with long-term follow-up and targeting self-identity for hoarding disorder: an open trial. Clin Psychol Psychother 25(5):701–709, 2018 29961961

Petry NM: Contingency management treatments: controversies and challenges. Addiction 105(9):1507–1509, 2010 20707772

St-Pierre-Delorme M-E, O'Connor K: Using virtual reality in the inference-based treatment of compulsive hoarding. Front Public Health 4:149, 2016 27486574

St-Pierre-Delorme M-E, Lalonde M, Perreault V, et al: Inference-based therapy for compulsive hoarding: a clinical case study. Clin Case Stud 10:291–303, 2011

Steketee G, Frost R: Compulsive hoarding: current status of the research. Clin Psychol Rev 23(7):905–927, 2003 14624821

Steketee G, Frost RO: Treatment for Hoarding Disorder: Therapist Guide, 2nd Edition. New York, Oxford University Press, 2013

Steketee G, Frost RO, Tolin DF, et al: Waitlist-controlled trial of cognitive behavior therapy for hoarding disorder. Depress Anxiety 27(5):476–484, 2010 20336804

Tolin DF, Frost RO, Steketee G: An open trial of cognitive-behavioral therapy for compulsive hoarding. Behav Res Ther 45(7):1461–1470, 2007 17306221

Tolin DF, Frost RO, Steketee G: Buried in Treasures: Help for Compulsive Acquiring, Saving, and Hoarding, 2nd Edition. Oxford, UK, Oxford University Press, 2014

Tolin DF, Frost RO, Steketee G, Muroff J: Cognitive behavioral therapy for hoarding disorder: a meta-analysis. Depress Anxiety 32(3):158–166, 2015 25639467

Tolin DF, Worden BL, Wootton BM, Gilliam CM: CBT for Hoarding Disorder: A Group Therapy Program: Therapist's Guide. Hoboken, NJ, Wiley Blackwell, 2017

Tolin DF, Wootton BM, Levy HC, et al: Efficacy and mediators of a group cognitive-behavioral therapy for hoarding disorder: a randomized trial. J Consult Clin Psychol 87(7):590–602, 2019 31008633

Twamley EW, Vella L, Burton CZ, et al: Compensatory cognitive training for psychosis: effects in a randomized controlled trial. J Clin Psychiatry 73(9):1212–1219, 2012 22939029

Woody SR, Kellman-McFarlane K, Welsted A: Review of cognitive performance in hoarding disorder. Clin Psychol Rev 34(4):324–336, 2014 24794835

Worden B, Bowe W, Tolin D: An open trial of cognitive behavioral therapy with
    contingency management for hoarding disorder. J Obsessive Compuls Relat
    Disord 12:78–86, 2017
Zakrzewski JJ, Gillett DA, Vigil OR, et al: Visually mediated functioning improves
    following treatment of hoarding disorder. J Affect Disord 264:310–317, 2020
    32056766

CHAPTER 8
Pharmacotherapy

To date, there are no medications approved by the U.S. FDA for hoarding disorder. This is due, in part, to the fact that hoarding disorder only relatively recently was added to DSM in 2013 (American Psychiatric Association 2013). The majority of what we know about pharmacotherapy for hoarding disorder comes from drug studies in individuals with obsessive-compulsive disorder (OCD) who have hoarding disorder symptoms, assessed by variable means (Saxena 2008, 2011; Saxena and Maidment 2004; Thompson et al. 2017). There are only a few small open-label studies in individuals whose symptoms meet diagnostic criteria for hoarding disorder (Grassi et al. 2016; Rodriguez et al. 2013; Saxena and Sumner 2014; Saxena et al. 2007). Although the results are promising, they can only be described as preliminary, since they derive from open trials or case series without control groups and based on small samples. There are no randomized controlled trials or meta-analyses to provide adequate support for these approaches. Patients need to be informed that the evidence level of the studies to date is low. Nevertheless, a trial with one of these drugs may be of some benefit. In this chapter, we examine pharmacological treatment approaches and strategies and their use in special contexts (patients with comorbid depression, inattention), the available efficacy evidence, and considerations for managing side effects and drug-drug interactions.

Goals of Treatment

The goals of treatment are to diminish hoarding symptoms and improve the patient's interpersonal, work, and social functioning. A modest proportion of patients will achieve freedom from significant symptoms with treatment. The clinician can use the assessment tools referred to in Chapter 3 (e.g., Clutter Image Rating [CIR], Saving Inventory—Revised [SI-R], Hoarding Rating Scale [HRS]; see Appendices B–D in this volume) to obtain a record of the patient's current and past symptoms.

Treatment planning depends on careful evaluation, as outlined in Chapters 2 and 3. As noted earlier, comorbid major depression and anxiety disorders will commonly be present. These comorbid conditions may not respond to the treatment prescribed for the patient's hoarding disorder, in which case treatment approaches to target comorbid conditions should be added. If the patient is abusing alcohol or drugs to alleviate depressive or anxious symptoms, this must be addressed before or in parallel to the other elements of the treatment plan. The presence of a personal or family history of hypomania, mania, or psychotic disorder should be explored, because these would influence therapy choices.

To maximize the usefulness of a comprehensive treatment plan, a clinician will need to get to know the patient and their situation to tailor the plan to the patient's needs, history, preferences, and level of functioning. For a patient with comorbid hoarding disorder and mild to moderate major depression (as in Case Example 1 later in this chapter), starting pharmacotherapy and cognitive-behavioral therapy (CBT) for hoarding disorder is a reasonable initial strategy. Many such patients will respond to CBT alone. In certain situations, such as when a patient has low energy and motivation that is secondary to moderate to severe major depression (as in Case Example 2 presented later in this chapter), medications alone may be preferable. In other cases, medications may be needed to decrease the intensity of the symptoms so that the patient can fully engage in CBT. Individuals with predominant inattention symptoms (as in Case Example 1) may consider a trial of a stimulant. There is evidence for the efficacy of CBT alone for hoarding in the form of randomized clinical trials (see Chapter 7). However, there is insufficient evidence to guide clinical decisions about the relative efficacy of medications alone, CBT alone, and their combination. Initial studies on compulsive hoarding suggest that symptom improvement from pharmacotherapy may be at least as great as that resulting from CBT (Saxena 2011). However, many experienced clinicians believe that the combination may be more effective than either treatment alone (Saxena 2011). All patients should be encouraged to contact the International OCD Foundation (https://hoarding.iocdf.org) and given other sources for educational material and support groups.

Pharmacotherapy

Treatment of hoarding disorder with serotonin reuptake inhibitors (SRIs) originated from the consideration of hoarding symptoms as part of OCD. Serotonergic neurotransmission was initially hypothesized to underlie OCD based on observations that clomipramine—which inhibits both serotonin and norepinephrine reuptake—relieved symptoms, whereas drugs with other targets (e.g., noradrenergic reuptake inhibitors) did not. To date, there have been no definitive studies to suggest serotonergic abnormalities are the root cause of OCD (Ahmari and Dougherty 2015). Although hoarding disorder was first considered a distinct diagnostic entity in 2013 because of its unique symptom profile and pathophysiology relative to OCD, pharmacotherapy for hoarding disorder has continued to focus primarily on SRIs.

Efficacy Studies

Several retrospective studies examining the role of OCD symptom factors in OCD treatment response found that hoarding symptoms were associated with poor response to SRI medications (Black et al. 1998; Mataix-Cols et al. 1999; Salomoni et al. 2009; Stein et al. 2007, 2008; Winsberg et al. 1999), but others have not replicated this association (Alonso et al. 2001; Erzegovesi et al. 2001; Ferrão et al. 2006; Landeros-Weisenberger et al. 2010; Shetti et al. 2005). In general, these studies have relied on inadequate measures of hoarding symptoms and samples not representative of most hoarding cases. Only a handful of prospective open-label studies have sought to specifically study hoarding disorder symptoms using more recently developed hoarding rating scales (see Chapter 3) and representative samples of patients with hoarding. As we review below, the effects of two medications—one selective serotonin reuptake inhibitor (paroxetine) and one serotonin-norepinephrine reuptake inhibitor (venlafaxine)—have been evaluated in patients assessed for hoarding disorder. Because attention is one of the executive functions found to be affected in hoarding disorder, trials have been conducted with medications typically used for ADHD, including psychostimulants (amphetamine salts, methylphenidate) and one norepinephrine reuptake inhibitor (atomoxetine). None of the medications reviewed below have been FDA approved for hoarding disorder.

Paroxetine

In an open-label trial, 79 patients with OCD (32 with comorbid hoarding disorder and 47 without hoarding symptoms) were treated with paroxetine for 12 weeks (mean dose=41.6±12.8 mg/day) (Saxena et al. 2007). Paroxetine was titrated by 10 mg/day increments every 4 days to a target dosage of 40 mg/day, as tolerated, and participants continued to take this dose for the first 8 weeks of treatment. In weeks 8–12, the dose could be increased to a maximum of 60 mg/day as tolerated. No other psychoactive medications, CBT, or treatments were allowed during the study period. OCD patients with hoarding symptoms (e.g., compulsive hoarding syndrome) responded as well to paroxetine treatment as those OCD patients without hoarding symptoms. Specifically, both groups had significant improvements in OCD symptoms, depression, anxiety, and overall functioning. Both groups had a similar proportion of responders (28% vs. 32%) and dropouts (12% vs. 15%). Hoarding symptoms improved as much as nonhoarding OCD symptoms. It is not clear whether these results would be generalizable to patients with hoarding symptoms who do not have comorbid OCD.

Use of paroxetine may be complicated by anticholinergic side effects. In this open-label study of paroxetine in hoarding (Saxena et al. 2007), only 16 of the 79 patients in the study could tolerate the target dose of 60 mg/day. Less than half reached the 40 mg/day dose, and 12 could not tolerate more than 30 mg/day.

Venlafaxine Extended-Release

In an open trial, 24 patients with symptoms meeting DSM-5 criteria for hoarding disorder were treated with venlafaxine extended-release for 12 weeks (mean dose=204±72 mg/day) (Saxena and Sumner 2014). One patient had comorbid OCD, but the hoarding symptoms were independent of the OCD symptoms. Venlafaxine was titrated by 37.5 mg/day increments every 4 days to a target of 225 mg/day, as tolerated, and participants continued to take this dose for the first 8 weeks of treatment. In weeks 9–12, the dose could be increased to a maximum of 300 mg/day as tolerated. No other psychoactive medications, CBT, or treatments were allowed during the study period, including assistance from professional organizers or other third parties. Hoarding symptoms decreased significantly, with a mean 36% decrease on the UCLA Hoarding Severity Scale (UHSS) and a 32% decrease on the SI-R. Sixteen of 23 completers (70%) were classified as responders, with response defined as at least 30% reduction in UHSS and SI-R scores, as well as a rating of at least "much improved" on the Clinical Global Impression—Improvement (CGI-I) scale.

This open-label study of extended-release venlafaxine in adults with hoarding disorder (Saxena and Sumner 2014) showed an improved tolerability profile in a sample similar to that studied by Saxena et al. (2007), (middle-age and older adults with hoarding disorder), with 20 of the 23 patients tolerating a dose of 150 mg/day, 16 tolerating at least 225 mg/day, and 4 reaching the target dose of 300 mg/day. In the study, no patients dropped out of the study because of side effects or lack of efficacy.

Atomoxetine

In an open-label study, 12 adults with symptoms meeting criteria for DSM-5 hoarding disorder were treated with atomoxetine for 12 weeks (mean dose 62.72 mg/day) (Grassi et al. 2016). Atomoxetine was started at 25 mg/day for 1 week, and the dose was then increased to 40 mg/day and remained there until week 4. The dose was increased again to a flexible target dose of 40–80 mg/day, as tolerated. No changes in psychoactive medications, CBT, or treatments were allowed during the study period. Of the 11 completers, 1 had comorbid OCD, but the hoarding symptoms were independent from the OCD; 3 had comorbid depression; and none had symptoms that met criteria for ADHD. Hoarding symptoms decreased significantly, with a mean 41% decrease on the UHSS and a 40% decrease on the SI-R. Six of 11 completers (55%) were classified as responders—with response defined as at least a 35% reduction of symptoms, as well as a rating of at least "much improved" on the CGI-I. No patients dropped out because of side effects or lack of efficacy; one dropped out because they moved out of state.

Methylphenidate Extended-Release

In an open-label case series, four adults with presentations meeting criteria for DSM-5 hoarding disorder—and with at least moderate attention problems (self-reported)—were treated with methylphenidate extended-release for 4 weeks (mean dose = 50±9 mg/day) (Rodriguez et al. 2013). Methylphenidate extended-release was titrated by 18 mg/day increments every week to a target dosage of 72 mg/day, as tolerated. No other psychoactive medications, CBT, or treatments were allowed during the study period. One patient had comorbid OCD, but hoarding symptoms were independent from the OCD. None had symptoms that met criteria for ADHD. Of the four participants, two had a reduction in hoarding symptoms (25% and 32%), as measured by the SI-R. None of the four participants chose to continue taking methylphenidate extended-release after study end because of difficulties tolerating the side effects (e.g., insomnia, palpitations).

Fluvoxamine

Vilaverde et al. (2017) treated a patient with hoarding disorder, depressive symptoms, and insomnia with fluvoxamine 100 mg daily, trazodone 150 mg daily, and a concurrent psychotherapy plan consisting of several sessions of psychoeducation, cognitive restructuring of beliefs, and exposure to non-acquiring. The trazodone was quickly discontinued because of side effects, and the patient continued to buy and collect objects over the first 6 months of treatment. Over the next 9 months, as fluvoxamine was gradually titrated up to 100 mg three times daily with quetiapine augmentation (200 mg), the patient's symptoms improved and he was able to unclutter and organize his living spaces (Vilaverde et al. 2017).

Risperidone

In a patient with schizophrenia and hoarding behaviors, augmentation of clozapine (200 mg/day) with risperidone resulted in worsened hoarding behaviors as the risperidone dose was gradually increased from 1 mg to 6 mg daily. The hoarding behaviors improved when risperidone was discontinued (Chong et al. 1996).

Augmentation Treatments

In the case of a 56-year-old male with OCD and hoarding symptoms, ADHD, and schizotypal personality disorder, Kaplan and Hollander (2004) described treatment with fluvoxamine followed by a trial augmentation of fluvoxamine 250 mg/day with risperidone 1 mg daily. They observed improved insight into hoarding symptoms. In the same case report, the patient's regimen was initially augmented with methylphenidate 5 mg twice a day (10 mg daily), which initially improved procrastination; however, the methylphenidate was discontinued because of agitation, and no other effects on hoarding symptoms were reported by the authors (see Kaplan and Hollander 2004). The authors also reported that augmentation with the psychostimulant amphetamine salts 2.5 mg twice a day (5 mg daily) was helpful in ameliorating some aspects of hoarding disorder, such as procrastination and distress when discarding. Hoarding disorder symptoms scales were not reported for this case, but the authors described the patient's continued hoarding behaviors.

In a pilot open-label trial of minocycline augmentation pharmacotherapy for 12 weeks, OCD patients as a group ($n=9$) showed no significant differences in symptoms or rate of improvement over time; however, one individual who reported hoarding as their only OCD symptom dimension had a 39% reduction in Yale-Brown Obsessive Compulsive Scale (Y-BOCS) score (from 33 to 20) from pre- to posttreatment (Rodriguez et al. 2010). Although the Y-BOCS does not capture the full spectrum of hoarding behaviors as do the hoarding-specific scales described in Chapter 3, the data for this one patient—without any other OCD symptoms—suggest minocycline augmentation of SRI pharmacotherapy may improve symptoms in individuals with primary hoarding behaviors. Replication of this initial finding in a larger sample of individuals with DSM-5 hoarding disorder is needed.

Strength of Evidence

Studies of hoarding disorder psychopharmacology tend to be small and open-label. These characteristics limit the conclusions that can be drawn from this literature. To date, there are no controlled trials to support efficacy. Despite this, there is some evidence of benefit from paroxetine, venlafaxine extended-release, amphetamine salts, methylphenidate, methylphenidate extended-release, and atomoxetine. Two case reports of risperidone augmentation and hoarding behaviors have been mixed. There are also no data on comparative efficacy between these drugs. These drugs should be considered only after better-proven treatments, including CBT for hoarding disorder, have been attempted (Tolin et al. 2015) (see Chapter 7 for an overview of CBT).

Management of Side Effects

Medication side effects may limit the maximum tolerated dose. Abrupt discontinuation of SRIs may lead to withdrawal symptoms (Coupland et al. 1996; Jha et al. 2018). Building a strong alliance and shared decision-making are critical in order to maximize pharmacotherapy outcomes.

Successful side effect management involves the application of a few general principles and continued attention to the specific needs of the patient (McElroy et al. 1995). The clinician should take time to educate the patient about the medication's most frequent side effects. This not only will reduce anxiety but also may enhance compliance. Patients should also be educated on ways to proactively minimize side effects, such as taking medications with meals and taking stimulant medications in the morning and sedating medications at nighttime. It should be explained that one cannot predict who will experience a given side effect and that it is important to reach out before the next visit, should an unwanted side effect occur. Patients should be asked whether they have any questions or concerns, and common examples should be provided, such as "Will it be addicting?," "Do I need to take this for the rest of my life?," and "Do I need to stop the medication if I become pregnant?" The patient should be asked about side effects at each visit. Finally, one can start at half the recommended starting dose, increase the dose slowly, reduce the dose, or cross-titrate to prevent or manage side effects.

Interactions With Other Drugs and Warnings

Patients who have comorbid conditions or who are unresponsive to one agent alone may require more than one psychotropic medication. Providers must take into account multiple drug-drug interactions, which may be pharmacokinetic, pharmacodynamic, or both. *Pharmacokinetics*—sometimes described as what the body does to a drug—refers to the time course of drug absorption, distribution, transport to and away from receptors, metabolism, and excretion. *Pharmacodynamics*—sometimes described as the effects of drugs on the body —refers to the mechanism of drug action at receptors and to the receptor effects on physiology. In addition, factors such as the patient's age, sex, diet, comorbid medical conditions, and concomitant prescription and nonprescription medications may also influence the likelihood of pharmacokinetic or pharmacodynamic drug interactions.

Case Examples

Case Example 1: Comorbid Hoarding Disorder and Mild Major Depression

Daphne was a 54-year-old, college-educated white woman who reported having struggled with hoarding symptoms and major depression since she was in high school. She never married, lived alone, and worked as a librarian. Prompted by members of her book club to host a meeting at her home and knowing this would not be possible without help, she joined an online support group, but she still struggled with clutter that impaired her ability to use her kitchen and living room. She initially avoided seeing a psychiatrist because of her reluctance to take medication for fear of side effects. On assessment, her assessment results met DSM-5 criteria for hoarding disorder and major depression. Hoarding-specific rating scales were used to rate her current symptoms. Her Hoarding Rating Scale—Interview (HRS-I) score was 21, which was well above the hoarding disorder cutoff of 14, and her SI-R total score of 67 was also well above the recommended maximum of 39 for her age cohort. Daphne's self-rated CIR was 5 for the living room and kitchen. The most significant clutter was in the bedroom, with a CIR score of 6. A CIR rating of 6 reflects clutter that would make any activity in the room extremely difficult. Her depression was rated in the mild range by the Hamilton Depression Rating Scale. Her symptoms did not meet criteria for hypomania, bipolar disorder, psychosis, substance use disorder, or other psychiatric disorders.

Together, Daphne and her psychiatrist decided to start paroxetine at 10 mg/day given that her sister, who suffered from depression, had used it successfully to manage her symptoms. Daphne increased the dose by 10 mg/ day each week until a dose of 40 mg/day was reached. Given the improvements she experienced in her mood and hoarding symptoms over 8 weeks, they decided to increase the medication by 10 mg/day per week to a target dose of 60 mg/day. Although Daphne experienced continued benefit, she also began to experience headaches, sedation, fatigue, constipation, and sexual side effects. Given these anticholinergic side effects, which are common with paroxetine, Daphne and her psychiatrist decided to reduce the dose back to 40 mg/day. Although her symptoms did not fully remit, Daphne experienced improved mood and energy and a 25% reduction in her hoarding symptoms. Daphne then began CBT for hoarding disorder. Over the next year, with encouragement from her therapist, Daphne worked slowly to unclutter her home, focusing first on her living room and kitchen. She found it motivating to think about hosting her book club as the goal as she uncluttered. Clutter was decreased, with her CIR clutter level at 2–3 in the living room and kitchen, she managed to reach her goal of hosting her first book club event. She continued to take paroxetine 40 mg/day and set aside time each weekend to declutter with her sister.

Discussion

This case example illustrates that for a patient with comorbid hoarding disorder and mild to moderate major depression, starting pharmacotherapy and CBT for hoarding disorder is a reasonable initial strategy. Many such patients will respond to CBT alone. As we noted earlier, in certain situations, such as when a patient has low energy and motivation secondary to moderate to severe major depression (as in Case Example 2 below), medications alone may be preferable. In other cases, medications may be needed to decrease the intensity of the symptoms so that the patient can fully engage in CBT. For individuals with predominant inattention symptoms (as in Case Example 3 below), a trial of a stimulant may be considered.

This case also highlights the importance of titrating medication to the maximum tolerated dose while monitoring for side effects. As noted previously, in an open-label study of paroxetine in hoarding disorder (Saxena et al. 2007), only 16 of the 79 patients in the study could tolerate the target dose of 60 mg/day, but 67 patients were able to tolerate 30 mg/day. If the side effects of paroxetine limit the maximally tolerated dose, an alternative strategy to consider is extended-release venlafaxine.

Case Example 2: Comorbid Hoarding Disorder and Severe Major Depression

Peter was a 61-year-old, married Asian man who reported struggling with hoarding and depression for much of his life. Peter had a high school education. He had worked for 40 years as a mechanic and was now on disability, with an income of less than $18,000 per year. Hoarding-specific rating scales were used to rate his current symptoms. His HRS-I score was 17, which was above the hoarding disorder cutoff of 14, and his SI-R total score of 55 was also above the recommended maximum of 39. His self-rated CIR was 5 for the bedroom, living room, and kitchen.

Peter had been in therapy for mild to moderate depression for more than 10 years and was also taking fluoxetine 40 mg/day, his maximum tolerated dose. He reported low mood, energy, appetite, and motivation; daily tearfulness; hopelessness; worthlessness; insomnia; and anhedonia for the past month. His symptoms did not meet criteria for hypomania, bipolar disorder, psychosis, substance use disorder, or other psychiatric disorders. On speaking to his psychiatrist, he reported being in bed for most of the day and night, unable to sleep, and without energy to take care of his hygiene, let alone unclutter his home. After a careful review for drug-drug interactions, the psychiatrist recommended cross-tapering with venlafaxine extended-release, starting at 37.5 mg/day and increasing by 37.5 mg/day increments every 4 days to 225 mg/day. His mood began to improve and his energy increased. Additional titration to 300 mg/day improved both depression and hoarding symptoms (by 30%) but resulted in side effects, including sexual dysfunction. He discussed with his psychiatrist several approaches for the management of sexual side effects, including decreasing the dose, trying drug holidays (i.e., skipping a day's medication), and waiting for the body to accommodate to the medication. For Peter, a trial of reducing the drug dose avoided sexual side effects but did not maintain the therapeutic effect. Peter went back to 300 mg/day and then noted a shift over several months from anorgasmia to normal orgasm as his body accommodated. Once he was on a stable medication regimen with improved mood and energy, he was referred for CBT for hoarding disorder.

Discussion

This case illustrates that in certain situations, such as when a patient has low energy and motivation due to major depression, medications alone may be preferable. In other cases, medications may be needed to decrease the intensity of the symptoms so that the patient can fully engage in CBT. Regardless of the specific details of the case, it is important to maximally treat comorbid conditions, including major depression.

With added comorbidities and potential for cross-titration or augmentation, it is also important to highlight drug-drug interactions, which may be pharmacokinetic, pharmacodynamic, or both. Pharmacodynamic interactions can take place when drugs have similar or opposing effects at the same receptor or when their effects on different receptors have adverse consequences (e.g., combining an SRI with a monoamine oxidase inhibitor may produce serotonin syndrome). The drug interactions considered here are primarily pharmacokinetic (e.g., effects of drugs on the metabolism of other drugs). Drug metabolism is primarily carried out by the cytochrome P450 (CYP) isoenzyme system. The degree to which one drug interferes with another's metabolism depends on the activity of the enzyme metabolizing the target drug, each drug's affinity for this enzyme, the concentrations of the drugs, and the availability of alternative metabolic pathways. Certain substances, like alcohol, are CYP isoenzyme inducers (i.e., increase rates of drug metabolism). Others, like paroxetine, inhibit CYP2D6, and combining it with any drug metabolized by CYP2D6 should be approached with caution. About 5%–10% of white individuals possess little or no CYP2D6 activity and hence are slow metabolizers of the many drugs this enzyme metabolizes. On the other hand, higher doses of SRIs are sometimes used for rapid metabolizers or for individuals who have an inadequate response after 4 weeks.

In 2004, the FDA placed a "black box" warning on antidepressant medications, including SRIs, reporting a twofold increased risk for spontaneously reported suicidal thinking or behavior in children and adolescents taking these medications (2% vs. 4%). However, no signal of increased suicidal thinking was detected on structured assessment using clinical rating scales in these same trials. Using SRIs in adolescents requires careful balancing of the benefits and risks.

Case Example 3: Comorbid Hoarding Disorder and Inattention

Sasha was a 50-year-old white woman living in a rural area who reported difficulty parting with possessions and challenges organizing her clutter. On assessment, her presentation met DSM-5 criteria for hoarding disorder but not ADHD, despite inattention being one of her main difficulties. Hoarding-specific rating scales were used to rate her current symptoms. Her HRS-I score was 20, which was well above the hoarding disorder cutoff of 14, and her SI-R total score of 67 was also well above the recommended maximum of 39 for her age cohort. Sasha's self-rated CIR was 4 for the living room. The most significant clutter was in the kitchen and bedroom, with a CIR score of 6. Her symptoms did not meet criteria for depression, hypomania, bipolar disorder, psychosis, substance abuse/dependence, or other psychiatric disorders.

Sasha did not want treatment with SRIs. She feared the potential side effects and also the possibility of having to continue taking a medication for an extended time. She was not able to meaningfully engage in CBT psychotherapy because of inattention. She and her psychiatrist decided together to begin a trial of a psychostimulant. She started methylphenidate extended-release at 18 mg/day in the morning. She reported improvement in attention and focus with the initial dose and did not want further titration. Sasha took the medication on days she wanted to dedicate to decluttering. Her hoarding symptoms reduced by 25% as measured by the SI-R, and she was able to clear her kitchen so that she could start cooking meals again. At the same time, her difficulty with hoarding disorder persisted, so her psychiatrist recommended augmentation with CBT therapy. Sasha found that with her improved attention, she was able to engage in CBT, and her hoarding symptoms continued to improve (e.g., reduced by 35% compared with her baseline as measured by the SI-R).

Discussion

This case illustrates that individuals with predominant inattention symptoms may consider a trial of a stimulant. Alternatives to (or augmentation strategies for) reducing hoarding disorder symptoms include treatment of the inattention domain with a trial of a psychostimulant, such as amphetamine salts, methylphenidate, methylphenidate extended-release, or atomoxetine. For those with continued symptoms, augmentation with CBT is recommended. Some patients find that by improving attention, they are better able to engage in CBT.

Conclusion

Hoarding disorder is a severe and debilitating illness. Whether patients are treated with medication or CBT therapy, there are several common issues and limitations across treatments. First, the dosage and management of medication side effects are important to achieving optimal symptom reduction. Although the open-label studies reviewed in this chapter are promising, further efficacy studies are needed for all of the agents discussed in the previous section. Once efficacy is more clearly established, mechanistic studies examining the correlates of therapeutic benefit will be important. Second, understanding and further refining descriptions of the features of hoarding disorder (e.g., excessive acquiring) will not only improve the chances of finding underlying genetic and neurobiological mechanisms but also allow for identification of characteristics that can guide prognosis and treatment. Exciting avenues for future work include personalized medicine, in which patients with specific, definable clinical characteristics could be prescribed tailored medication on the basis of their predicted treatment response. A third common theme is that we know little about how our treatments work at the level of the nervous system. Although we are starting to understand the neurobiological basis of hoarding disorder (see Chapter 6), much more research needs to be done to elucidate the etiology and pathophysiology. New horizons for research include development of clinical correlates—or endophenotypes—of hoarding symptoms in order to understand the underlying mechanism of disease. Translational approaches, such as developing mouse models of hoarding and neuroimaging of the neurotransmitter systems, will help us to understand how neural substrates are linked to symptom reduction. Taken together, these lines of research may also lead to predictive markers of response to help guide strategies for individualized treatment.

KEY CLINICAL POINTS

- Studies of hoarding disorder psychopharmacology have been small and open-label, and this limits the conclusions that can be drawn from this literature. To date, there are no controlled trials to support efficacy.

- Despite the lack of larger, controlled medication trials in hoarding disorder, there is some evidence of benefit from paroxetine, venlafaxine extended-release, amphetamine salts, methylphenidate, methylphenidate extended-release, and atomoxetine. No data on comparative efficacy between these drugs are available as of this writing.

- Drugs with known benefit should be considered only after better-proven treatments—including cognitive-behavioral therapy for hoarding disorder—have been attempted.

- Medication side effects may limit the maximum tolerated dose.

- Abrupt discontinuation of serotonin reuptake inhibitors may lead to withdrawal symptoms.

- Building a strong alliance and shared decision-making are critical to maximizing pharmacotherapy outcomes.

- Patients with comorbid conditions or who are unresponsive to one agent alone may require more than one psychotropic medication.

- Providers must take into account multiple drug-drug interactions, which may be pharmacokinetic, pharmacodynamic, or both.

References

Ahmari SE, Dougherty DD: Dissecting OCD circuits: from animal models to targeted treatments. Depress Anxiety 32(8):550–562, 2015 25952989

Alonso P, Menchon JM, Pifarre J, et al: Long-term follow-up and predictors of clinical outcome in obsessive-compulsive patients treated with serotonin reuptake inhibitors and behavioral therapy. J Clin Psychiatry 62(7):535–540, 2001 11488364

American Psychiatric Association: Diagnostic and Statistical Manual of Mental Disorders, 5th Edition. Arlington, VA, American Psychiatric Association, 2013

Black DW, Monahan P, Gable J, et al: Hoarding and treatment response in 38 nondepressed subjects with obsessive-compulsive disorder. J Clin Psychiatry 59(8):420–425, 1998 9721822

Chong SA, Tan CH, Lee HS: Hoarding and clozapine-risperidone combination. Can J Psychiatry 41(5):315–316, 1996 8793152

Coupland NJ, Bell CJ, Potokar JP: Serotonin reuptake inhibitor withdrawal. J Clin Psychopharmacol 16(5):356–362, 1996 8889907

Erzegovesi S, Cavallini MC, Cavedini P, et al: Clinical predictors of drug response in obsessive-compulsive disorder. J Clin Psychopharmacol 21(5):488–492, 2001 11593074

Ferrão YA, Shavitt RG, Bedin NR, et al: Clinical features associated to refractory obsessive-compulsive disorder. J Affect Disord 94(1–3):199–209, 2006 16764938

Grassi G, Micheli L, Di Cesare Mannelli L, et al: Atomoxetine for hoarding disorder: a pre-clinical and clinical investigation. J Psychiatr Res 83:240–248, 2016 27665536

Jha MK, Rush AJ, Trivedi MH: When discontinuing SSRI antidepressants is a challenge: management tips. Am J Psychiatry 175(12):1176–1184, 2018 30501420

Kaplan A, Hollander E: Comorbidity in compulsive hoarding: a case report. CNS Spectr 9(1):71–73, 2004 14999178

Landeros-Weisenberger A, Bloch MH, Kelmendi B, et al: Dimensional predictors of response to SRI pharmacotherapy in obsessive-compulsive disorder. J Affect Disord 121(1–2):175–179, 2010 19577308

Mataix-Cols D, Rauch SL, Manzo PA, et al: Use of factor-analyzed symptom dimensions to predict outcome with serotonin reuptake inhibitors and placebo in the treatment of obsessive-compulsive disorder. Am J Psychiatry 156(9):1409–1416, 1999 10484953

McElroy SL, Keck PE Jr, Friedman LM: Minimizing and managing antidepressant side effects. J Clin Psychiatry 56 (suppl 2):49–55, 1995 7844107

Rodriguez CI, Bender J Jr, Marcus SM, et al: Minocycline augmentation of pharmacotherapy in obsessive-compulsive disorder: an open-label trial. J Clin Psychiatry 71(9):1247–1249, 2010 20923629

Rodriguez CI, Bender J Jr, Morrison S, et al: Does extended release methylphenidate help adults with hoarding disorder? A case series. J Clin Psychopharmacol 33(3):444–447, 2013 23609401

Salomoni G, Grassi M, Mosini P, et al: Artificial neural network model for the prediction of obsessive-compulsive disorder treatment response. J Clin Psychopharmacol 29(4):343–349, 2009 19593173

Saxena S: Recent advances in compulsive hoarding. Curr Psychiatry Rep 10(4):297–303, 2008 18627667

Saxena S: Pharmacotherapy of compulsive hoarding. J Clin Psychol 67(5):477–484, 2011 21404273

Saxena S, Maidment KM: Treatment of compulsive hoarding. J Clin Psychol 60(11):1143–1154, 2004 15389621

Saxena S, Sumner J: Venlafaxine extended-release treatment of hoarding disorder. Int Clin Psychopharmacol 29(5):266–273, 2014 24722633

Saxena S, Brody AL, Maidment KM, Baxter LR Jr: Paroxetine treatment of compulsive hoarding. J Psychiatr Res 41(6):481–487, 2007 16790250

Shetti CN, Reddy YC, Kandavel T, et al: Clinical predictors of drug nonresponse in obsessive-compulsive disorder. J Clin Psychiatry 66(12):1517–1523, 2005 16401151

Stein DJ, Andersen EW, Overo KF: Response of symptom dimensions in obsessive-compulsive disorder to treatment with citalopram or placebo. Br J Psychiatry 29(4):303–307, 2007 18200396

Stein DJ, Carey PD, Lochner C, et al: Escitalopram in obsessive-compulsive disorder: response of symptom dimensions to pharmacotherapy. CNS Spectr 13(6):492–498, 2008 18567973

Thompson C, Fernández de la Cruz L, Mataix-Cols D, Onwumere J: A systematic review and quality assessment of psychological, pharmacological, and family-based interventions for hoarding disorder. Asian J Psychiatr 27:53–66, 2017 28558897

Tolin DF, Frost RO, Steketee G, Muroff J: Cognitive behavioral therapy for hoarding disorder: a meta-analysis. Depress Anxiety 32(3):158–166, 2015 25639467

Vilaverde D, Gonçalves J, Morgado P: Hoarding disorder: a case report. Front Psychiatry 8:112, 2017 28701963

Winsberg ME, Cassic KS, Koran LM: Hoarding in obsessive-compulsive disorder: a report of 20 cases. J Clin Psychiatry 60(9):591–597, 1999 10520977

CHAPTER 9
Harm Reduction

When an individual is unable or unwilling to engage in treatment for hoarding, their family, neighbors, and landlord may feel helpless, overwhelmed, frustrated, or angry. The expression of these intense feelings to the person with hoarding disorder may inadvertently add to the individual's mistrust and isolation (Tompkins and Hartl 2009). One strategy to consider in these cases is harm reduction—an intervention based on a set of pragmatic principles, strategies, and applications designed to minimize the risk caused by problematic effects of behaviors (Logan and Marlatt 2010; Marlatt 1998). This intervention was adapted for hoarding, with a focus on engaging the patient, building a team, assessing the harm and risks, and creating and implementing a plan to minimize those risks (Tompkins 2011, 2015).

Harm reduction is not a treatment for hoarding disorder. The primary goal of harm reduction is to manage symptoms to decrease risk, whereas the goal of treatment is to reduce symptoms, distress, and impairment. Furthermore, harm reduction does not target the thoughts, beliefs, and behavioral patterns that underpin hoarding disorder behaviors, whereas treatments such as cognitive-behavioral therapy (CBT) for hoarding do (see Chapter 7). Harm reduction assumes that the individual is not open to treating their underlying disorder but that they may accept help from others to manage the hoarding problem; in contrast, treatment relies, to some extent, on the individual's desire to engage in skill building and to decrease hoarding symptoms. Examples of harm reduction strategies in the context of hoarding dis-order include putting a basket behind the front door to hold the individual's wallet, eyeglasses, and other important items, or labeling food with an ex-piration date and asking the individual to allow a family member to discard the food on that date. Another difference between harm reduction and treat-ment is that in harm reduction the clinician is typically in a consultation role within a larger harm reduction team—which may include family, friends, professional organizers, visiting nurses, and/or in-home health aides—whereas in a treatment model, the clinician is typically the one responsible for the treatment plan in partnership with the client. When applied to hoard-ing disorder, harm reduction strategies can help family members, clinicians, human service professionals, and others support the individual in maintain-ing a safe home environment.

Harm Reduction Model

The harm reduction approach originated in the Netherlands in the late 1970s as an alternative to abstinence-only interventions for adults with sub-stance abuse problems. It included reversing a ban on needles and proac-tively providing clean needles, which dramatically reduced drug-related deaths (Tompkins 2015). In the 1980s, the British government in Liverpool expanded the approach and introduced a comprehensive program termed "harm reduction" that included offering medical care, clean needles, and safe injection education. In response to the AIDS epidemic, harm reduction emerged in the United States to mitigate the risk associated with active sub-stance use, including reducing the spread of HIV (Des Jarlais and Friedman 1993). Harm reduction has been applied to nicotine use, sexually transmit-ted diseases, and other public health problems (Ball 2007; Emmanuelli and Desenclos 2005; Ferguson et al. 2006; Wilson et al. 2007).

Denning and colleagues (Denning 2000; Denning et al. 2004) set out to describe a set of guiding principles, values, and assumptions for harm re-duction that have since been applied to hoarding disorder and termed the "harm reduction attitude" (Tompkins 2015). These principles include the following (Tompkins 2015):

a. The therapist should do no harm (e.g., give thoughtful consideration of the risks and benefits of a cleanout or relocation).
b. It is not necessary to stop all hoarding behavior.
c. No two hoarding situations are identical.
d. The client who hoards is an essential member of the harm reduction team.
e. Change is slow.

f. Agreement failures do not mean the harm reduction approach is failing.
g. The client who hoards may have other more pressing problems than hoarding (i.e., the pressing problems should be incorporated into the harm reduction plan).

These principles guide the harm reduction approach and process, which has two phases (initial and ongoing) and several features (initiation, engagement, assessment of harm, team building, planning, and ongoing management).

In the initial phase, the primary objective is to assess the risk level and whether the client needs an intervention or whether they can continue living in their home without an intervention. If an intervention is needed, the content, degree, and timeline for the intervention will be informed by the severity and immediacy of the risk. The clinician will prepare the client for the ongoing phase by engaging them in the selection of their harm reduction team and determining the level of intervention and plan needed to meet the minimum standards of safety for the client. This initial phase can also include court-established benchmarks (e.g., immediate removal of flammable materials, clearing fire escapes, repairing toilet).

In the ongoing phase, the primary objective is to continue to reassess the harm risk level over time in the context of planned interventions developed during the initial phase. Harm risk may be dynamic based on the results of the interventions or changes in the client's functional capacity. The second objective is to maintain an effective harm reduction team to implement and manage the harm reduction plan. This phase includes monitoring the adherence and helping with compliance—which requires retaining access to the home. Often it is helpful during the ongoing phase for the court to order this—specifying that the client meet with the clinician in the home and reach health and safety standards within a designated timeline (Tompkins 2015). Each feature of the harm reduction process is summarized in the sections that follow.

Features of the Harm Reduction Process
Initiation

Cases surface in many ways, including via a family member seeking help from a clinician with their loved one's clutter or through awareness from community agencies (e.g., police, fire department, code enforcement, animal control), landlords or property managers, professional organizers, visiting nurse services, neighbors, Adult Protective Services (APS), Child Protective Services, or a local hoarding task force. See the handbook by Bratiotis et al. (2011) for a detailed description of the role of task forces in hoarding disorder; see also Chapter 10 for further description of community-based interventions.

Engagement

Engagement of both the client and the potential harm reduction team members begins early in the process and includes 1) emphasizing that the goal is managing the problem so that the client can remain in their home, 2) de-emphasizing discarding, and 3) providing context that if a modified cleanout is necessary, it is part of a larger plan to help the patient live more comfortably and safely in their home. Team members may also need engagement, since some may have their own specific reasons for resistance (e.g., a property manager would rather evict the client, family members want client to move to a supported living facility to alleviate the ongoing stress).

For some clients, decades of pressure from family, clinicians, or other community members may have resulted in erosion of trusted relationships. For others, court-mandated cleanouts have elicited fear and lack of autonomy. Other challenges in engaging clients include poor insight and low motivation, which hinder the kind of behavioral change needed to reduce risk. Behavioral change has been proposed to occur in stages such as precontemplation, contemplation, preparation, change, and maintenance (Prochaska and Velicer 1997). This framework may be used in the context of clients with hoarding who have low motivation and are not willing to accept assistance. Motivational interviewing is an evidence-based approach to behavior change; specifically, it is a client-centered, goal-oriented method used to explore and resolve ambivalence and enhance intrinsic motivation to change (Miller 2006; Miller and Rollnick 2002, 2013). The four fundamental principles include expressing empathy, developing discrepancy (e.g., helping the client see how clutter is inconsistent with their personal goals), rolling with resistance, and supporting self-efficacy (Miller and Rollnick 2002). Motivational interviewing techniques may be used to elicit change in clients with hoarding disorder and can be more formally learned by the clinician and other members of the harm reduction team through training courses.

Motivational interviewing has an evidence base as a brief intervention for reducing substance use and as an adjunct to other treatments, including CBT (Burke et al. 2003; Hettema et al. 2005; Maltby and Tolin 2005; Simpson et al. 2008; Westra and Dozois 2006). In a trial of 12 patients with obsessive-compulsive disorder (OCD), Maltby and Tolin (2005) combined motivational interviewing with other strategies in a multimodal four-session intervention prelude to standard CBT and found that this intervention increased CBT with exposure and response prevention entry among OCD patients who had previously refused exposure and response prevention. In an open-label trial of six OCD patients, Simpson and colleagues (2008) integrated motivational interviewing with exposure and response prevention and reported increased retention and adherence. Although motivational interviewing alone has not been tested among hoarding patients as it has for other disorders, CBT for hoarding disorder utilizes motivational principles and techniques, which are often employed when clients express ambivalence. Similarly, motivational interviewing can decrease defensiveness and motivate efforts to engage in the harm reduction approach.

Assessment

It is recommended that assessment be divided into two parts: the initial assessment and assessment of harm potential (Tompkins 2015). As described previously, the initial assessment can be done quickly (e.g., assessing if clutter in the home poses an imminent risk and if a modified cleanout is necessary); the client may appreciate spending less time in the home, which will allow for more time to engage the client in the harm reduction process. If a modified cleanout is necessary, it is important to prepare the client and have a document in which each person's role and responsibility are detailed—with documentation of the pre-cleanout phase, onsite support plan, features, possessions plan, and post-cleanout phase (Tompkins 2015). This planning is critical, given that cleanout interventions can result in strong emotional responses ranging from loss and despair to anger. In some cases in which clients were away on vacation or purposely excluded from the planning process and then surprised by a forced cleanout, there have been reports of hospitalization and death by suicide (Brace 2007).

Assessment of harm potential involves assessing environmental risks with standardized scales. In Chapter 3, we described helpful measures for this, including the Clutter Image Rating (Frost et al. 2008) to measure the level of clutter in standard rooms of the home, the Home Environment Index (Rasmussen et al. 2014), and the HOMES Multi-Disciplinary Hoarding Risk Assessment (Bratiotis 2009). The next type of assessment is for physical and mental capacity to care for oneself—done through administering the Activities of Daily Living Scale (Frost et al. 2013), evaluating medical conditions with a physical exam by a primary care doctor, evaluating psychiatric conditions through a psychiatrist, and, if needed, meeting with a neurologist for assessment of dementia or other neurological conditions.

Personal safety of the evaluator is also important. If there is a foul odor at the door or visible feces, mold, or other contaminants, or if the clutter is above shoulder level, it is wise to consider whether it is safe to enter the home, or whether additional professional services are needed. For professional cleaners, entering may require wearing a respirator, gloves, and protective equipment. A good practice is to enter the home accompanied by another member of the team rather than alone.

Important considerations include maintaining rapport with the client, asking permission if items must be touched, and giving the client as much control as possible during the visit. Failing to do so can thwart ongoing cooperation. For example, a plan for one of our clients included having a trusted family friend assist with attempts to organize. On his first visit, however, he picked up a gum wrapper off of the floor and discarded it without asking the client. After the incident, the client refused to allow the helper back into her home.

Finally, setting up a return visit and/or call may help to create space for a follow-up meeting and reinforce that harm reduction is an ongoing process.

Harm Reduction Team

Because hoarding and clutter can overwhelm an individual provider, a team-based approach is highly recommended to reduce burnout and maximize information sharing of multiple areas of expertise. The clinician and client both serve as members of the harm reduction team, along with family members, supports, code enforcement, and any other representatives that are important for the process. Important considerations within the team include privacy—as most clinicians are bound by the Health Insurance Portability and Accountability Act (HIPAA), which states that clinical information can only be shared with the patient's written approval or if mandated by law (Drogin 2019). Within the team it is important to articulate the bounds of what can be disclosed, which is not the same for each team member, but is instead guided by their profession (e.g., APS will differ from fire and police). Whenever possible, the ethical and boundary issues should be discussed proactively early in the process and a plan documented. For example, most professions have codes for protecting the essential rights of individuals, including autonomy and privacy, as well as respecting their dignity and not taking advantage of the client for personal or financial gain. Another consideration is that when clinicians, social workers, and other mandated reporters enter the home, they may be in a position to report child neglect and abuse, which supersedes the client's right to privacy. As these issues come up, they should also be documented, and the ethical plan should be adjusted as necessary.

Harm Reduction Plan

After a core harm reduction team has been established, the team can begin the process of creating a harm reduction plan, which minimizes confusion and misunderstandings. These plans are formalized (e.g., crafted by the team and signed) and highly customized for the individual, depending on their level of insight and engagement and the circumstances surrounding the condition of the home. Establishing harm reduction targets that are specific, measurable, attainable, relevant, and time-bound (SMART goals) is important (Doran 1981). An example of a nonspecific goal would be to "discard moldy food." Exactly when a food has turned "moldy" can be up for debate, as the client's definition may be different from the observer's. A more specific goal would be to "discard food that is beyond the expiration date." Measurable goals could include a maximum number of inches tall that a stack should be or a function that can be easily seen (e.g., ability to swing the front door fully open and have the ground in this zone fully clutter-free). At the same time, the goal must be attainable and personalized to what the individual can do, including the target date. Finally, the target must be relevant to the client and contribute to improvement in situations of safety, functional capacity, health, and so forth. An example of a relevant goal would be increasing the client's safety in the home (via tasks such as removing flammable items from the oven). (For more in-depth examples and harm reduction planning worksheets, see Tompkins 2015.) Once the targets are identified, another important component of the plan includes the monitoring plan (e.g., who will visit, how frequently will they visit, what will be the goals for the visit). A minimum starting plan will contain at least one in-home visit per month (with weekly visits for the first few months), with the frequency titrated as needed (Tompkins 2015). The plan should also specify the team members and their roles, as well as flexibility—reminding the team that this agreement will fluctuate depending on the client's level of risk. Having a structured plan that is signed by all parties may increase the likelihood of adherence; indeed, public commitments have been recommended as a way to increase adherence to behavioral plans (Shelton and Levy 1981). If the client is unable or unwilling to sign and honor a public plan, the clinician can shift into motivational interviewing strategies to explore the client's ambivalence.

Maintenance, Home Visits, and Agreement Failures

Key elements include regularly scheduled meetings of the entire team. Tompkins (2015) recommends that the initial meeting be 2 hours in length and subsequent meetings 90 minutes in length. Shorter meetings may not allow adequate time for all the agenda items to be discussed, whereas longer meeting times risk fatigue of team members and scheduling difficulty. The meeting begins with eliciting agenda items and prioritizing them in terms of importance. Other important components of the meeting include reviewing progress on the goals and planning for the next team meeting and in-home visit. Praising the group members (including the client) is vital to continuing engagement. Another important aspect is anticipating and working through agreement failures. Agreement failures should be tracked to see how often they are occurring, and the team should engage in dialogue about what led up to these. Some of the most common reasons for treatment failure include not setting up the agreement collaboratively, not having effective harm reduction targets, not having an effective monitoring plan, not managing overinvolved or underinvolved team members, and not addressing comorbid conditions to ensure they are optimally treated. Aspects of managing these expected treatment failures include taking time to understand what led up the failure, empathic listening, and collaborative problem-solving. Successful navigation of the agreement failures may strengthen the alliance and can be an opportunity for even more inroads toward harm reduction.

Case Examples

Case Example 1

Marge, a 28-year-old woman, told her primary care doctor she was suffering from tension headaches. When asked about recent stressors, Marge described concerns for the safety of her 57-year-old mother because of a hoarding problem. She reported almost daily heated arguments with her mother about her collecting and saving. Marge reported that she was "at her wit's end" and felt helpless and fearful for her mother's safety.

Although her mother had always been a collector of dolls and antiques, she had recently started collecting almost anything she could get her hands on. Now she had run out of room in her small apartment, yet she refused to stop accumulating items, which were mainly from flea markets and thrift stores. Her bed was covered with so much stuff that Marge's mother slept in a recliner in the living room. There were only narrow pathways throughout the apartment, and in the kitchen, even the pathway had cans, papers, magazines, and other items covering the floor. One of her bathrooms could not be used because of the clutter, and the sink in the other one was clogged and could not be used.

Marge could not understand how her mother didn't see this behavior as a problem. When Marge confronted her about it, she complained that Marge was violating her rights. Marge wondered whether she needed to call APS or seek a court-appointed guardian. Marge consulted with her mother's primary care doctor about the problem, and he recommended a harm reduction approach. Rather than trying to get her to get rid of her possessions, the focus was on how to manage the health and safety risks faced by Marge's mother. In the initial phase, the plan was to assess risk level and what level of intervention was needed, and to continue preparing Marge's mother for the ongoing phase.

Marge's mother balked at the mention of assessing the risk level in the home and stopped answering phone calls from Marge or her primary care doctor. The primary care doctor helped assemble a team of people, including Marge (with some coaxing), several other family members, her mother's primary care doctor, and a nurse practitioner with some experience in this area.

The team's next step was for the nurse practitioner to call Marge's mother daily at the same time and inquire about her physical health and well-being. Initially, Marge's mother did not answer the calls, though she did listen to the messages the nurse practitioner left. One day, just before the call, Marge's mother slipped on a pile of magazines, twisting her ankle and falling hard on her arm. She agreed to allow the nurse practitioner to come over immediately to examine her ankle and wrist. After that, Marge's mother began answering the nurse practitioner's calls, and they were able to establish a warm and trusting relationship largely based on her medical care. Before long, Marge's mother allowed the nurse practitioner to visit her regularly in her home. On her first visit, the nurse practitioner did not comment on the clutter or problems with it. Instead, she commented on how many wonderful treasures were there. Marge's mother seemed delighted by the attention and engaged in animated conversations about the things she had collected. The nurse practitioner even suggested that she might figure out a way to show off her things to others. At that suggestion, Marge's mother opened up about how difficult that would be and elaborated on some of the negative consequences of her collecting behavior (e.g., embarrassment, not being able to have visitors). This allowed the nurse practitioner to employ a motivational interviewing approach in the discussions about these difficulties. Although she was initially reluctant, over the course of several months, Marge's mother agreed to join the harm reduction team and became engaged in selecting harm reduction targets and establishing a plan for managing the clutter. The key feature was that the efforts were not to be focused on the removal of her possessions; instead, the immediate objective was to arrange them to ensure her health and safety.

Discussion

This case highlights several important issues. First, hoarding also affects family members and the community. Family may feel overwhelmed when their loved one with hoarding disorder refuses help. This situation can result in relationship conflicts and social withdrawal (Frost and Hartl 1996; Tolin et al. 2008), as well as stress, worry, and physical manifestations (e.g., tension headaches). At times, the situation can deteriorate to a complete lack of trust and avoidance. Although not present in this case, another challenge stems from a clinician's countertransference (e.g., feelings of anxiety or being overwhelmed) when working with individuals with hoarding disorder, which—if not identified—may manifest in suboptimal care (Millen et al. 2017). A neutral third party who can approach the situation from a medical perspective (without discussing the clutter) may be a way to reestablish a trusting connection with the client. Second, each client's individual autonomy should be upheld to the extent possible while weighing this factor against minimizing risk to their health and well-being (National Commission for the Protection of Human Subjects of Biomedical and Behavioral Research 1979). Individuals who have the capacity to make informed decisions or who are in no danger of harming themselves or others have a right to the particular level of clutter in their homes. In this case, although the mother was having difficulty managing clutter and had a rupture in the relationship with her daughter, she was willing to accept third-party help to keep her environment safe. The harm reduction approach allowed the mother the opportunity to keep the majority of her collections and other items. At the same time, if Marge's mother had not been able to engage with a third party or exhibited an inability to care for herself with a demonstrated lack of capacity for decision-making, she would have been referred for a higher level of intervention like APS or a court-appointed guardian.

Case Example 2

Tina, a single 55-year-old librarian living in New York City, was frantically looking for help. Her landlord had served her with a 3-day Notice to Cure, which is issued in cases where the tenant has violated a term or condition of the lease. In this case, Tina's landlord was concerned that the apartment complex's maintenance worker was unable to enter the apartment to replace the smoke alarm due to the sheer volume of items in the home. The landlord required the home to have clear pathways between entries/exits so that the smoke alarm could be installed. Concerned about eviction and the possibility of losing all of her possessions, she reached out to her local eviction prevention agency, who engaged the local hoarding task force. After initial discussion about her options, Tina declined referrals for treatment but was open to learning more about harm reduction approaches employed by the hoarding task force. The initial assessment confirmed the difficulties the maintenance worker had installing the fire alarm. Together with the harm reduction team, the task force was able to identify harm reduction targets to meet the minimum standards of safety (e.g., clear paths between the front door and the fire escape and smoke alarm, removal of flammable materials from the stove) that were consistent with the terms of the lease. In parallel, the team reached out to the landlord to describe the plan and to ask for an extension.

The harm reduction team continued to meet regularly to implement and manage the harm reduction plan, monitor Tina's adherence, help with compliance, and regularly reassess the harm risk level. The plan included home visits by the hoarding task force members to add transparency and accountability to the goals for harm reduction. During one of the home visits in the ongoing phase, Tina told one of the team members her suspicions that she was being robbed by her neighbors at night. She described putting down an important item before bed, and then in the morning she could not locate it. The more uncluttered her home was, the more suspicious she became. Tina's landlord refused to provide an extension, and Tina was unsuccessful in meeting her landlord's rapid deadline, triggering an eviction notice. The team was able to provide Tina with referrals for a pro bono lawyer and recommended medical and psychiatric evaluations because of her increased suspiciousness. She was found to be physically healthy except for obesity, with normal labs and neuroimaging. She endorsed symptoms of hoarding disorder and denied symptoms of major depression, bipolar disorder, eating disorders, anxiety disorders, psychosis, substance use disorders, or other mental illnesses. Tina was referred to group CBT for hoarding disorder. Ultimately, Tina and her lawyer were able to request accommodation because of disability from hoarding disorder, resulting in additional time for Tina to continue the harm reduction plan—creating paths in her home, allowing installation of the smoke alarm, and being in compliance with the lease. As Tina's stress level decreased, her suspicions about her neighbors also subsided.

Discussion

This case highlights several important issues. First, when a client receives any kind of communication from a landlord or legal notice, consultation with a legal representative is recommended to protect the individual's rights in these cases. Individuals who are threatened with eviction because of clutter have the legal right to request accommodation because of disability from hoarding. Second, when the client has a very limited time frame to get their home in compliance, a harm reduction approach should be considered, especially since treatment for hoarding disorder can take many months. Even though Tina's hoarding behaviors may be maladaptive to some degree (e.g., inability to have the smoke alarm installed), the information in the case did not indicate that she was in imminent danger. Thus, her individual autonomy should be upheld and every attempt should be made to engage her in the decision-making process. Third, Tina's progress was aided by transparency and accountability from the hoarding task force (e.g., home visits) for continued progress in decluttering efforts. Fourth, it is important to recommend that clients receive a medical and psychiatric evaluation to ensure the diagnosis of hoarding disorder and recommendation of treatment, including for comorbid conditions.

Conclusion

The harm reduction model is a useful framework to consider when patients lack awareness of their illness, when they lack motivation toward recovery, when family relationships have deteriorated, or when change is needed in a short period of time. Harm reduction has been successful in other disorders characterized by lack of recognition or motivation. This model focuses on reducing the potential harm from hoarding behaviors rather than resolving symptoms. It begins with an assessment of harm potential, followed by the creation of a harm reduction team, then collaborative development and implementation of a harm reduction plan. The plan includes specification of goals, home visits, inspections, and problem solving of difficulties. More research is needed to determine the effectiveness of this approach.

KEY CLINICAL POINTS

- Harm reduction is an intervention based on a set of pragmatic principles, strategies, and applications designed to minimize the risk caused by problematic effects of behaviors.

- Harm reduction intervention has been adapted for hoarding disorder—with a focus on engaging the patient, building a team, assessing the harm and risks, and creating and implementing a plan to minimize those risks.

- Harm reduction is not a treatment for hoarding disorder.

- The primary goal of harm reduction is to manage symptoms in order to decrease risk; whereas the goal of treatment is to reduce symptoms, distress, and impairment.

- The harm reduction approach for hoarding behaviors consists of two phases (initial and ongoing) and several features (initiation, engagement, assessment of harm, team building, planning, and ongoing management).

- In the initial phase, the primary objective is to assess the risk level and whether the client needs an intervention.

- In the ongoing phase, the primary objective is to continue to reassess the harm risk level over time in the context of carrying out the planned interventions developed during the initial phase.

- The second objective of the ongoing phase is to maintain an effective harm reduction team to implement and manage the harm reduction plan.

References

Ball AL: HIV, injecting drug use and harm reduction: a public health response. Addiction 102(5):684–690, 2007 17506148

Brace PB: Hoarding becomes a health, safety issue. The Nantucket Independent, November 21, 2007

Bratiotis C: HOMES Multi-Disciplinary Hoarding Risk Assessment. 2009. Available at: https://vet.tufts.edu/wp-content/uploads/HOMES_SCALE.pdf. Accessed February 27, 2020.

Bratiotis C, Schmalisch CS, Steketee G: The Hoarding Handbook: A Guide for Human Service Professionals. Oxford, UK, Oxford University Press, 2011

Burke BL, Arkowitz H, Menchola M: The efficacy of motivational interviewing: a meta-analysis of controlled clinical trials. J Consult Clin Psychol 71(5):843–861, 2003 14516234

Denning P: Practicing Harm Reduction Psychotherapy: An Alternative Approach to Addictions. New York, Guilford, 2000

Denning P, Little J, Glickman A: Over the Influence: The Harm Reduction Guide for Managing Drugs and Alcohol. New York, Guilford, 2004

Des Jarlais DC, Friedman SR: AIDS, injecting drug use, and harm reduction, in Psychoactive Drugs and Harm Reduction: From Faith to Science. Edited by Heather N. London, Whurr Publishers, 1993, pp 297–309

Doran GT: There's a S.M.A.R.T. way to write management's goals and objectives. Manage Rev 70(11):35–36, 1981

Drogin EY: Ethical Conflicts in Psychology, 5th Edition. Washington, DC, American Psychological Association, 2019

Emmanuelli J, Desenclos JC: Harm reduction interventions, behaviours and associated health outcomes in France, 1996-2003. Addiction 100(11):1690–1700, 2005 16277629

Ferguson SG, Shiffman S, Gwaltney CJ: Does reducing withdrawal severity mediate nicotine patch efficacy? A randomized clinical trial. J Consult Clin Psychol 74(6):1153–1161, 2006 17154744

Frost RO, Hartl TL: A cognitive-behavioral model of compulsive hoarding. Behav Res Ther 34(4):341–350, 1996 8871366

Frost R, Steketee G, Tolin D, Renaud S: Development and Validation of the Clutter Image Rating. J Psychopathol Behav Assess 30(3):193–203, 2008

Frost RO, Hristova V, Steketee G, Tolin DF: Activities of Daily Living Scale in hoarding disorder. J Obsessive Compuls Relat Disord 2(2):85–90, 2013 23482436

Hettema J, Steele J, Miller WR: Motivational interviewing. Annu Rev Clin Psychol 1:91–111, 2005 17716083

Logan DE, Marlatt GA: Harm reduction therapy: a practice-friendly review of research. J Clin Psychol 66(2):201–214, 2010 20049923

Maltby N, Tolin DF: A brief motivational intervention for treatment-refusing OCD patients. Cogn Behav Ther 34(3):176–184, 2005 16195056

Marlatt GA: Harm Reduction: Pragmatic Strategies for Managing High-Risk Behaviors. New York, Guilford, 1998

Millen A, Linkovski O, Dunn LB, Rodriguez CI: Ethical challenges in treating hoarding disorder: two primary care clinical case studies. Focus Am Psychiatr Publ 15(2):185–189, 2017 31975851

Miller WR: Motivational factors in addictive behaviors, in Rethinking Substance Abuse: What the Science Shows, and What We Should Do About It. Edited by Miller WR, Carroll KM. New York, Guilford, 2006, pp 134–150

Miller WR, Rollnick S: Motivational Interviewing: Preparing People for Change, 2nd Edition. New York, Guilford, 2002

Miller WR, Rollnick S: Motivational Interviewing: Helping People Change, 3rd Edition. New York, Guilford, 2013

National Commission for the Protection of Human Subjects of Biomedical and Behavioral Research: The Belmont Report: Ethical Principles and Guidelines for the Protection of Human Subjects of Research. Washington, DC, U.S. Department of Health, Education, and Welfare, April 18, 1979, pp 4–13

Prochaska JO, Velicer WF: The transtheoretical model of health behavior change. Am J Health Promot 12(1):38–48, 1997 10170434

Rasmussen JL, Steketee G, Frost RO, et al: Assessing squalor in hoarding: the Home Environment Index. Community Ment Health J 50(5):591–596, 2014 24292497

Shelton JL, Levy RL: Behavioral Assignments and Treatment Compliance: A Handbook of Clinical Strategies. Champaign, IL, Research Press, 1981

Simpson HB, Zuckoff A, Page JR, et al: Adding motivational interviewing to exposure and ritual prevention for obsessive-compulsive disorder: an open pilot trial. Cogn Behav Ther 37(1):38–49, 2008 18365797

Tolin DF, Frost RO, Steketee G, Fitch KE: Family burden of compulsive hoarding: results of an internet survey. Behav Res Ther 46(3):334–344, 2008 18275935

Tompkins MA: Working with families of people who hoard: a harm reduction approach. J Clin Psychol 67(5):497–506, 2011 21360706

Tompkins MA: Clinician's Guide to Severe Hoarding: A Harm Reduction Approach. New York, Springer, 2015

Tompkins MA, Hartl TL: Digging Out: Helping Your Loved One Manage Clutter, Hoarding & Compulsive Acquiring. Oakland, CA, New Harbinger Publications, 2009

Westra H, Dozois D: Preparing clients for cognitive behavioral therapy: a randomized pilot study of motivational interviewing for anxiety. Cognit Ther Res 30:481–498, 2006

Wilson GT, Grilo CM, Vitousek KM: Psychological treatment of eating disorders. Am Psychol 62(3):199–216, 2007 17469898

CHAPTER 10
Community

The negative impact of hoarding disorder is far-reaching, including substantial risk to the health and safety of individuals, their families, neighbors, and the community. The complex needs of individuals with hoarding disorder can be overwhelming for a single human service agency or individual, particularly when cases involve the housing, health, legal, and adult/child protective systems. Most such cases need immediate resolution of problems created by clutter. At the same time, individuals with hoarding disorder often display limited insight and perceive decluttering efforts under threat of eviction as "inhuman" and "threatening" (Gibson 2015). These conditions create a critical need for education, engagement, and effective coordination of the community members.

In this chapter, we describe community partnerships, including hoarding task forces, public-academic collaborations, and partnerships initiated by individuals with lived experiences of hoarding disorder (Bratiotis et al. 2011; Kysow et al. 2020; Woody et al. 2020). These community partnerships can take many shapes, and we provide examples below on how they can be useful to shape policy and provide education and other resources in situations in which outcomes depend on multiple complex factors (Koelen et al. 2008). They involve thoughtful coordination efforts and engagement that may involve human service professionals or agencies who encounter clients with hoarding symptoms, including housing staff (e.g., landlords, code inspectors), public health and safety officials (e.g., police and fire department), those in the legal field (e.g., lawyers, judges), eviction prevention agency workers, agency officials from adult and child protective services, health care providers (e.g., visiting nurses, paramedics, occupational therapists, home health aides), professional organizers, and mental health professionals.

Hoarding Task Force Intervention Model

Task forces are thought to have been introduced in the 1920s by the United States military as temporary units established to work on a defined activity or objective under one leader (Merriam-Webster n.d.). The term expanded beyond the armed forces during World War II—first to a business context and then to many another sectors. Task forces are involved in a wide range of activities, including community development, organizing, and policy advocacy (Conrad and Schneider 2010; Roussos and Fawcett 2000). In 1999 in Virginia, the Fairfax County Hoarding Task Force was formed; this task force is thought to be the first hoarding task force in the United States (Bratiotis 2009). Since then, these groups have proliferated throughout the country.

Hoarding disorder is resource-intensive (San Francisco Task Force on Compulsive Hoarding 2009), and addressing all of the needs of a client—ranging from mental health to structural and fire risk to determining whether children can stay in the home—can easily overwhelm any one single provider or agency. Further, working with high-need individuals at high risk for poor outcomes, such as eviction, is taxing and can elicit strong emotions. To mitigate these issues, the task force team provides coordinated intervention across multiple systems, case consultation, and education. This mechanism has advantages, including optimizing resource allocation, mitigating overwork by sharing the workload, serving as a space for human service professionals to xchange valuable knowledge and experience honed through their fieldwork, d providing emotional support for team members (Bratiotis 2009, 2013). Although there is relatively little empirical evidence on the effectiveness oarding task forces, qualitative data have been generated on their for- n and operation within the United States (Bratiotis 2009, 2013). A rative case study of 5 task forces—a sampling from the more than 50 g task forces operating in the United States in 2009—captured the ts of human service providers (in mental health, social services, alth, housing, fire and police, and legal) to elucidate the hoarding sk force process (e.g., composition, organization, funding, policies). lso examined the process by which task forces organize and op- policy and practice changes that emerge. Specifically, three of the five task forces were organized because of a precipitating event (e.g., public attention to a community case of hoarding), suggesting initiation was a grassroots process started by concerned frontline workers (Bratiotis 2013). Additional issues reported that motivated task force formation included inadequate resources, lack of knowledge, and lack of interagency coordination. For four of the five task forces, the leadership/chair role was rotated among the different agencies every 3–4 years, with initial leadership by a staff member from the fire department or a mental health, adult protection, or housing agency (Bratiotis 2013). The majority of agencies did not compensate staff effort, and individuals performed their task force service as an addition to their regular work duties. Meetings were typically between 1 and 2 hours, with structured agendas (Bratiotis 2013). As a result of participation in the task force, two agencies began tracking their cases for outcome and quality improvements. The authors found that a primary function of hoarding task forces was case consultation and that member agencies participating in a hoarding task force influenced hoarding policy and decisions made within their organization (Bratiotis 2013). Another primary function is community education. The local task force for one of us (R.F.) offered 1-day workshops on hoarding every 1–2 years for the first 15 years of its existence. The efforts were successful in drawing hundreds of attendees for each workshop. Although task forces as originally conceived were intended to be a time-limited effort to identify, define, and provide a model for problem-solving, most task forces on hoarding represent ongoing, long-term efforts. Partly for this reason, some groups have changed the name from "Hoarding Task Force" to something more encompassing. For instance, in western Massachusetts, the local group changed their name to the Western Massachusetts Hoarding Resource Network.

Hoarding task forces often begin with the efforts of one or two highly motivated individuals who have some experience dealing with hoarding cases. The task forces often falter when these individuals give up their leadership role. To help with this problem, Bratiotis (2009, 2013) recommends expanding the social work role in these task forces—given their unique training and skill set—and viewing task forces as agents for furthering hoarding policies within the community. The authors further posit that future research should focus on viability of hoarding task force operations.

Challenges and Opportunities

There are both challenges and opportunities from the perspective of each of these human service professionals/agencies in helping clients struggling with clutter (see Bratiotis et al. 2011 for further discussion). In this section, we provide examples across agencies.

Housing and Legal Systems

Hoarding behaviors may first be detected by housing staff, including land-lords, housing associations, subsidized housing providers, property manag-ers, and those employed by housing agencies (inspectors or maintenance workers). These individuals may need to involve the legal system to access the home or intervene when tenants cannot comply with housing codes. One of the challenges of housing legal interventions for hoarding behaviors is the lack of attention to treatment for the underlying mental disorder and the overemphasis on the consequences of hoarding, like removing clutter. If the underlying condition is not treated, hoarding may precipitate homelessness by placing individuals at risk for eviction. Even if individuals find another home, they may continue to accumulate clutter and be evicted again and re-peatedly re-enter the legal system.

Indeed, evictions are a cause of homelessness (Crane et al. 2005; Van Laere et al. 2009). In one study of the economic and social burden of hoard-ing disorder (N=864), the team found that 2% of individuals with hoarding reported being evicted and 6% endorsed being threatened with eviction be-cause of their hoarding (Tolin et al. 2008). In the United Kingdom, among randomly selected homeless individuals (N=78) newly admitted to Salvation Army shelters, 21% endorsed hoarding symptoms and 8% reported that hoarding problems directly contributed to their homelessness (D. Mataix-Cols, L. Grayton, A. Bonner, et al., "A Putative Link Between Compulsive Hoarding and Homlessness: A Pilot Study," unpublished manuscript, 2009). In another study, individuals seeking help from a not-for-profit eviction in-tervention agency in New York City (N=115) were screened for hoarding disorder; of those seeking help who had symptoms that met the criteria for hoarding disorder (n=25), 32% were currently in legal eviction proceedings (i.e., threatened with imminent eviction), 44% had a history of previous legal eviction proceedings, and 20% had been evicted from their home one or more times (Rodriguez et al. 2012). Taken together, these studies suggest a link be-tween hoarding disorder, homelessness, and eviction. The fact that only 48% of these individuals were currently seeking mental health treatment represents an opportunity for intervention. Further prospective research is needed to determine whether identifying and treating hoarding disorder early may decrease risk of eviction and homelessness.

There are several opportunities for legal system involvement in hoard-ing cases (Bratiotis et al. 2011). The first is playing a role in granting right-of-entry permission for authorities to enter a home and remove vulnerable individuals and animals from a harmful situation. Another is playing a key role in enforcing an existing right-of-entry (e.g., consequences of summons to appear in court, fines) to allow housing agencies to inspect conditions relevant to a lease or rental property. Public health officials may also need to seek a warrant to enter a private home when there is visible evidence of a situation that could cause a public health problem. An additional role is to enforce mandated change (e.g., orders for—or warning notices of potential— eviction, condemnation of a house, loss of legal custody of a minor, loss of guardianship of an elder). There has been increasing awareness around mental illness and hoarding behaviors, and more judges and lawyers are sophisticated in recommending a plan with benchmarks and a timeline with reasonable expectations to achieve safety through reducing clutter, alongside mental health evaluation and support (Volunteer Lawyers Project 2008). These suggestions have raised the level of discourse and problem-solving, rather than tackling the issues with surface changes of eviction and mandated cleanouts, which can negatively impact mental health.

Public health codes vary by state and geographic region in the United States. For example, the responsibility for keeping the property in compliance may be primarily assigned to the landlord or the tenant, depending on where they live. Furthermore, each city or town can further amend or adapt international code (Bratiotis et al. 2011; International Code Council 2020). Another consideration is that private property is protected, and the individual has the right to determine how the space is used. If there are no safety issues, health issues, or code violations, a person is entitled to keep as many items as they wish, even if their friends or relatives disagree. Thus, a homeowner may decline a property inspection by the Board of Health (however, in some states, such as Massachusetts, this decision can be overridden by a court-issued warrant) (Bratiotis et al. 2011). Since laws vary by state, the scope of a warrant may vary (e.g., limited to the exterior of the home only). In contrast to private ownership, property managers have a right to enter renters' homes. Further, regular inspection may be a condition of residence for subsidized housing, although, again, this may vary across specific agreements and programs.

The federal Fair Housing Act (see 42 U.S.C. §§3601-3619, and specifically subsection 42 U.S.C. §3604[f][3] on discrimination) promotes equal access to housing. It prohibits discrimination on the basis of characteristics such as race, religion, gender, familial status, and disability (including mental disability) and, among other things, requires that a housing owner/manager provide reasonable accommodation upon a tenant's request. In cases of hoarding disorder, reasonable accommodation could take the form of allowing time for a tenant to engage with mental health services. Of note, compliance timelines and laws around eviction vary by state (Bratiotis et al. 2011).

For individuals with hoarding behaviors who enter the court system, having scales to document progress can be helpful. These scales are discussed in detail in Chapters 3 and 4 and include the Clutter Image Rating (see Appendix B in this volume) to assess clutter volume, the Home Environment Index to rate squalid conditions, and the Activities of Daily Living—Hoarding Scale (see Appendix E in this volume) to inform the impact of hoarding on the client's life. In addition, housing-specific recommended measures include the Hoarding Referral Sheet (developed by Jesse Edsell-Vetter, Metropolitan Housing Partnership, Boston, Massachusetts) and the Inspections Hoarding Referral Tool (Metropolitan Boston Housing Partnership 2014)—which allows drawings of clutter and tracking of blocked exits (Bratiotis et al. 2011). In addition, the Institute for Challenging Disorganization (ICD; www.challengingdisorganization.org) has made the ICD Clutter-Hoarding Scale available in eight different languages on their website (National Study Group on Chronic Disorganization; www.challenging-disorganization.org/clutter-hoarding-scale-). Geared toward professional organizers, these measures allow for objective tracking of progress. The Clutter Image Rating in particular, which can be rated by the inspector and the client (if they are willing), allows for an opportunity for discussion and a window into the client's insight by seeing how closely the two assessments align.

Safety Personnel: Emergency Medical Team and Fire Response

In addition to the health and safety risks to the client (e.g., fire, falls, mold, pest infestation), excessive clutter can also make it hard for emergency services to enter a home to respond to a cardiac emergency or put personnel in danger due to the risk of being trapped in the clutter.

In a study of residential fires in hoarding homes in Melbourne, Australia, fewer than half these homes had operating smoke detectors (Harris 2010; Lucini et al. 2009). The study also reported that fires did not exclusively happen in homes with severe clutter; moderate clutter (as assessed on the Clutter Image Rating) was also a fire hazard. Fires that begin in the homes of individuals with hoarding behaviors are more difficult to extinguish and more likely to spread to neighbors' homes (Harris 2010; Lucini et al. 2009). This study also found that despite the fact that relatively few residential house fires involved hoarding conditions (0.025%), the ones that did accounted for 24% of fire-related fatalities (Lucini et al. 2009). In one case familiar to us (recounted by a local fire captain), a valued firefighter lost his life while entering a building to rescue a tenant with hoarding disorder. He became disoriented in the narrow passageways, and his coworkers could not get to him when several piles collapsed around him as the flames engulfed the room.

Two hoarding-related fire deaths in 2010 and 2011 motivated the local health authority to establish the City of Vancouver's Hoarding Action Response Team (HART), a hoarding task force that enabled a coordinated effort between several nonprofit human service organizations and provided a budget for staff salaries and infrastructure (e.g., office space and IT resources). This funded collaboration between the local health authority and the city fire prevention branch was composed of a full-time fire prevention officer, a full-time psychiatric nurse, a fire captain, and a clinical health supervisor. A research team collected the data on 82 cases involving hoarding conditions (using HART's case tracking systems containing health and team intervention records) from 2016 to 2018 (Kysow et al. 2020). Results indicate that HART's model of a community-based intervention was associated with clutter reduction and preservation of tenancy, with the majority of cases successfully closed within six home visits. The team also experienced challenges, including clients not responding to phone or email contact (causing delays to the initial home visits), client disengagement (canceled and missed appointments), and low resources (e.g., no team budget for decluttering services or maintenance visits to monitor for setbacks). Despite these barriers, the cross-disciplinary and committed nature of the team enabled it to reduce clutter and keep at-risk clients in their homes.

Adult and Child Protective Services

Adult Protective Services (APS) and Child Protective Services may be called upon by mandated (or nonmandated) reporters who hear or observe situations that violate the rights of vulnerable individuals (e.g., < age 18, > age 60, mentally or physically disabled) or violate health and safety codes (42 U.S.C. Ch. 132 and Ch. 35, §3002). In cases of potential child abuse or neglect due to hoarding, the court appoints a *guardian ad litem* in the service of protecting the child's welfare. The guardian ad litem will conduct an independent assessment of the family and home. Of note, definitions of eligibility for elder abuse prevention services vary by state. One of the most challenging aspects for these agencies is establishing trust with the client and family. Starting by offering help and approaching the situation from a harm reduction lens may build rapport and lead to the client accepting help on more difficult decluttering/code-related tasks. Protective service professionals can play a critical part in court proceedings—acting as both advocate and liaison to the court in detailing intervention efforts and progress on hoarding behaviors over time (Bratiotis et al. 2011). APS and the courts recognize that adults have the right to make decisions for themselves and that they cannot force a client to accept help or leave the home, even if they are being abused or neglected because of hoarding behaviors. An exception is in cases when the client is not competent to make their own decisions (typically ascertained by a competency evaluation). In these cases, the court can appoint a guardian to safeguard the client.

Professional Organizers

Professional organizers help improve organization in work and home spaces (Kolberg 2007), and a subset of professional organizers have additional specialized training to work with individuals with hoarding behaviors, including education on issues of inattention, indecision, excessive acquiring, and attachment to possessions (Kolberg 2009; Kolberg and Nadeau 2016). One of the benefits for clients working with professional organizers is that they may feel less stigma (Bratiotis et al. 2011). Indeed, an online study of acceptability of treatment and services of individuals with clinically significant hoarding behaviors (N=203; Saving Inventory—Revised>40) reported that a professional organizing service was the second-most acceptable (out of 11 treatments and services for hoarding) (Rodriguez et al. 2016). Of note, only 3 of 11 treatments and services were deemed acceptable (the first was individual cognitive-behavioral therapy [CBT], and the third was use of a self-help book). The most acceptable aspects of these included the domains of personalized care, being held accountable, and belief the treatment/service works (Rodriguez et al. 2016). Given that treatment acceptability may underlie preferences for behavioral treatments (Sidani et al. 2009), and preferences have been reported to be indicators of treatment initiation and retention (Dwight-Johnson et al. 2001; Raue et al. 2009), clients' initial connection with professional organizers may be an important way to maximize outcomes for individuals and their communities.

Referral listings by region can be found through the National Association of Productivity and Organizing Professionals (www.napo.net) and ICD, two groups within the field of professional organizing that work with individuals with hoarding behavior (Bratiotis et al. 2011). One note to clarify a term used by members of ICD: *chronic disorganization* is defined as disorganization that a) occurs over a long period of time, b) leads to impaired quality of life, and c) recurs despite repeated self-help attempts (Kolberg 2007). The ICD community acknowledges that chronic disorganization may be present in many conditions, including ADHD, hoarding disorder, PTSD, anxiety, depression, and traumatic brain injury. Although many individuals with hoarding disorder have problems with disorganization, the strength of attachment to possessions is the hallmark of those who hoard, in contrast to people who suffer disorganization without hoarding (Grisham et al. 2009). Other possible differences include that individuals with hoarding have a great sense of shame and have an excessive number of objects that others may deem of little value, whereas individuals with chronic disorganization without hoarding disorder have objects that others would deem as useful or valuable (Bratiotis et al. 2011). However, further research is needed to understand and clarify these relationships beyond observations. Recognition of these differences (including strong emotional attachment to objects) will inform useful strategies, including asking permission to touch a client's possessions, being prepared for a client's strong emotions (e.g., grief, anxiety, anger) while sorting and parting with possessions, teaching decision-making strategies, and using the client's own word choices to refer to their possessions, which they may view as treasures (Bratiotis et al. 2011).

Public-Academic Partnerships

Because of the stigma associated with hoarding (Chasson et al. 2018), individuals with hoarding behaviors may keep their disorder hidden until an emergency like a fire or threat of eviction attracts the attention of family and landlords (Rodriguez et al. 2010). State mental health agencies are particularly interested in home evictions due to code violations, because these actions can cause homelessness in the populations they serve. One opportunity to bridge the gap between mental illness and public agencies is to build capacity for mental health researchers to pursue policy-relevant research. One example is the New York State Office of Mental Health (OMH) Policy Scholars program, which provides small grants to early-career researchers to grow their skills in identifying needs and their knowledge in navigating the complexities of large public mental health systems (Millen et al. 2020; Rodriguez et al. 2010, 2013; Wilson et al. 2017). Challenges include a tight project timeline, with the goal being to design and deliver a project with a prompt payoff for the public partners within 1 year. OMH mentors are critical in addressing another challenge: working effectively with OMH policymakers to ensure the scholars' research is helpful to the programs hosting the research. Opportunities include having experts from state agencies and academia shape the research projects toward practical utility while advancing the scholars' research efforts. Scholars also develop fluency with the language of both policymaking and research that serves to foster communication and collaboration between partner health system administrators and researchers as they generate timely improvements and transform mental health services (Rodriguez et al. 2013).

One example of this approach was an OMH project exploring the hypothesis that the population seeking help from a community agency that serves individuals with housing problems would have a high prevalence of hoarding disorder, given that the threat of eviction—and potential loss of all possessions—may trigger contact with the agency. Indeed, a study of 115 clients seeking the agency's help confirmed a 5- to 10-fold higher rate of hoarding disorder than in the general population (e.g., 22% clinician-rated and 23% self-rated prevalence in the population served by the agency vs. 1.5%–6% prevalence in the general population; see Chapter 1) (Rodriguez et al. 2012). The authors reported that of the 25 clients with symptoms that met criteria for hoarding disorder, 32% were in legal eviction proceedings, yet only 48% were currently seeking mental health treatment. This project highlighted that community eviction prevention agencies may be a site for identifying individuals with hoarding disorder who may be open to treatment during a critical time.

Building upon this finding, the next step was pilot-testing an adaptation of critical time intervention (CTI)—an evidence-based, time-limited care coordination model that helps ensure continuity of support for clients with severe mental illness during critical transition points (Herman et al. 2011)—with individuals at risk for eviction. Originally conceived to prevent previously homeless men with mental illnesses from returning to homelessness, CTI focuses on the difficult transition from institutional living (e.g., hospital, shelter) to community living (Susser et al. 1997). The adapted version of CTI for individuals with hoarding disorder (CTI-HD) focused on the critical time period of the threat of eviction, during which an individual experiences concern about eviction or receives an eviction notice (Millen et al. 2020). Case managers were trained in delivering the 9-month CTI-HD model in three phases. In Phase 1 (3 months), case managers had weekly face-to-face meetings in the client's home, weekly phone check-ins, engagement, rapport building, risk assessment, assessment of mental health needs, referral to free legal counseling, entitlement registration, reconnection to their support networks, and referral to evidence-based CBT skills groups. In Phase 2 (4 months), the case manger's involvement was titrated down to one check-in every 2 weeks, at which time adjustments to the client's support network, mental health needs, and other resources were made as required to meet their needs and prepare for anticipated relapse risk factors. In Phase 3 (2 months), the case manager's involvement consisted of one check-in per month, optimization of supports, and planning for termination. Of the 14 adults with severe symptoms of hoarding disorder at risk for eviction who enrolled, 11 participants (80%) completed the 9-month intervention, and no participant was evicted. All participants enrolled in the facilitated CBT skills group (the Buried in Treasures Workshop [Frost et al. 2012]). Completers reported a modest decrease in hoarding severity (25% reduction as measured by the Saving Inventory—Revised) and in clutter (an average reduction from 6 to 5, as measured by the Clutter Image Rating), but the level of clutter was still severe enough to put clients at continued risk for eviction (Millen et al. 2020). Taken together, the data suggest that while helpful, CTI-HD alone is unlikely to eliminate the risk of eviction for individuals with severe symptoms of hoarding disorder.

In another example, a team of researchers engaged local community partners (including APS, hoarding task force participants, case managers, social workers, and community leaders) in San Mateo and Santa Clara counties in California to assess the needs of first responders and individuals with hoarding disorder (Wilson et al. 2017). Identified areas of high need included the availability of local providers trained in low-cost, evidence-based treatments and the resolve to engage and empower the community stakeholders themselves to increase their skill base and improve access to care. In a pilot study, the team tested the feasibility and efficacy of a 1-day multimedia educational workshop for community stakeholders, which included hands-on experiential activities, didactics, a prerecorded lecture from a peer facilitator, and a question-and-answer session with an individual with hoarding disorder (Wilson et al. 2017). The interest level was high, with all 20 available workshop spaces reserved within 48 hours of launch (with a waiting list of 32 individuals). Among the 17 individuals who completed the workshop, knowledge of the subject matter improved by 29%, and the interest in running a group increased from 6% to 59% after the workshop. After completion of the workshop, two members of the workshop ended up volunteering to serve clients with hoarding (either by leading a Buried in Treasures Workshop or by providing in-home uncluttering coaching sessions), and the rest did not start a group in their communities because they did not have time for an unreimbursed activity. These results, along with the event's low cost ($40 per participant), showed that offering an educational community workshop to improve access is a feasible and cost-effective strategy to engage community stakeholders.

In yet another highly successful public-academic partnership, the Metropolitan Boston Housing Partnership—in conjunction with the Tenancy Preservation Program and with assistance from the Boston University School for Social Work—developed a program to prevent eviction of hoarding clients in public housing (Metropolitan Boston Housing Partnership 2014, 2015). The program was developed with four specific goals: reduce the frequency of eviction and condemnation due to excessive hoarding; educate public housing professionals regarding hoarding; assist agencies, courts, and the legislature in the development of better approaches to hoarding problems; and collect data to better understand the problem. The effort resulted in an individualized case management protocol based on existing knowledge about hoarding disorder and included regular home visits to assist with decluttering, exercises borrowed from CBT for hoarding, and ongoing monitoring and help with other associated problems. Over the 3-year period under study, 175 case participants came through the program. The cases all involved public housing tenants at risk of eviction for their hoarding behaviors. Only two of the participants lost their housing as a result of hoarding, which represented a vast improvement over the typical outcomes. Across all of the cases was a significant decline in the Clutter Image Rating scores (from 3.7 to 2.4) (Metropolitan Boston Housing Partnership 2015). Of significance is the fact that none of these case participants sought help for their hoarding, so they may represent a different sample from those seen in typical treatment studies. Nevertheless, the condition of their homes substantially improved. These findings indicate that even in cases where clients have little intrinsic motivation, improvement is possible.

Community Partnerships Initiated by Clients With Lived Experiences

Another example of a research, community, and social services collaboration for hoarding disorder is a partnership in Montreal initiated in 2011 by four clients with hoarding disorder (Bodryzlova et al. 2020). Identifying the lack of hoarding services in their outpatient clinic, they enlisted the help of a local community organizer at a primary care clinic to organize a meeting with individuals with lived experience of hoarding behaviors and social service professionals. They identified that social service professionals felt ill-equipped to help clients in crisis situations and that clients could not find adequate mental health services or help for uncluttering (Bodryzlova et al. 2020). That led to the development of the Montreal Compulsive Hoarding Enlarged Committee (MCHEC) in 2015, composed of 30 partners—including clients with lived experience, health care professionals, researchers, municipal services providers, and representatives from Montreal's Public Health Department and Montreal City Hall. With funding from the Montreal City Council and Canadian Institutes of Health Research, the MCHEC increased awareness of hoarding disorder, created a specialized intervention team, and published the results of a survey depicting factors affecting referral rate for hoarding disorder at primary mental health care in Quebec (Bodryzlova and O'Connor 2018). The group has created trainings, colloquia, and peer-led support groups for clients with hoarding disorder and their families, as well as offered peer-assisted help with uncluttering. Challenges for the MCHEC include the need for sustainability and reliance on the objectives of the hosting health care facilities and individual leadership. Opportunities include incorporation of these efforts sustainably into health care systems, with paid specialists with backgrounds in education and conflict management skills to facilitate communication between stakeholders; compensation for peer leadership and training activities; and consultations. The authors state that even though MCHEC is not generalizable to scale (Bodryzlova and O'Connor 2018), these efforts show that individuals with lived experience of hoarding disorder can drive change by bridging the gap between their own need and mental and health care services.

Case Example

A local task force made up of representatives from the local health department, city code enforcement, elder services, mental health, a housing authority, and disability services, as well as several people with lived experience of hoarding disorder, provided case management for difficult cases. The guardian for a 73-year-old woman brought her case to the attention of the task force. The house she had lived in all of her life was in such bad shape that the local health department was considering condemnation. Her home was filled with possessions to the point that it prevented her from being able to carry out the basic activities of daily living. For instance, the exits were blocked with objects and piles of magazines. Stacks of papers were piled throughout the home, with some next to her furnace and on her stovetop. There were only very narrow pathways through each room, and some rooms were completely impassable. Her bathroom was barely functional, and her kitchen sink was filled with objects. Because of a disability, the woman had a guardian who was responsible for the woman's financial and personal well-being. In addition to the condition of the home, the woman was out of money, and the guardian was considering selling the house in order to give her enough money to live on. Unfortunately, sale of the home would require a home inspection, and since parts of the house were virtually inaccessible, this was not possible. Additionally, most of the woman's social life centered on neighbors and the local community. Moving her to a different location would have a negative impact on her social life.

Since the woman reported willingness to work with the task force to save her home, a plan was created to help her in the process of meeting requirements to avoid condemnation and to allow inspection by the bank. As a first step, the task force recommended pursuing a reverse mortgage to allow the woman to remain in her home. The second step was to secure a 30-day grace period related to the code violations. Third, members of the task force met with her and reviewed the condition of her home in order to complete the Uniform Inspection Checklist (www.centerforhoardingandcluttering.com/uniform-inspection-checklist-2), a shorthand and simplified checklist of conditions that must be met in order to avoid condemnation and eviction. This document lays out in layman's terms exactly what needs to be done to meet the minimum requirements of the health and code enforcement departments and allow inspection by the bank. The checklist was carefully reviewed by a task force representative to make sure the conditions covered the necessary improvements. Representatives helped the woman develop a plan for doing the work outlined in the checklist. With her approval, the task force trained and arranged for a member of her church to assist her in making the improvements. At the end of the 30-day extension, the woman had met all the conditions laid out in the checklist and was able to set up an inspection prior to the granting of a reverse mortgage.

Discussion

This case points out several things that are important from the perspective of a community approach. First, the focus was on allowing the woman to remain in her home and part of her local community. As she had lived in her home for all of her life, moving to an unfamiliar environment surrounded by people she did not know would seriously affect her quality of life. Second, most often when hoarding cases such as this arise, the individual is given a 30-day notice to clean up the property. Seldom is the instruction more specific, though sometimes the order is to get rid of rubbish or trash. For people with hoarding disorder, the definition of rubbish or trash is different. We have seen cases in which the individual believes they have complied because they have gotten rid of what they consider trash, only to be accused of noncompliance. The task force was instrumental in defining very specifically what needed to change for the home to be compliant. Furthermore, the emphasis was on meeting the conditions "spelled out above" and not on "getting rid of stuff"—consistent with a harm reduction approach. Finally, the work of the task force was largely organizational and did not include any of the physical labor involved. Including help from a trusted acquaintance was crucial and part of the community effort to assist.

Conclusion

Community interventions are critical when clients fall between the cracks of health systems. A single provider or agency can become overwhelmed, whereas a task force can serve as a much-needed safety net for the client and a source of support for the task force members. Beyond hoarding disorder, task forces may be a process and a tool to shape policy for other issues facing communities.

Given that the infrastructure for community interventions is lacking, areas of great need include structural and financial investment in paid positions for hoarding-specific practitioners to deliver collaborative hoarding interventions. Evidence-based intervention trainings for mental health and human health service professionals are needed to expand the workforce delivering care. Advocacy is needed for reimbursement for hoarding disorder services—at the health insurance level as well as at the government level regarding legislature for mental health insurance coverage. By generating data on best practices, public-academic partnerships provide ways to study community interventions, shape interventions and best practices, and encourage the next generation of researchers to invest in hoarding disorder intervention research. Involvement of clients with lived experience with hoarding disorder in interventions and research will enhance the generation of client-centered approaches, which may improve the likelihood of engagement in services and applicability of findings.

KEY CLINICAL POINTS

- The consequences of hoarding behavior may be time-consuming and costly for communities.

- In addition to the health and safety risks to the client, excessive clutter can also make it hard for emergency services to enter a home to respond to a cardiac emergency or put personnel in danger due to risk of being trapped in the clutter.

- Effective management of cases may require intervention and coordination across multiple human service systems.

- Models for community partnerships include hoarding task forces, public-academic collaborations, and partnerships initiated by individuals with lived experiences of hoarding disorder.

- Studies of hoarding task forces highlight their primary functions, including case consultation and community education.

- There has been increasing awareness around mental illness and hoarding behaviors, and more judges and lawyers are sophisticated in recommending a plan with benchmarks and a timeline with reasonable expectations to achieve safety through reducing clutter, alongside mental health evaluation and support.

- More structural and financial infrastructure is needed to ensure hoarding disorder treatments are accessible (available in the community where the person lives), acceptable (they are offered in a way that the person will participate in the treatment), and effective (the person gets better and is no longer disabled by hoarding behaviors).

References

Bodryzlova Y, O'Connor K: Factors affecting the referral rate of the hoarding disorder at primary mental health care in Quebec. Community Ment Health J 54(6):773–781, 2018 29353402

Bodryzlova Y, O'Connor K, Vallée V, et al: Community partnership in response to hoarding disorder in Montreal. Psychiatr Serv 71(6):631–634, 2020 32114943

Bratiotis C: Task force community response to compulsive hoarding cases. Doctoral dissertation, Boston University, Boston, MA, 2009

Bratiotis C: Community hoarding task forces: a comparative case study of five task forces in the United States. Health Soc Care Community 21(3):245–253, 2013 23199135

Bratiotis C, Schmalisch CS, Steketee G: The Hoarding Handbook: A Guide for Human Service Professionals. Oxford, UK, Oxford University Press, 2011

Chasson GS, Guy AA, Bates S, Corrigan PW: They aren't like me, they are bad, and they are to blame: a theoretically-informed study of stigma of hoarding disorder and obsessive-compulsive disorder. J Obsessive Compuls Relat Disord 16:56–65, 2018

Conrad P, Schneider JW: Deviance and Medicalization: From Badness to Sickness. Philadelphia, PA, Temple University Press, 2010

Crane M, Byrne K, Fu R, et al: The causes of homelessness in later life: findings from a 3-nation study. J Gerontol B Psychol Sci Soc Sci 60(3):S152–S159, 2005 15860792

Dwight-Johnson M, Unutzer J, Sherbourne C, et al: Can quality improvement programs for depression in primary care address patient preferences for treatment? Med Care 39(9):934–944, 2001 11502951

Frost RO, Ruby D, Shuer LJ: The Buried in Treasures Workshop: waitlist control trial of facilitated support groups for hoarding. Behav Res Ther 50(11):661–667, 2012 22982080

Gibson EJ: Perceptions of Determining Factors: A Case Study of Eviction Risks of People Who Hoard in Waterloo Region. Waterloo, Ontario, Canada, Wilfrid Laurier University, 2015

Grisham JR, Frost RO, Steketee G, et al: Formation of attachment to possessions in compulsive hoarding. J Anxiety Disord 23(3):357–361, 2009 19201154

Harris J: Household hoarding and residential fires. Presentation at the International Congress of Applied Psychology, Melbourne, Australia, 2010

Herman DB, Conover S, Gorroochurn P, et al: Randomized trial of critical time intervention to prevent homelessness after hospital discharge. Psychiatr Serv 62(7):713–719, 2011 21724782

International Code Council: 2021 International Property Maintenance Code. Washington, DC, International Code Council, 2020

Koelen MA, Vaandrager L, Wagemakers A: What is needed for coordinated action for health? Fam Pract 25 (suppl 1):i25–i31, 2008 18936114

Kolberg J: Conquering Chronic Disorganization. Decatur, GA, Squall Press, 2007

Kolberg J: What Every Professional Organizer Needs to Know About Hoarding. Decatur, GA, Squall Press, 2009

Kolberg J, Nadeau K: ADD-Friendly Ways to Organize Your Life: Strategies That Work From an Acclaimed Professional Organizer and a Renowned ADD Clinician. New York, Routledge/Taylor and Francis Group, 2016

Kysow K, Bratiotis C, Lauster N, Woody SR: How can cities tackle hoarding? Examining an intervention program bringing together fire and health authorities in Vancouver. Health Soc Care Community 28(4):1160–1169, 2020 31984612

Lucini G, Monk I, Szlatenyi C: An analysis of fire incidents involving hoarding households. Report to Worcester Polytechnic Institute. Worcester, MA, 2009

Merriam-Webster: A brief history of the "task force." Available at: www.merriam-webster.com/words-at-play/a-brief-history-of-the-task-force. Accessed July 14, 2021.

Metropolitan Boston Housing Partnership: A New Approach to Hoarding Intervention: Preliminary Data From the Hoarding Intervention and Tenancy Preservation Project. 2014. Available at: www.metrohousingboston.org/wp-content/uploads/2017/10/Hoarding-Report-2014-FINAL.pdf. Accessed July 14, 2021.

Metropolitan Boston Housing Partnership: Rethinking Hoarding Intervention: MBHP's Analysis of the Hoarding Intervention and Tenancy Preservation Project. 2015. Available at: www.metrohousingboston.org/wp-content/uploads/2017/10/Hoarding-Report-2015_FINAL.pdf. Accessed July 14, 2021.

Millen AM, Levinson A, Linkovski O, et al: Pilot study evaluating critical time intervention for individuals with hoarding disorder at risk for eviction. Psychiatr Serv 71(4):405–408, 2020 31910750

Raue PJ, Schulberg HC, Heo M, et al: Patients' depression treatment preferences and initiation, adherence, and outcome: a randomized primary care study. Psychiatr Serv 60(3):337–343, 2009 19252046

Rodriguez C, Panero L, Tannen A: Personalized intervention for hoarders at risk of eviction. Psychiatr Serv 61(2):205, 2010 20123831

Rodriguez CI, Herman D, Alcon J, et al: Prevalence of hoarding disorder in individuals at potential risk of eviction in New York City: a pilot study. J Nerv Ment Dis 200(1):91–94, 2012 22210369

Rodriguez CI, Arbuckle MR, Simpson HB, et al: Public-academic partnerships: a rapid small-grant program for policy-relevant research: motivating public-academic partnerships. Psychiatr Serv 64(2):106–108, 2013 23370621

Rodriguez CI, Levinson A, Patel SR, et al: Acceptability of treatments and services for individuals with hoarding behaviors. J Obsessive Compuls Relat Disord 11:1–8, 2016 28163996

Roussos ST, Fawcett SB: A review of collaborative partnerships as a strategy for improving community health. Annu Rev Public Health 21:369–402, 2000 10884958

San Francisco Task Force on Compulsive Hoarding: Beyond Overwhelmed: The Impact of Compulsive Hoarding and Cluttering in San Francisco and Recommendations to Reduce Negative Impacts and Improve Care. San Francisco, CA, Mental Health Association of San Francisco, 2009

Sidani S, Miranda J, Epstein DR, et al: Relationships between personal beliefs and treatment acceptability, and preferences for behavioral treatments. Behav Res Ther 47(10):823–829, 2009 19604500

Susser E, Valencia E, Conover S, et al: Preventing recurrent homelessness among mentally ill men: a "critical time" intervention after discharge from a shelter. Am J Public Health 87(2):256–262, 1997 9103106

Tolin DF, Frost RO, Steketee G, et al: The economic and social burden of compulsive hoarding. Psychiatry Res 160(2):200–211, 2008 18597855

Van Laere I, De Wit M, Klazinga N: Preventing evictions as a potential public health intervention; characteristics and social medical risk factors of households at risk in Amsterdam. Scand J Public Health 37(7):697–705, 2009 19666669

Volunteer Lawyers Project: Hoarding and the Law (white paper). Boston, MA, Volunteer Lawyers Project, 2008

Wilson J, Wilkerson E, Filippou-Frye M, Rodriguez C: A workshop to engage community stakeholders to deliver evidence-based treatment for hoarding disorder: a pilot study. Psychiatr Serv 68(12):1325–1326, 2017 29191148

Woody SR, Lenkic P, Bratiotis C, et al: How well do hoarding research samples represent cases that rise to community attention? Behav Res Ther 126:103555, 2020 32044474

PART IV
Challenges

CHAPTER 11
Elders

Hoarding behaviors first appear early in life, as summarized in Chapter 2, with the typical age at onset between 15 and 19 years (Zaboski et al. 2019). Although late onset of hoarding disorder has been reported, it appears to occur only in small numbers (Tolin et al. 2010). Late onset of hoarding behaviors (after age 40) may reflect an underlying medical condition, such as focal brain lesions due to cardiovascular disease or herpes simplex encephalitis (Anderson et al. 2005), and should be investigated. Research on the course of hoarding behavior suggests that it takes decades after the appearance of early hoarding symptoms before they become prominent (Grisham et al. 2006; Tolin et al. 2010). Despite the early onset, much of the research on prevalence and severity seems to suggest that hoarding is most problematic among older adults (Ayers et al. 2015). In this chapter, we review the research related to hoarding in the elderly.

Hoarding Prevalence and Severity in the Elderly

Findings on the role of aging in hoarding have been conflicting. The earliest accounts suggested a greater prevalence among older adults, yet those came from community agencies dealing with the issue. For instance, Frost et al. (2000) surveyed health departments in Massachusetts regarding their experiences with hoarding cases. Among the identified cases, 40% also in-volved departments of aging. High rates of acquiring, saving, and hiding behaviors in nursing homes (15%) and adult day care centers (25%) have also been reported (Marx and Cohen-Mansfield 2003). Social service staff of elder services and similar agencies report large numbers of hoarding cases among older adults each year (McGuire et al. 2013). Greater prevalence among older adults might also explain why attempts to recruit hoarding sam-ples for study routinely generate a larger number of older participants than recruitments for community controls or for other mental disorders (Frost et al. 1998, 2011).

Three studies have examined retrospective reports given by people with hoarding problems on their personal history of hoarding behaviors. In a large survey of people with hoarding problems (N=751), Tolin et al. (2010) asked participants to rate the severity of hoarding behaviors for each 5-year period of their lives. Over 90% of the participants reported an increasing or chronic course not reaching moderate severity until about age 40. By age 40, 82% of the sample felt they had moderate or even more severe hoarding symptoms. By age 50, 89% did so. Once hoarding symptoms appeared, fewer than 1% showed a course of declining symptoms. Using a similar strat-egy, Ayers et al. (2010) found that hoarding severity increased with each de-cade of life, based on the recollections of a small sample of late-life hoarding participants (N=18). Dozier et al. (2016a) also found increasing severity for all hoarding symptoms across the life span of those with hoarding disorder. Clutter increased with each decade of life, while difficulty discarding stabi-lized around age 50. There were no reported remissions or decreases in symptoms among the 82 participants. Over 60% of the sample reached the most extreme severity rating by age 50.

Several population-based prevalence studies reported higher rates among older adults. In the largest such study to date, Cath et al. (2017) sur-veyed a random sample of more than 15,000 people from the Netherlands Twins Registry regarding the presence of hoarding and obsessive-compulsive disorder (OCD) symptoms. Using individual items from the Hoarding Rat-ing Scale selected to map onto the DSM-5 criteria, they found an overall prevalence rate of 2.12%. More specifically, the prevalence of hoarding rose by 20% for every 5 years of age. Around age 35, there was a sharp increase in severity, continuing in subsequent years, which appeared to be due largely to increases in difficulty discarding. Younger participants in the Cath et al. study had the lowest prevalence rate (below 2%), while those over 70 years of age had a prevalence rate of over 6%. For older males, the severity of hoarding symptoms increased more rapidly than for older females.

Similarly, Samuels et al. (2008) found a prevalence rate for hoarding of 6.2% among adults 55 to 94 years old, but only 2.3% among 34- to 44-year-olds, and 2.9% among those 45 to 52 years old. In contrast, two studies failed to find differences in prevalence across similar age groupings. Fullana et al. (2010) found no difference in hoarding symptoms among those ages 18–24, 25–49, and 50 and over in a study across six European countries. Mueller et al. (2009), using slightly different age groupings (18–39, 40–59, ≥60) in a German sample, failed to find differences in the proportion of hoarding cases between these age groupings. The age groupings in these studies may have obscured the relationship between age and hoarding symptoms, particularly if, as is suggested by other studies, hoarding severity peaks around age 50 and levels off.

Among a sample of community controls, Reid et al. (2011) found that older adults had more hoarding symptoms (excessive acquisition, difficulty discarding, clutter) than did younger adults. However, two studies using hoarding disorder samples failed to find correlations between age and hoarding symptoms. Dozier et al. (2016a) failed to find correlations between age and Saving Inventory—Revised scores among 122 people with hoarding disorder. Although the age range for the sample was large, the median age was 63, suggesting that the distribution was skewed. Diefenbach et al. (2013) also failed to find a correlation between age and Saving Inventory—Revised scores, although they did find a correlation between age and therapist-rated global symptom severity. In both of these studies, the range of hoarding severity scores was severely restricted, which may have resulted in the failure to find a relationship. The general conclusion to be drawn from these studies is that older adults are at higher risk for having hoarding problems that meet criteria for hoarding disorder, though the hoarding severity level may not correlate with age or may reach a peak at age 50 before leveling off.

Most studies have shown elevated levels of all three dimensions of hoarding problems (excessive acquisition, difficulty discarding, clutter) among cases of elderly individuals with hoarding compared with nonclinical controls. However, Steketee et al. (2012) found somewhat lower excessive acquisition in their older hoarding adults compared with other hoarding samples, though the severity on this dimension was still greater than that seen in the nonhoarding control group. Cath et al. (2017) found that while the severity of clutter leveled off somewhat after age 40–44, excessive acquisition severity continued to slowly worsen and difficulty discarding dramatically increased after age 35. These authors reported that the sharp increase in hoarding prevalence after age 35 seen in their study was driven primarily by increases in difficulty discarding.

Other features of hoarding appear similar between younger and older adults who hoard. The types of items saved among the elderly who hoard appear similar to the types of items saved by younger people with hoarding problems (Kim et al. 2001). Lack of insight has been observed in a large percentage of the elderly who hoard, but this has also been observed in similar studies with younger samples. Elder service agency officials indicated that only 15% of the elderly hoarding cohort in the Kim et al. (2001) study "definitely acknowledged the irrationality of their hoarding behavior." Similarly, in the McGuire et al. (2013) study, social service staff reported that fewer than 10% of their mostly elderly cases were "insightful about their hoarding." While very low, these figures are comparable to the judgments of family and friends of hoarding loved ones across the full age spectrum who indicated excellent or good insight in the Tolin et al. (2008) study (see Chapter 4).

Functional Impairments Associated With Late-Life Hoarding

Hoarding behaviors among the elderly pose special risks. Interviews of older adults who hoard have revealed a number of ways in which age influences hoarding severity and impairment (Eckfield and Wallhagen 2013). New and worsening health conditions are prominent causes of impairment (Eckfield and Wallhagen 2013; Tolin et al. 2008). Reduced strength, stamina, energy, and mobility from health declines reduce the ability to manage clutter and create barriers to discarding. Reductions in mobility and flexibility can also increase the risk of falling if floors are covered with objects that must be stepped on or over. Stairways that are congested with objects increase the risk of more serious falls. Risk of death in house fires (Lucini et al. 2009) is also elevated when mobility is limited by infirmities associated with aging.

Changes in the social context of older adults' lives can contribute to the impairment experienced by people with hoarding problems (Eckfield and Wallhagen 2013). A common occurrence among the elderly is the transition to living alone following the death of a spouse. This event removes someone who may have played a significant role in managing the condition of the home. When people live alone, the clutter in their home tends to be more severe (Frost and Steketee 2010). A complicating factor is that as people with hoarding disorder age, their relationships with family and friends often fracture following failed attempts at helping (Frost and Steketee 2010). This further increases their isolation and loneliness (Burgess et al. 2018; McGuire et al. 2013). Some (perhaps those with abuse history or paranoia) may want social isolation, and their clutter serves as a barrier to interactions. Limited social contact eliminates the possibility of social feedback related to self-care and clutter. Another change in social context occurs when older relatives die and their belongings are inherited. Not only is the emotional meaning of the possessions often overwhelming, but also the sheer logistics of managing a household worth of stuff are as well. As older adults stop working, they must forge new roles and identities for themselves. This was cited by a number of individuals in the Eckfield and Wallhagen (2013) study. Many of the participants described a lack of purpose and boredom without a job to go to or a family to raise. Under such circumstances, the meaning of possessions may gain more significance, making discarding more difficult.

Yet another feature of life among older adults is insecurity regarding financial stability. Hoarding behaviors are more common among people with lower incomes and fewer financial resources (Samuels et al. 2008). Participants in the Eckfield and Wallhagen (2013) study cited worries about finances as leading them to hang onto items they thought they might need in the future. This is consistent with some theorizing that humans are biologically driven to respond to uncertainty with accumulation of resources (Vickers and Preston 2014).

Age-related changes in the home setting are important events that influence the ability to manage possessions (Eckfield and Wallhagen 2013). The buildup of possessions over a lifetime in the same home is substantial for most people. For people who have had hoarding problems for most of their lives, the problem is magnified. Moving from such a home into assisted living or downsizing creates considerable stress regarding decisions that must be made about possessions. Most often the result is moving many items into storage and taking more possessions than can reasonably fit into a new home. Most of those items remain in the bags or boxes in which they were moved, often resulting in the purchase of new replacements when searched-for items can't be found.

Kim et al. (2001) interviewed elder service workers about the conditions in the homes of their hoarding clients. Nearly two-thirds of the elderly who hoarded had difficulties with self-care. Clutter interfered with the use of bathtubs, sinks, and showers. Often, bathroom features (e.g., toilet) were nonfunctional. Only 10% of the residences were described as clean, and a third were described as extremely dirty or filthy. In 32% of the homes (of elderly clients with hoarding behaviors), service providers reported overpowering odors from rotten food and animal or human feces. The hoarding interfered with the ability to maintain personal hygiene to at least a moderate degree in 60% of cases. Body odor and disheveled personal appearance were observed as well, including blackened skin, filthy hair, and soiled clothes. Unsanitary conditions in the home, odor in the home, body odor, unkempt appearance, and perceived physical danger were all significantly correlated with the amount of clutter in the home (Kim et al. 2001).

Clark et al. (1975) labeled people living in such conditions as suffering from "Diogenes syndrome." They described Diogenes syndrome as a condition of the elderly characterized by gross self-neglect, domestic squalor, hoarding of rubbish, social isolation, and lack of insight. The condition was named after the fourth century B.C. cynic philosopher Diogenes of Sinope, who lived in isolation—neglecting hygiene and violating social conventions. The term *Diogenes syndrome* is a misnomer, because the behavior of the ancient philosopher has only a superficial resemblance to severe self-neglect in the elderly (Marcos and Gómez-Pellín 2008). Nevertheless, hoarding is often associated with the existence of squalor or unsanitary living conditions, especially among the elderly (Snowdon et al. 2007). In a review of research on severe domestic squalor, Snowdon et al. (2007) concluded that excessive accumulation of possessions occurred in over half of severe domestic squalor cases. Rasmussen et al. (2014) found that degree of squalor was associated with hoarding severity among a large sample of people who self-identified with hoarding problems. Although associated with hoarding, squalor characterizes the environment of only a small portion of people with hoarding disorder. Furthermore, many people who live in squalor do not hoard, and those who do may not do so in a manner consistent with hoarding disorder (Snowdon et al. 2007). Specifically, in many cases the accumulation of objects is not intentional, nor are there attachments to these objects. See Chapter 13 for more information on squalor.

Self-neglect, or the inability to carry out basic self-care and activities of daily living, is the most common abuse-related problem reported to social service agencies devoted to the protection of older adults (Hei and Dong 2017). Self-neglect in the elderly occurs in the context of cognitive impairment, psychological distress, and impaired physical functioning. Inability to complete basic activities of daily living is at the core of self-neglect in the elderly (Dong and Simon 2016). Hoarding is a core feature in current models of self-neglect among the elderly (Dong and Simon 2016) and a common occurrence among social service clientele. Among a large sample of community-dwelling older adults in Chicago, hoarding was associated with greater impairments in activities of daily living (Dong and Simon 2016).

Several studies have examined impairments in the ability to perform activities of daily living in hoarding samples. Older adults with hoarding problems showed significantly more impairment in activities of daily living due to hoarding than older adults without hoarding problems (Ayers et al. 2012b). Among hoarding elders, over 85% reported significant problems with finding important things, and many reported difficulties moving around in the house (61%), eating at a table (57%), using the kitchen sink (39%), preparing food (32%), and even sleeping in a bed (32%). None of the non-hoarding older adults reported problems in these areas. Diefenbach et al. (2013) also found that older adults with hoarding reported more impairment in activities of daily living than did a nonclinical sample of older adults. It should be noted, however, that the comparison groups in these studies were nonhoarding individuals and not younger adults with hoarding. Other research indicates that younger adults with hoarding demonstrate more impairment in activities of daily living compared with nonhoarding individuals as well (Ong et al. 2015). Only a few studies provide evidence regarding activities of daily living of older adults with hoarding compared with younger adults with hoarding. Two studies of participants with hoarding failed to find evidence of an association between age and impaired activities of daily living such as ability to move around the house, sit in chairs, or sleep in a bed (Diefenbach et al. 2013; Dozier et al. 2016b). However, older participants with hoarding behaviors did show greater impairment on a different measure of daily functioning, which included finances, communication, comprehension/planning, transportation, and household skills (Dozier et al. 2016b). Similarly, using a measure evaluating personal health care, household management, meal preparation, and keeping in touch with family and friends, Ayers et al. (2014b) found that hoarding severity predicted functional disability in older adults.

Medical Comorbidities in Elders Who Hoard

In a large study of self-identified hoarding cases, Tolin et al. (2008) found those with serious hoarding problems to have a significantly compromised health status. In over 60% of the cases in which criteria for moderate to severe hoarding were met, the individual reported at least one chronic and severe medical condition—a significantly higher percentage than among self-identified cases in which the severity criteria for hoarding were not met (<50% reported a chronic and severe medical condition). Individuals in this study with moderate to severe hoarding also reported more chronic and severe medical conditions than a matched sample from the National Comorbidity Survey (Kessler et al. 1994), including arthritis, asthma, hypertension, stroke, diabetes, heart problems, kidney/liver disease, lupus/thyroid disorder, autoimmune disease, chronic fatigue syndrome, ulcers, stomach and gallbladder problems, and cancer. In addition, individuals with moderate to severe hoarding, as well as those whose hoarding behaviors were judged to be subclinical, had significantly higher BMIs than family members who reported on a hoarding loved one. In fact, the average BMI for the individual with moderate to severe hoarding was 31.6, which is in the obese range (National Heart, Lung and Blood Institute and National Institute of Diabetes and Digestive and Kidney Diseases 1998). Timpano et al. (2011) replicated the finding of increased BMI in hoarding cases. Individuals in their hoarding group were more than twice as likely to be classified as obese than their nonhoarding participants. These findings were drawn from samples that included the full age range of hoarding case individuals.

Several studies have reported greater medical comorbidity among elderly hoarding individuals compared with nonpsychiatric controls. Diefenbach et al. (2013) found higher reports of medical problems in an elderly hoarding group compared with elder adults who did not hoard. Among a general sample of elderly adults reporting on health status, hoarding was more common among those reporting only fair or poor health (Dong et al. 2012). Relatedly, Ayers et al. (2010) reported high rates of hypertension, head injury, arthritis, gastric problems, and sleep apnea among older adults with hoarding. Ayers et al. (2014a) subsequently reported that 90% of elderly hoarding individuals in their study had at least one chronic or severe medical condition, whereas only 44% of the matched nonpsychiatric controls did so. Among the most frequent medical conditions affecting hoarding individuals at a higher rate than community controls in this study were cardiovascular conditions, arthritis, sleep apnea, head injury, and diabetes. Ayers et al. (2014a) also found that levels of hoarding severity were associated with the total number of medical problems. Specific medical conditions most strongly related to hoarding severity were sleep apnea, arthritis, and hematological conditions. The percentage of older adults with hoarding problems having at least one serious medical condition in the Ayers et al. (2014a) study (90%) is substantially greater than the 61% having such a medical condition among the full range of ages of those with hoarding from the Tolin et al. (2008) study. This suggests that although all hoarding individuals appear to be at increased risk for severe health problems, the risk is especially acute for older adults.

The reason for the association of hoarding disorder with chronic and serious medical conditions, especially among older adults, is unknown. The wide variety of conditions related to hoarding might suggest some type of broader systemic problem common to both hoarding and poor health. Just what that systemic problem might be is unknown. Other possible causes have to do with behaviors associated with hoarding that might affect health. Social isolation, particularly among the elderly, might affect help-seeking for medical issues. Ayers et al. (2014a) found that older adults with hoarding visited their primary care doctor only once every 18 months. This frequency is far less than the average for nonhoarding adults older than 65 (Schappert and Rechtsteiner 2008). Lack of insight among some with hoarding symptoms may extend to physical problems as well, leading to underutilization of health care services. Hoarding may also be associated with poor health habits such as overeating, poor nutrition, and a sedentary lifestyle. If the individual is unable to use cooking facilities, they may be more likely to rely on fast foods with limited nutritional value. Squalor or lack of sanitation may contribute to more frequent and chronic bacterial and viral infections. In some hoarding cases, individuals save and even eat rotting food, which may affect gastrointestinal disorders.

Poor health may drive the development and worsening of hoarding symptoms. Decreases in energy and stamina may influence attempts to gain control over clutter (Eckfield and Wallhagen 2013). Sleep apnea and cardiovascular problems may reduce the capacity to deal with clutter. Regardless of the reason for the association between hoarding and poor health in older adults, careful evaluation of the medical condition of hoarding patients is extremely important and requires further investigation.

Psychiatric Comorbidity and Associated Features of Late-Life Hoarding

In samples of elderly individuals, evidence of higher than typical rates of psychiatric disorders—such as generalized anxiety disorder, depression, and anxiety disorders—suggests that the mental health status of elderly hoarding individuals may be even more compromised (Proctor et al. 2003; Richardson et al. 2011; Wetherell et al. 2010). Depression has been found to be a frequent disorder among people diagnosed with hoarding (Frost et al. 2011). This relationship appears to be true among older hoarding disorder samples as well. Depression, social anxiety, and worry were strongly correlated with hoarding severity in one sample of nonclinical elderly individuals (Reid et al. 2011). Yet, the study found that depression does not appear to increase or remain high in elderly hoarding individuals. Dozier et al. (2016b) found depression to be negatively correlated with age in other samples of elderly hoarding disorder cases. In fact, among a large sample of people with hoarding, Diefenbach et al. (2013) reported that older age was associated with less severe anxiety and anxiety sensitivity, and fewer current mood and anxiety disorders. For individuals with hoarding who are depressed, however, the presence of hoarding may be associated with additional problems. Mackin et al. (2011) found that individuals with late-life depression and hoarding performed poorly on measures of categorization/problem-solving, verbal memory, and information processing speed than people with late-life depression without hoarding symptoms.

Interventions for Hoarding in the Elderly

Until recently, most interventions in hoarding cases involved community agencies cleaning out homes of hoarding individuals. In a survey of health departments in Massachusetts, Kim et al. (2001) found that clearing out the entire house was the most frequent intervention, despite the fact that in 43% of cases, it did not improve the hoarding behaviors, in 15% the behaviors actually got worse, and in 8% conditions improved initially only to relapse. In only 15% of cases was there any sort of sustained improvement. These negative findings, along with the fact that most cases of elderly hoarding involve multiple social service agencies (e.g., elder services, housing agency, health department), have led to the development of hoarding task forces coordinating the efforts of all stakeholders (Bratiotis and Woody 2014). Despite these efforts, recent evidence suggests that most social service agencies are woefully unprepared to deal with hoarding cases. In a study of social service workers, McGuire et al. (2013) reported that few caseworkers had received any kind of training related to hoarding and no standard protocols existed for how to deal with such cases.

Relatively little research has explored clients' response to cognitive-behavioral treatment in geriatric hoarding cases. Turner et al. (2010) treated a small sample ($N=6$) of individuals with hoarding disorder using cognitive-behavioral therapy (CBT) (Steketee and Frost 2007), which included both office and in-home sessions. The format was somewhat flexible, with the number of sessions varying from 28 to 41. The average age of the sample was 72. Significant improvement was observed, with declines in clutter (28%), difficulty discarding (34%), and excessive acquisition (>50%). Improvement in activities of daily living was 24%.

Ayers et al. (2011) had less success with a small sample ($N=12$) of older clients (mean age=73) with hoarding disorder. They found a relatively poor response to the existing treatment for hoarding (Steketee and Frost 2007). While there were significant declines in hoarding symptoms at posttest and follow-up, there were no declines in therapists' overall symptom severity ratings. Also, relatively few patients were considered treatment responders, and several of the responders relapsed by 6-month follow-up. Treatment response was defined as at least a 35% improvement in hoarding symptom measures and a score of minimally improved or better on the Clinical Global Impression—Improvement rating. Importantly, homework completion was strongly correlated with decreases in hoarding symptoms at both posttest and follow-up.

In a follow-up study, Ayers et al. (2012a) examined session feedback from clients, therapists' session notes, and follow-up interviews with the therapists to gain a sense of what happened in treatment. Therapists indicated that lack of homework compliance was a major factor in the therapy process and outcomes. Few patients completed homework between sessions. Patients were somewhat better at completing the discarding and nonacquiring tasks at home than they were at cognitive exercises. Explanations for failure to complete homework included forgetfulness, level of difficulty, and competing demands. Rather than suggesting a motivational problem, Ayers et al. (2011) suggested that the poor homework compliance resulted from cognitive deficits that impeded clients' ability to complete homework on their own. Therapists also concluded that cognitive skill deficits—such as prospective memory, planning, problem-solving, and cognitive flexibility—were major impediments to homework completion and overall outcome. Clients also reported that they found exposures to discarding and nonacquiring helpful but did not feel the same about cognitive strategies. Interestingly, clients did not find the time spent on case formulation helpful. This might suggest that clients did not approach the therapy with a clear understanding of the rationale for treatment. However, clients did find the home visits by the therapist to be helpful. Both therapists and clients found their relationship to be an important part of therapy.

In light of the possible influence of cognitive deficits on treatment response, Ayers et al. (2014c) modified the standard CBT for hoarding disorder to include a heavier emphasis on cognitive skills training. They expanded work on problem-solving and organizational skills from the two to three sessions in the standard manual to six sessions. They also added modules on prospective memory and cognitive flexibility. With a small number of elderly clients ($n=11$, average age=66), they found more substantial reductions in hoarding symptoms (38%–41%) than in the earlier investigation. Seventy-three percent of participants qualified as full treatment responders, while the rest were partial responders. Neurocognitive impairments like those seen in hoarding disorder have been found to be associated with poor response to CBT among other geriatric mental health patients (Mohlman 2005). The heavy emphasis on these skills may substantially improve treatment outcome in geriatric hoarding cases.

Conclusion

The relative paucity of research on geriatric hoarding makes drawing conclusions difficult. The severity of hoarding seems to increase across the decades and reach moderate to severe levels after age 50, and then either levels off or continues to get worse throughout the life span. There is little evidence that the symptoms of hoarding are qualitatively different among the elderly than among younger cohorts. Executive function and neurocognitive deficits are clearly evident among elders with hoarding, but these are also prevalent among younger individuals with hoarding as well. No studies have shown differential severity of hoarding or neurocognitive functioning between older and younger individuals with hoarding.

Hoarding behaviors are associated with interference in activities of daily living, such as the ability to sit on a chair or sleep in a bed. However, it is not clear that impairments of these types of daily living activities are worse among older individuals who hoard than they are in younger individuals who hoard. There is some evidence that different kinds of impairment in daily functioning may be worse among older hoarding patients, particularly those related to finances, household skills, and keeping in touch with friends and family. In addition to these types of impairments, age-related physical changes and cognitive problems may make the consequences of hoarding more severe. For instance, the risk of injury from falling may increase with age even more in dwellings that remain at a constantly high level of clutter. Decreased mobility may make it more difficult to declutter as well as exit a dwelling in case of emergency. Also, as people age, changes in needed health behaviors—such as taking medication in a consistent manner—may be impaired by clutter and disorganization that might not have been as problematic before the new activities were required. Therefore, while the severity of symptoms may not be different from that for younger hoarding cohorts, symptoms may result in more impairment because of aging factors.

The minimal research on treatment of geriatric hoarding suggests that the addition of cognitive skills training may be of substantial benefit. This may be true in the treatment of younger hoarding cohorts as well, since we see the same neurocognitive deficits in both younger and older individuals with hoarding disorder. Modifying the standard treatment for hoarding disorder to include cognitive rehabilitation certainly deserves further study.

KEY CLINICAL POINTS

- Hoarding disorder appears to be more prevalent among the elderly.

- Age-related cognitive decline may affect the ability to benefit from cognitive-behavioral therapy for hoarding disorder.

- Hoarding symptoms do not appear to be qualitatively different for elderly versus younger individuals with hoarding disorder.

- Isolation and loneliness are significant problems for elderly people with hoarding disorder.

- Hoarding is a common problem among the clientele of social service agencies that serve the elderly.

References

Anderson SW, Damasio H, Damasio AR: A neural basis for collecting behaviour in humans. Brain 128 (Pt 1):201–212, 2005 15548551

Ayers CR, Saxena S, Golshan S, Wetherell JL: Age at onset and clinical features of late life compulsive hoarding. Int J Geriatr Psychiatry 25(2):142–149, 2010 19548272

Ayers CR, Wetherell JL, Golshan S, Saxena S: Cognitive-behavioral therapy for geriatric compulsive hoarding. Behav Res Ther 49(10):689–694, 2011 21784412

Ayers CR, Bratiotis C, Saxena S, Wetherell JL: Therapist and patient perspectives on cognitive-behavioral therapy for older adults with hoarding disorder: a collective case study. Aging Ment Health 16(7):915–921, 2012a 22548463

Ayers CR, Schiehser D, Liu L, Wetherell J: Functional impairment in geriatric hoarding participants. J Obsessive Compuls Relat Disord 1:263–266, 2012b

Ayers CR, Iqbal Y, Strickland K: Medical conditions in geriatric hoarding disorder patients. Aging Ment Health 18(2):148–151, 2014a 23863040

Ayers CR, Ly P, Howard I, et al: Hoarding severity predicts functional disability in late-life hoarding disorder patients. Int J Geriatr Psychiatry 29(7):741–746, 2014b 24343998

Ayers CR, Saxena S, Espejo E, et al: Novel treatment for geriatric hoarding disorder: an open trial of cognitive rehabilitation paired with behavior therapy. Am J Geriatr Psychiatry 22(3):248–252, 2014c 23831173

Ayers CR, Najmi S, Mayes TL, Dozier ME: Hoarding disorder in older adulthood. Am J Geriatr Psychiatry 23(4):416–422, 2015 24953872

Bratiotis C, Woody S: Community interventions for hoarding, in The Oxford Handbook of Hoarding and Acquiring. Edited by Frost RO, Steketee G. Oxford, UK, Oxford University Press, 2014, pp 316–328

Burgess AM, Graves LM, Frost RO: My possessions need me: anthropomorphism and hoarding. Scand J Psychol 59(3):340–348, 2018 29608213

Cath DC, Nizar K, Boomsma D, Mathews CA: Age-specific prevalence of hoarding and obsessive compulsive disorder: a population-based study. Am J Geriatr Psychiatry 25(3):245–255, 2017 27939851

Clark AN, Mankikar GD, Gray I: Diogenes syndrome: a clinical study of gross neglect in old age. Lancet 1(7903):366–368, 1975 46514

Diefenbach GJ, DiMauro J, Frost R, et al: Characteristics of hoarding in older adults. Am J Geriatr Psychiatry 21(10):1043–1047, 2013 23567383

Dong X, Simon M: Prevalence of elder self-neglect in a Chicago Chinese population: the role of cognitive physical and mental health. Geriatr Gerontol Int 16(9):1051–1062, 2016 26337031

Dong X, Simon MA, Evans DA: Prevalence of self-neglect across gender, race, and socioeconomic status: findings from the Chicago Health and Aging Project. Gerontology 58(3):258–268, 2012 22189358

Dozier ME, Porter B, Ayers CR: Age of onset and progression of hoarding symptoms in older adults with hoarding disorder. Aging Ment Health 20(7):736–742, 2016a 25909628

Dozier ME, Wetherell JL, Twamley EW, et al: The relationship between age and neurocognitive and daily functioning in adults with hoarding disorder. Int J Geriatr Psychiatry 31(12):1329–1336, 2016b 26876803

Eckfield MB, Wallhagen MI: The synergistic effect of growing older with hoarding behaviors. Clin Nurs Res 22(4):475–491, 2013 23960251

Frost RO, Steketee G: Stuff: Compulsive Hoarding and the Meaning of Things. Boston, MA, Houghton Mifflin Harcourt, 2010

Frost RO, Kim HJ, Morris C, et al: Hoarding, compulsive buying and reasons for saving. Behav Res Ther 36(7–8):657–664, 1998 9682522

Frost RO, Steketee G, Williams L: Hoarding: a community health problem. Health Soc Care Community 8(4):229–234, 2000 11560692

Frost RO, Steketee G, Tolin DF: Comorbidity in hoarding disorder. Depress Anxiety 28(10):876–884, 2011 21770000

Fullana MA, Vilagut G, Rojas-Farreras S, et al; ESEMeD/MHEDEA 2000 investigators: Obsessive-compulsive symptom dimensions in the general population: results from an epidemiological study in six European countries. J Affect Disord 124(3):291–299, 2010 20022382

Grisham JR, Frost RO, Steketee G, et al: Age of onset of compulsive hoarding. J Anxiety Disord 20(5):675–686, 2006 16112837

Hei A, Dong X: Association between neighborhood cohesion and self-neglect in Chinese-American older adults. J Am Geriatr Soc 65(12):2720–2726, 2017 29044477

Kessler RC, McGonagle KA, Zhao S, et al: Lifetime and 12-month prevalence of DSM-III-R psychiatric disorders in the United States: results from the National Comorbidity Survey. Arch Gen Psychiatry 51(1):8–19, 1994 8279933

Kim HJ, Steketee G, Frost RO: Hoarding by elderly people. Health Soc Work 26(3):176–184, 2001 11531193

Lucini G, Monk I, Szlatenyi C: An analysis of fire incidents involving hoarding households. Report to Worcester Polytechnic Institute. Worcester, MA, 2009

Mackin RS, Areán PA, Delucchi KL, Mathews CA: Cognitive functioning in individuals with severe compulsive hoarding behaviors and late life depression. Int J Geriatr Psychiatry 26(3):314–321, 2011 21319334

Marcos M, Gómez-Pellín M de la Cruz: A tale of a misnamed eponym: Diogenes syndrome. Int J Geriatr Psychiatry 23(9):990–991, 2008 18752218

Marx MS, Cohen-Mansfield J: Hoarding behavior in the elderly: a comparison between community-dwelling persons and nursing home residents. Int Psychogeriatr 15(3):289–306, 2003 14756164

McGuire J, Kaercher L, Park J, Storch E: Hoarding in the community: a code enforcement and social service perspective. J Soc Serv Res 39:335–344, 2013

Mohlman J: Does executive dysfunction affect treatment outcome in late-life mood and anxiety disorders? J Geriatr Psychiatry Neurol 18(2):97–108, 2005 15911938

Mueller A, Mitchell JE, Crosby RD, et al: The prevalence of compulsive hoarding and its association with compulsive buying in a German population-based sample. Behav Res Ther 47(8):705–709, 2009 19457476

National Heart, Lung and Blood Institute and National Institute of Diabetes and Digestive and Kidney Diseases: Clinical Guidelines on the Identification, Evaluation, and Treatment of Overweight and Obesity in Adults: The Evidence Report. Bethesda, MD, National Institutes of Health, National Heart, Lung and Blood Institute, 1998

Ong C, Pang S, Sagayadevan V, et al: Functioning and quality of life in hoarding: a systematic review. J Anxiety Disord 32:17–30, 2015 25847547

Proctor EK, Morrow-Howell NL, Dore P, et al: Comorbid medical conditions among depressed elderly patients discharged home after acute psychiatric care. Am J Geriatr Psychiatry 11(3):329–338, 2003 12724112

Rasmussen JL, Steketee G, Frost RO, et al: Assessing squalor in hoarding: the Home Environment Index. Community Ment Health J 50(5):591–596, 2014 24292497

Reid JM, Arnold E, Rosen S, et al: Hoarding behaviors among nonclinical elderly adults: correlations with hoarding cognitions, obsessive-compulsive symptoms, and measures of general psychopathology. J Anxiety Disord 25(8):1116–1122, 2011 21889875

Richardson TM, Simning A, He H, Conwell Y: Anxiety and its correlates among older adults accessing aging services. Int J Geriatr Psychiatry 26(1):31–38, 2011 20066684

Samuels JF, Bienvenu OJ, Grados MA, et al: Prevalence and correlates of hoarding behavior in a community-based sample. Behav Res Ther 46(7):836–844, 2008 18495084

Schappert SM, Rechtsteiner EA: Ambulatory medical care utilization estimates for 2006. Natl Health Stat Report (8):1–29, 2008 18958997

Snowdon J, Shah A, Halliday G: Severe domestic squalor: a review. Int Psychogeriatr 19(1):37–51, 2007 16973099

Steketee G, Frost RO: Compulsive Hoarding and Acquiring. New York, Oxford University Press, 2007

Steketee G, Schmalisch C, Dierberger A, et al: Symptoms and history of hoarding in older adults. J Obsessive Compuls Relat Disord 1:1–7, 2012

Timpano KR, Schmidt NB, Wheaton MG, et al: Consideration of the BDNF gene in relation to two phenotypes: hoarding and obesity. J Abnorm Psychol 120(3):700–707, 2011 21668081

Tolin DF, Frost RO, Steketee G, et al: The economic and social burden of compulsive hoarding. Psychiatry Res 160(2):200–211, 2008 18597855

Tolin DF, Meunier SA, Frost RO, Steketee G: Course of compulsive hoarding and its relationship to life events. Depress Anxiety 27(9):829–838, 2010 20336803

Turner K, Steketee G, Nauth L: Treating elders with compulsive hoarding: a pilot program. Cognit Behav Pract 17:449–457, 2010

Vickers BD, Preston SD: The economics of hoarding, in The Oxford Handbook of Hoarding and Acquiring. Edited by Frost RO, Steketee G. Oxford, UK, Oxford University Press, 2014, pp 221–232

Wetherell JL, Ayers CR, Nuevo R, et al: Medical conditions and depressive, anxiety, and somatic symptoms in older adults with and without generalized anxiety disorder. Aging Ment Health 14(6):764–768, 2010 20635235

Zaboski BA II, Merritt OA, Schrack AP, et al: Hoarding: a meta-analysis of age of onset. Depress Anxiety 36(6):552–564, 2019 30958911

CHAPTER 12
Animal Hoarding

From our review of the phenomenology and etiology of hoarding so far, it is clear that the disorder is complex and multifaceted. Despite some effort (Meyer et al. 2013), there has been very little evidence that subtypes of hoarding exist, with one exception. There are clear indications that animal hoarding forms a distinct but related subtype of hoarding disorder (Frost et al. 2011). In this chapter, we describe existing research on the phenomenology of animal hoarding, summarize current theorizing about its etiology, and address what exists with respect to interventions. At the same time, research on this topic is hobbled by difficulties in soliciting research participants. Most animal hoarding cases are only discovered when the individual is in legal trouble for abuse or neglect of animals. The accompanying media coverage and legal proceedings deter participation in research projects. All but a few animal hoarding studies consist of reviews of existing court or agency records rather than direct interviews or observations of individual sufferers. Nevertheless, a picture of the phenomena is emerging.

In 1997 a small group of individuals began collaborating on a plan to develop a clearer understanding of and approach to people who hoard animals. The Hoarding of Animals Research Consortium (HARC) included a sociologist, a psychologist, a psychiatrist, several social workers, a veterinarian, and an animal welfare law enforcement specialist. HARC developed a definition of animal hoarding that included four features in addition to the larger-than-normal number of companion animals (Patronek et al. 2006):

1. Failure to provide minimal standards of sanitation, space, nutrition, and veterinary care for the animals
2. Inability to recognize the effects of this failure on the welfare of the animals, human members of the household, and the environment
3. Obsessive attempts to accumulate or maintain a collection of animals in the face of progressively deteriorating conditions
4. Denial or minimization of problems and living conditions for people and animals

DSM-5 and Animal Hoarding

While animal hoarding is not an official subtype of hoarding disorder, the text accompanying the diagnostic criteria contains a description of it. Borrowing from the HARC definition, DSM-5 describes animal hoarding as "the accumulation of a large number of animals and a failure to provide minimal standards of nutrition, sanitation, and veterinary care as well as failure to act on the deteriorating condition of the animals (including disease, starvation, or death) and the environment (e.g., severe overcrowding, extremely unsanitary conditions). Animal hoarding may be a special manifestation of hoarding disorder" (American Psychiatric Association 2013, p. 249).

The DSM-5 diagnostic criteria for hoarding disorder do not specify the types of possessions necessary to qualify for a diagnosis. Since animals are considered property, animal hoarding would appear to qualify for a hoarding disorder diagnosis. Descriptive accounts of animal hoarding appear to fit as well. People who hoard animals display great reluctance to let them go— even to shelters or veterinary clinics that would provide them with better care. Furthermore, the carcasses of dead animals often litter the floors of affected homes. The individuals' attachments to animals are extreme and rigid, sometimes appearing to reflect delusional thinking, particularly with regard to the perceived need to "save" the animals. The urges to save—and the distress experienced when animals are taken away—are extreme. The results of these symptoms are that active living areas inside the homes of people who hoard animals are cluttered with animals and assorted possessions, are extremely disorganized, and cannot be used for their intended purposes. Finally, animal hoarding cases clearly cause significant impairment in social, occupational, and other important areas of functioning. Particularly acute is the absence of a safe and healthy environment for the animals as well as the people living in the home. Based on these similarities, animal hoarding appears to meet all four of the inclusion criteria for hoarding disorder.

Hoarding disorder diagnoses are not made if the symptoms can be attributed to another mental disorder. Hoarding behavior is sometimes due to schizophrenia, dementia, or obsessive-compulsive disorder (OCD), along with a few other disorders (American Psychiatric Association 2013). Animal hoarding may be attributable to other severe mental illnesses as well, though no empirical evidence exists to test this hypothesis. However, Patronek (1999) found that over one-quarter of animal hoarding case files described resolutions that involved institutional care or guardianship, suggesting problems in addition to the hoarding of animals. A variety of other psychiatric diagnoses have been suggested to account for or contribute to animal hoarding including dementia, substance abuse, delusional disorder, social anxiety, and obsessive-compulsive disorder, among others. Mental health problems are frequent in this population (Patronek 1999). Snowdon et al. (2020) found that mental health problems were judged to be significant contributors to the issue in more than half of the animal hoarding cases reported on. In describing her 9 years of clinical work with animal hoarding cases, Nathanson (2009) suggested that the most frequently observed mental disorders are addiction, anxiety, dissociative disorder, complicated grief, and some form of attachment disorder. Others have similarly suggested themes of anxiety, grief, and attachment problems (Patronek and Nathanson 2009; Steketee et al. 2011). As of this writing, there are no other disorders that have been clearly tied to the development of animal hoarding, nor have there been any medical conditions tied to animal hoarding.

DSM-5 specifiers for hoarding disorder are also relevant for animal hoarding cases. Excessive acquisition is present in the majority of both forms of hoarding. Consistent findings indicate that over 90% of individuals who hoard objects acquire actively rather than passively. The frequency of active versus passive acquisition in animal hoarding may be more evenly balanced. Many of the animals in animal hoarding cases derive from a passive failure to spay or neuter animals, resulting in excessive breeding (Patronek 1999; Worth and Beck 1981). More active acquisitions of animals involve responding to advertising for animals or adopting from animal shelters or the internet. Some accumulate animals because they become known in the community as someone who will take in unwanted pets if they are dropped off nearby. More active acquisition appears to be characteristic of those animal hoarding cases in which the motivation is to rescue animals (Patronek et al. 2006)

Poor insight appears to be present in a small percentage of object hoarding cases (Mataix-Cols et al. 2013). However, poor insight has been widely reported in animal hoarding cases. Frost et al. (2000) found that among individuals reported to health departments for health code violations, a smaller percentage of people who hoarded animals willingly cooperated with authorities (6%) compared with people who hoarded only possessions (43%). In their sample, over 50% of the individuals in animal hoarding cases refused to cooperate, and an additional 40% only reluctantly cooperated. Ferreira et al. (2017) reported that only 27% of the people who hoarded animals in their study recognized difficulties due to their hoarding. Other studies have observed low insight in animal hoarding cases as well (Campos-Lima et al. 2015; Dozier et al. 2019). However, most individuals who hoard animals appear to see themselves as caregivers who have the best interest of the animals at heart, which suggests that the behaviors are ego-syntonic (Patronek and Nathanson 2009).

The stark contrast between others' perceptions of the home and hoarding and individuals' insistence that nothing is wrong and that the animals are happy and well cared for—when there are clearly sick, dying, and dead animals in the home, with significant levels of feces and urine throughout—has led to speculation that animal hoarding may be a form of delusional disorder (HARC 2000; Lockwood 2018). Some evidence suggests possible dissociation in animal hoarding. Brown and Katcher (1997, 2001) found significant associations between levels of pet attachment and dissociation. People with high levels of pet attachment were three times more likely to display clinical levels of dissociation. These findings suggest that dissociation could be a prominent feature of animal hoarding.

Ferreira et al. (2017) have suggested more formal diagnostic criteria—gauged to match DSM-5 criteria for hoarding disorder, but more detailed and specifically tied to the suffering of animals and difficulty donating them. Proposed inclusion criteria include hoarding of many animals (number not specified), failure to care for them, suffering of animals along with refusal to donate any of them, interference with normal activities of daily living, impaired social functioning, and impaired executive functioning. These criteria have yet to be examined further.

Associated Features

While object hoarding is closely tied to the volume of possessions that clutter the living areas of the home, animal hoarding is more complex. Individuals who hoard animals have more than the typical number of companion animals, but how the animals are cared for defines the problem to a greater extent than does the number of animals kept. A relatively small number of animals, if uncared for, can create uninhabitable living conditions more extreme than in most cases of object hoarding. Consequently, animal hoarding poses more of a public health threat than object hoarding. Not only is the individual's health and well-being impaired, but the health and well-being of the animals are compromised, and there are serious consequences for the community as well. The financial burden of resolving animal hoarding cases can be enormous. Community agencies are usually faced with the costs associated with removal of the animals and their care (HARC 2002; Ockenden et al. 2014; Saldarriaga-Cantillo and Rivas Nieto 2015). In some cases that also include criminal proceedings, the animals become evidence that must be maintained throughout the legal proceedings (Lockwood 2018), the costs of which can be enormous.

Many people who hoard animals hoard inanimate objects as well. When all case reports of animal hoarding are considered, it appears that approximately 50% of individuals who hoard animals also hoard inanimate objects (range 31%–100%) (Calvo et al. 2014; Cunha et al. 2017; Elliott et al. 2019; Ferreira et al. 2017; HARC 2000, 2002; Ockenden et al. 2014; Patronek 1999). In addition, Ramos et al. (2013) found that individuals who owned more than 20 cats and were potentially in the early stages of animal hoarding scored higher on the Saving Inventory—Revised than individuals who owned just one or two. The types of possessions found in animal hoarding homes resemble those of object hoarding homes (e.g., newspapers, books, clothing, containers) (HARC 2002). Whether the motives for saving these items are the same as those seen in cases of object hoarding only is not clear. Mixed among these items is animal waste as well as rotting food and garbage, which is seen in only a minority of object hoarding cases.

As in severe cases of object hoarding, activities of daily living are compromised in the majority of animal hoarding cases—especially the ability to prepare food, sit at a table, use sinks, and maintain even basic personal hygiene. These activities are more impaired if the individual lives alone than if there is someone else living there (HARC 2002). In addition, essential utilities and appliances—such as water, laundry facilities, and even toilets—are not functional in many such homes. In a review of health department complaints related to hoarding behaviors, the homes that included animal hoarding were rated as significantly less sanitary, posing significantly greater risk to public health, causing more difficulties for the agency, and tending to involve more agencies than the homes of people who only hoarded objects (Frost et al. 2000). Extreme squalor and lack of sanitation characterize nearly 100% of animal hoarding cases, yet they characterize only a small percentage of object hoarding cases (Frost et al. 2000, 2011). In more severe cases, animal feces and urine—sometimes several inches deep—cover the floors and walls. Houses may be condemned and demolished because of the damage done by these conditions. High levels of animal feces and urine in the home generate toxic levels of ammonia harmful to both animals and humans, as well as intensify the spread of zoonotic diseases (Castrodale et al. 2010; Strong et al. 2019).

The number of animals in reported cases varies widely. In the HARC (2002) study of 71 animal hoarding cases, the number of animals ranged from 10 to 918. The average animal census in hoarding cases ranges from 30 to 60. The condition of the animals in most studies of animal hoarding is poor—with many of them malnourished, obviously injured, and/or diseased (e.g., respiratory infections, dermatological disease). In many cases, dead animals litter the floors (Jacobson et al. 2020; Patronek 1999).

In the U.S., the most commonly hoarded animals are cats, followed by dogs, birds, and small mammals (Lockwood 2018), although among males and individuals prosecuted for animal abuse, dogs may be more frequently hoarded than cats (Berry et al. 2005; Worth and Beck 1981). Occasional cases of wild or large farm animals have been reported. No clear data on the prevalence of animal hoarding exist. However, extrapolation from case reports from humane societies and health and animal control agencies suggests more than 5,000 reported cases per year in the United States (Lockwood 2018). Recently collected data on animal abuse suggest that there was a substantial increase in the prevalence of animal hoarding cases from 2009 to 2011 (Ramos et al. 2013). This increase in prevalence might be attributable to better record keeping, however.

Culture

Animal hoarding is not just a U.S. phenomenon. Cases have been reported throughout the world, with only slight differences in expression. For instance, in Spain and Brazil, dogs are more frequently hoarded than cats, which might be explained by the larger ratio of dog to cat ownership in those countries compared with the United States (Cunha et al. 2017). Little information is available on socioeconomic status. However, HARC (2002) reported that over half of the individuals in their animal hoarding sample were unemployed, though many of those who were employed held white-collar or professional positions. Similarly, Patronek (1999) reported that 72% of those for whom such data were available were on disability, retired, or unemployed.

Demographics and Course

Although epidemiological studies are lacking, most studies reporting on larger sample sizes indicate that 70%–85% of people who hoard animals are female (Ferreira et al. 2017; HARC 2002; Patronek 1999; Worth and Beck 1981). Among individuals who hoard animals, there is some indication that women have more animals than do men (HARC 2002; Reinisch 2009). Most are single, divorced, or widowed (Ferreira et al. 2017; HARC 2002; Patronek 1999). This is consistent with most accounts of animal hoarding cases—where individuals are described as socially isolated and frequently estranged from family and friends (Patronek and Nathanson 2009). However, those whose motivation is mission-driven (see the following section) appear to be networked with enablers who facilitate acquisition (Patronek and Nathanson 2009). The median age of individuals in identified animal hoarding cases is mid-50s to 60s (HARC 2002). The usual age at onset of animal hoarding problems is unknown, but relatively few cases among individuals younger than 30 can be found in the literature. Animal hoarding problems are typically diagnosed in middle or older age (Frost et al. 2011). Ferreira et al. (2017) reported an average duration of animal hoarding to be greater than 20 years. Some reports indicate a greater prevalence of animal hoarding among the poor and less educated (Ferreira et al. 2017). Like object hoarding, animal hoarding appears to be chronic, with high recidivism following removal of the animals by authorities (Frost et al. 2011; Strong et al. 2019).

Animal Hoarding Subtypes

On the basis of the experiences of animal control officers in trying to resolve animal hoarding cases, Patronek and HARC have hypothesized that there are three types of animal hoarding cases: "overwhelmed caregiver," "rescuer," and "exploiter." These are based largely on the nature of the attachments to animals and flexibility of thinking about their care (Patronek et al. 2006). Overwhelmed caregivers represent the least severe and easiest type of animal hoarding cases to deal with. They are characterized by some degree of awareness of problems with the care they are providing to their animals. Before the onset of the hoarding, they appear to have adequate resources and capacity for caring for large numbers of animals. A change in circumstances precipitates a gradual decline in resources and capacity. The precipitating change is typically the death of a spouse, loss of income, illness, or a disability status. Once their resources are stretched, there is a slow decline in the condition of the home and animals. Eventually, they become overwhelmed and unable to provide adequate care. Individuals who fall into this category tend to be shy and socially isolated, which results in poor connections to available sources of help. They are less secretive than individuals with other animal hoarding subtypes and less resistant to the intervention of authorities—usually allowing access to their home and accepting help with improving conditions and releasing custody of animals. They are less likely to actively seek out animals to acquire. They display an intense, lifelong attachment to animals, and their caretaking role is part of their sense of self and self-worth.

Rescuers are individuals who believe it is their mission to rescue and care for animals that would otherwise suffer or die. They actively acquire animals, sometimes stealing them from legitimate owners. Although they may begin with adequate resources, the rapidly growing number of animals overwhelms them. They resist attempts by authorities to intervene and often avoid contact with animal care professionals, believing that they are the only one who can provide adequate care. Their beliefs in this regard can appear delusional, with insistence that starving, sick, and dying animals in their care are adequately cared for. Many believe themselves to have special abilities to communicate with animals in ways that other people don't. Such beliefs lead them to resist releasing animals to others for proper veterinary care. Rescuers often have extensive networks of people who enable their hoarding.

More serious is the exploiter. However, this subtype may not be a form of hoarding at all; rather, it may be a form of sociopathy or antisocial personality disorder. For these individuals, animals appear to serve their need for control. They appear to lack empathy for animals or people and are indifferent to harm they may cause. They also appear somewhat delusional in denying the extreme condition of their home or animals. They strongly reject any intervention from legitimate authorities and—like the rescuers—believe their knowledge far exceeds that of legitimate animal care professionals. Consistent with antisocial personality disorder, many exploiters are articulate, charismatic, and capable of presenting themselves in a way that conveys competence. They are manipulative and highly narcissistic but lack any sense of guilt or remorse for their suffering animals. Their lack of any emotional attachment to their animals sets them apart from the other forms of animal hoarding and suggests that they might be better characterized as suffering from antisocial personality disorder.

Snowdon et al. (2020) added two other categories: "breeders" and "incipient." Among 50 cases identified as animal hoarding, they judged 11 to involve rescuers, 12 overwhelmed caregivers, 5 exploiters, and 15 breeders, with 7 representing incipient or subclinical hoarding. Four of the incipient cases were judged to involve rescuers or overwhelmed caregivers. Whether the breeders' behavior would qualify for diagnosis of hoarding disorder is unclear, since their motivation appears to be financial rather than attachment-based. This is the only existing study that has attempted to determine the frequency of the different types of animal hoarding.

Etiology

Despite the lack of rigorous research on animal hoarding, some useful hypotheses have been developed about its etiology. Patronek and Nathanson (2009) speculate about the possible origins of the problem, based on their observations from over 20 years of experience working on these cases. They propose a three-part model for the development of animal hoarding. First, the development of consistent attachments early in life typically did not occur, because of dysfunctional or abusive parenting. As a result, the individual did not develop adequate adult functioning, and subsequently—without adequate human attachments and coping skills—comes to rely on animals for emotional comfort. Frost and Steketee (2010) describe an animal hoarding case that fits this model precisely. The woman endured significant abuse from a sadistic governess as a child and neglect from her parents. She described her parents as "not malicious, just neglectful." She said that she and her brother "were like seeds tossed over the fence' and expected to grow" (p. 120). She went on to reflect about her upbringing and her relationship to animals:

> Because I never got any love, any touching, feeling, love that you need to get—somebody once said, "You never bonded with your mother." Well, my mother was not a bad person; she was charming and nice. My friends loved her, but she was in la-la land. So with the animals, you always knew where you were with them, and they were pure love, all of them. And if they didn't like something you did, they told you right away, and they didn't hold any grudge, and they were just love. But I didn't understand that's what it was; I was just drawn to it. (p. 124)

There is some growing evidence to support this framework. In the most direct test of hypotheses related to this model, Steketee et al. (2011) found that individuals with documented animal hoarding reported more chaotic homelives during childhood, more negative family relationships during childhood, and more attachment problems with family members than did multiple pet owners who did not show hoarding tendencies. They also tended to experience more stressful life events during childhood.

The hypothesis that pets may provide security to children subjected to neglect, abuse, and trauma is not new, nor is the suggestion that in these circumstances pets can become a substitute for human relationships (Rynearson 1978). The extreme isolation seen in descriptions of animal hoarding cases (e.g., Frost et al. 2000; Steketee et al. 2011) is consistent with the difficulties in adult relationships that are also often described in animal hoarding cases. Adult functioning among animal hoarding individuals was significantly worse than for controls in the Steketee et al. (2011) study. Also revealed in the Steketee et al. (2011) study was the finding that animal hoarding individuals have significantly greater distrust of authorities.

The combination of their delusional-level beliefs in their ability to care for animals, social isolation, distrust of authorities, and dysfunctional attachment history makes it unlikely that these individuals would receive or benefit from feedback from others about their animal care capabilities.

In two studies, Brown and Katcher (1997, 2001) found high levels of dissociation to be correlated with pet attachment. Among the participants with the highest levels of pet attachment, a significantly greater percentage had clinical levels of dissociation than among those with lower levels of pet attachment. Brown (2011) argued that individuals who hoard animals may use dissociation to blunt the effects of trauma, which may explain the poor insight often seen in animal hoarding, such as the inability to recognize the poor condition of the animals.

Many people who hoard animals articulate beliefs about animals that may contribute to the development of this behavior. Some express what appears to observers to be a messianic urge to rescue or save all animals (Lockwood and Cassidy 1988; Worth and Beck 1981). A few researchers have suggested that this belief and the accompanying behaviors are attempts to repair their sense of self and to create a suitable identity (Brown 2011; Patronek and Nathanson 2009). Strong beliefs such as these lead sufferers to sometimes collect animals that belong to others and are already well cared for (Frost and Steketee 2010). Along with this belief is often a belief that the sufferers possess special abilities to empathize with, communicate with, and care for animals (Slyne et al. 2013). This is sometimes associated with a belief that they have special or psychic powers to discern when animals need help (Frost and Steketee 2010).

An intriguing line of research suggests a parasitic infection as a possible etiological conduit for animal hoarding. *Toxoplasma gondii* is a parasite that infects large numbers of warm-blooded animals, especially cats. Oocytes and parasitic material from infected animals are shed through feces and spread to other organisms. Toxoplasmosis cysts rapidly proliferate in infected organisms and produce changes in the brain—notably rapid increases in dopamine production—which are believed to trigger behavior changes in these newly infected organisms. For instance, infected rodents appear to lose their fear of—and, in fact, increase their preference for—the odor of cat urine. *T. gondii* infection is not uncommon in humans, with seroprevalence rates in the United States and United Kingdom ranging from 11% to 22% (Centers for Disease Control and Prevention 2020; Flegr 2007). Some evidence suggests that infected humans show behavior changes similar to those of mice. Flegr and colleagues (Flegr 2013; Flegr et al. 2011) found that male students who were seropositive for *T. gondii* rated the odor of diluted cat urine as more pleasant than did noninfected students, though the effect was not observed among female students. In homes with a large number of poorly cared for cats, the density of fecal material increases *T. gondii* infection (Cunha et al. 2019) and makes transmission to humans more likely. Olfactory perception changes that might result could explain the emotional bond and absence of disgust at unsanitary conditions observed among individuals who hoard animals. Brain changes produced by *T. gondii* have been linked to other mental disorders, including obsessive-compulsive disorder (Nayeri Chegeni et al. 2019). In addition, personality changes have been observed in seropositive humans (Flegr 2010; Flegr et al. 1996), including reduced novelty-seeking and increased impulsivity, both of which have been associated with hoarding individuals (Fullana et al. 2004; Grisham et al. 2007).

Interventions for Animal Hoarding

The outcomes of interventions for animal hoarding are typically worse than those in cases that involve the hoarding of objects only (Frost et al. 2000). Legal issues involving object hoarding consist of mostly code violations and are treated as misdemeanors. Although they may result in eviction, they seldom result in criminal prosecution. Animal hoarding, on the other hand, often leads to criminal prosecution for animal abuse, which is the most common form of intervention. Every state has criminal codes for animal abuse or neglect (Lockwood 2018). However, there are difficulties applying these laws to animal hoarding cases. Neglect is typically considered an act of omission—such as failure to provide adequate care due to ignorance, poverty, family crises, or similar situations. Penalties for neglect often do not deter hoarding behavior, particularly in cases involving lack of insight. Furthermore, such cases typically do not involve long-term monitoring or provision for mental health counseling. For this reason, many animal hoarding cases are tried under animal abuse or cruelty laws. Abuse is a potential felony carrying the possibility of severe punishment and/or incarceration. However, conviction requires proof of intent to harm or knowingly neglectful behavior. Proving intent in animal hoarding cases is difficult, given the frequent lack of insight, intense emotional attachments, and distorted beliefs about the ability to care for animals. Such cases are also complex and costly. Frequently, the animals themselves must be treated as evidence, and this means they must be cared for by heavily overloaded local shelters for the length of the trial. Costs for the care must be borne by the local community unless bonding laws permit charging the defendant for the care. Even in situations where the legal cases are resolved quickly, considerable time and effort are required to return the animals to a healthy state, if they survive at all (Jacobson et al. 2020). Finally, while these procedures may succeed in removing the animals, they do nothing to change the behavior of the individual. In a review of long-term outcomes in animal hoarding prosecutions, over 40% of individuals were sentenced to jail time, though most sentences were less than 6 months, and recidivism rates were near 100% (Berry et al. 2005).

Several states have attempted to draft laws specifically targeting animal hoarding. Illinois passed the Humane Care for Animals Act in 2001. It defined animal hoarding as one form of animal neglect that is specific to companion animals. According to the statute, animal neglect is a Class B misdemeanor, and subsequent violations are considered felonies. Other states, including Hawaii and Rhode Island, have attempted to criminalize animal hoarding but have run into heavy criticism for criminalizing behavior attributable to a mental health disorder (Lockwood 2018).

The outcome of a court proceeding may differ depending on the nature of the motivation behind the hoarding behavior. For overwhelmed caregivers, who are less likely to resist intervention and more likely to accept assistance as well as ongoing monitoring, a court-ordered resolution may be more successful. For the mission-driven (rescuer) or exploiter cases, removal of the animals does little to change the person's behavior, and future hoarding is likely. Most cases are negotiated out in order to gain custody of the animals, with little or no punishment (or rehabilitation) for the offenders. Long-term monitoring and counseling are sometimes ordered, but seldom is there any follow-up.

The court-based approaches to animal hoarding have been fragmented at best and have not been successful at limiting recidivism (Patronek et al. 2006). Several investigators have proposed changes to the way animal hoarding cases are handled. Muller-Harris (2011) proposed the creation of a special type of court to handle animal cruelty and hoarding cases. The court would focus on three objectives: caring for and protecting the animal victims, rehabilitating the offenders, and instituting long-term monitoring to ensure compliance. It remains to be seen if such a court will be helpful.

Patronek et al. (2006) proposed a "layered process," whereby efforts to curb animal hoarding would focus on stages of prevention. Primary prevention could begin with early signs of animal hoarding identified by veterinarians or personnel from animal shelters or rescue organizations. This would require an understanding of what we know or suspect about the development of hoarding, including experiences of childhood trauma, neglect, and attachment problems. Also, providing appropriate social contacts with animal care personnel might steer vulnerable individuals away from people or organizations that may "indulge or enable their preoccupation with animals" (Patronek et al. 2006). Secondary prevention could be instituted in acute cases to prevent the hoarding from becoming chronic or recurrent. Such approaches may depend on early identification of animal hoarding tendencies. Some evidence suggests that high animal ownership (e.g., more than 10 cats) is associated with decrements in the quality of life for the owner with respect to finances, job performance, social life, and sanitation (Slyne et al. 2013). High animal ownership also seems to be associated with exaggerated beliefs about being the only person who can adequately care for the animals (Slyne et al. 2013). Such beliefs may be precursors to the development of full-blown animal hoarding and could be interrupted by appropriate intervention. Tertiary prevention could be designed to prevent chronic cases from becoming more severe. Given the failures to prevent this with current approaches, the exact nature of this intervention has yet to be developed.

Recognition of animal hoarding as a form of hoarding disorder has raised awareness of the need for effective mental health interventions for the problem. Unfortunately, no such interventions have been developed or tested. However, several key principles can be derived from the existing literature. First, initial evaluation must include a home assessment. Even following removal of the animals, the physical condition of the home may be compromised (e.g., broken appliances, excessive clutter, sanitation problems). This must be incorporated into the treatment plan. Second, the forceful removal of animals will have been a traumatic experience for the hoarding client. The resulting grief will need to be addressed. Third, the anger and resentment toward authorities and resistance to counseling—especially if the counseling is ordered by the court—will have to be addressed first. Expertise in motivational interviewing will be an important component in dealing with this issue. Fourth, significant attachment-based problems in animal hoarding clients are likely, and the development of a good working relationship is crucial. People who hoard animals attach special significance to their ownership of animals. Their animals form much of their identity and sense of self (Patronek and Nathanson 2009). They also appear to be the most important emotional attachment figures in the individuals' lives. This phenomenon is magnified by the social isolation that characterizes most individuals who hoard animals. Therapy focusing on decreasing social isolation, expanding the basis for self-identity, and gaining more human attachments will likely pay the most dividends.

Conclusion

It appears that animal hoarding cases generally meet diagnostic criteria for hoarding disorder. Those who hoard animals display persistent difficulty letting go of animals—even those that are sick, dying, or sometimes already dead. The difficulty is due to the perceived need to save the animals or intense distress at letting them go. The accumulation of animals (and possessions) congests and clutters the living areas of the home, making them difficult or impossible to use for their intended purposes. The behavior causes extreme distress or impairments that are more extreme than those seen in object hoarding cases. In addition, there are no known medical or mental disorders that have been identified in reported cases that can account for the behavior.

Yet clear differences in symptomatology between typical object hoarding and animal hoarding exist, suggesting animal hoarding is a special manifestation of the disorder. First, a relatively small number of object hoarding cases involve squalid or extremely unsanitary homes (Rasmussen et al. 2014). In animal hoarding cases, however, the overwhelming majority would be considered squalid—with animal feces, urine, and often long-dead animals littering the floor. Undoubtedly this is because inanimate objects do not require any attention, whereas unattended animals can make a home uninhabitable in a short period of time. Second, the overwhelming majority of object hoarding cases involve the saving of a wide variety of objects, whereas animal hoarding cases frequently involve only a single species, although there are cases in which individuals hoard a variety of animal species. Furthermore, the defining feature is less about the number of animals and more about the inability to provide proper care. Third, acquisition may not be as active in animal hoarding, with a lot of animals coming from uncontrolled breeding (Jacobson et al. 2020). Fourth, people who hoard animals are less likely to recognize that there is a problem than those who hoard objects (Frost et al. 2000, 2011). Regardless of the relationship with object hoarding, it is clear that animal hoarding is a mental health problem in need of an understanding of etiology and the development of effective interventions.

KEY CLINICAL POINTS

- Animal hoarding may form a distinct subtype of hoarding disorder.

- People who hoard animals appear to have presentations that meet all of the DSM-5 criteria for hoarding disorder.

- Existing research suggests that those involved in animal hoarding cases are mostly female and between the ages of 50 and 80 years.

- Animal hoarding cases are found around the world, with only slight variations in case characteristics.

- People who hoard animals typically show limited insight regarding the problem.

- The homes of people who hoard animals are more likely to have squalid conditions than the homes of people who hoard objects.

- Researchers hypothesize three types of animal hoarding cases: those involving overwhelmed caregivers, rescuers, and exploiters.

References

American Psychiatric Association: Diagnostic and Statistical Manual of Mental Disorders, 5th Edition. Arlington, VA, American Psychiatric Association, 2013

Berry C, Patronek G, Lockwood R: Long-term outcomes in animal hoarding cases. Animal Law 11(167):167–194, 2005

Brown S: Theoretical concepts from self psychology applied to animal hoarding. Society & Animals 19:175–193, 2011

Brown S-E, Katcher AH: The contribution of attachment to pets and attachment to nature to dissociation and absorption. Dissociation: Progress in the Dissociative Disorders 10(2):125–129, 1997

Brown S-E, Katcher AH: Pet attachment and dissociation. Society & Animals 9(1):25–41, 2001

Calvo P, Duarte C, Bowen J, et al: Characteristics of 24 cases of animal hoarding in Spain. Animal Welfare 23:199–208, 2014

Campos-Lima AL, Torres AR, Yücel M, et al: Hoarding pet animals in obsessive-compulsive disorder. Acta Neuropsychiatr 27(1):8–13, 2015 25359656

Castrodale L, Bellay YM, Brown CM, et al: General public health considerations for responding to animal hoarding cases. J Environ Health 72(7):14–18, quiz 32, 2010 20235404

Centers for Disease Control and Prevention: Parasites—Toxoplasmosis (Toxoplasma infection). 2020. Available at: www.cdc.gov/parasites/toxoplasmosis. Accessed January 27, 2021.

Cunha GR, Martins CM, Ceccon-Valente MF, et al: Frequency and spatial distribution of animal and object hoarder behavior in Curitiba, Paraná State, Brazil. Cad Saude Publica 33(2):e00001316, 2017 28380121

Cunha G, Pellizzaro M, Marinelli Martins C, et al: Serological survey of Leptospira spp. and Toxoplasma gondii in companion animals rescued from hoarding behavior cases in Curitiba. Int J Dev Res 09:30683–30685, 2019

Dozier ME, Bratiotis C, Broadnax D, et al: A description of 17 animal hoarding case files from animal control and a humane society. Psychiatry Res 272:365–368, 2019 30599440

Elliott R, Snowdon J, Halliday G, et al: Characteristics of animal hoarding cases referred to the RSPCA in New South Wales, Australia. Aust Vet J 97(5):149–156, 2019 31025326

Ferreira EA, Paloski LH, Costa DB, et al: Animal hoarding disorder: a new psychopathology? Psychiatry Res 258:221–225, 2017 28843626

Flegr J: Effects of toxoplasma on human behavior. Schizophr Bull 33(3):757–760, 2007 17218612

Flegr J: Influence of latent toxoplasmosis on the phenotype of intermediate hosts. Folia Parasitol 57(2):81–87, 2010 20608469

Flegr J: How and why Toxoplasma makes us crazy. Trends Parasitol 29(4):156–163, 2013 23433494

Flegr J, Zitková S, Kodym P, Frynta D: Induction of changes in human behaviour by the parasitic protozoan Toxoplasma gondii. Parasitology 113 (Pt 1):49–54, 1996 8710414

Flegr J, Lenochová P, Hodný Z, Vondrová M: Fatal attraction phenomenon in humans: cat odour attractiveness increased for toxoplasma-infected men while decreased for infected women. PLoS Negl Trop Dis 5(11):e1389, 2011 22087345

Frost RO, Steketee G: Stuff: Compulsive Hoarding and the Meaning of Things. Boston, MA, Houghton Mifflin Harcourt, 2010

Frost RO, Steketee G, Williams L: Hoarding: a community health problem. Health Soc Care Community 8(4):229–234, 2000 11560692

Frost RO, Patronek G, Rosenfield E: Comparison of object and animal hoarding. Depress Anxiety 28(10):885–891, 2011 21608085

Fullana MA, Mataix-Cols D, Caseras X, et al: High sensitivity to punishment and low impulsivity in obsessive-compulsive patients with hoarding symptoms. Psychiatry Res 129(1):21–27, 2004 15572181

Grisham JR, Brown TA, Savage CR, et al: Neuropsychological impairment associated with compulsive hoarding. Behav Res Ther 45(7):1471–1483, 2007 17341416

HARC: People who hoard animals. Psychiatr Times 17(4):1–6, 2000

HARC: Health implications of animal hoarding. Health Soc Work 27(2):125–136, 2002 12079167

Jacobson LS, Giacinti JA, Robertson J: Medical conditions and outcomes in 371 hoarded cats from 14 sources: a retrospective study (2011-2014). J Feline Med Surg 22(6):484–491, 2020 31188057

Lockwood R: Animal hoarding: the challenge for mental health, law enforcement, and animal welfare professionals. Behav Sci Law 36(6):698–716, 2018 30191593

Lockwood R, Cassidy B: Killing with kindness. Humane Society News 33(3):14–18, 1988

Mataix-Cols D, Billotti D, Fernández de la Cruz L, Nordsletten AE: The London field trial for hoarding disorder. Psychol Med 43(4):837–847, 2013 22883395

Meyer JF, Frost RO, Brown TA, et al: A multitrait-multimethod matrix investigation of hoarding. J Obsessive Compuls Relat Disord 2(3):273–280, 2013 23814700

Muller-Harris DL: Animal violence court: a therapeutic jurisprudence-based problem-solving court for the adjudication of animal cruelty cases involving juvenile offenders and animal hoarders. Animal Law Review (Lewis & Clark Law School) 17:313–336, 2011

Nathanson JN: Animal hoarding: slipping into the darkness of comorbid animal and self-neglect. J Elder Abuse Negl 21(4):307–324, 2009 20183137

Nayeri Chegeni T, Sarvi S, Amouei A, et al: Relationship between toxoplasmosis and obsessive compulsive disorder: a systematic review and meta-analysis. PLoS Negl Trop Dis 13(4):e0007306, 2019 30969961

Ockenden E, De Groef B, Marston L: Animal hoarding in Victoria, Australia: an exploratory study. Anthrozoos 27:33–47, 2014

Patronek GJ: Hoarding of animals: an under-recognized public health problem in a difficult-to-study population. Public Health Rep 114(1):81–87, 1999 9925176

Patronek GJ, Nathanson JN: A theoretical perspective to inform assessment and treatment strategies for animal hoarders. Clin Psychol Rev 29(3):274–281, 2009 19254818

Patronek GJ, Loar L, Nathanson JN: Animal Hoarding: Structuring Interdisciplinary Responses to Help People, Animals and Communities at Risk. Report from 2004 Boston Forum Hosted by Hoarding of Animals Research Consortium (HARC). 2006. Available at: https://vet.tufts.edu/wp-content/uploads/Angell-Report.pdf. Accessed December 15, 2019.

Ramos D, Cruz N, Ellis S, et al: Early stage animal hoarders: are these owners of large numbers of adequately cared for cats? Hum Anim Interact Bull 1:55–69, 2013

Rasmussen JL, Steketee G, Frost RO, et al: Assessing squalor in hoarding: the Home Environment Index. Community Ment Health J 50(5):591–596, 2014 24292497

Reinisch AI: Characteristics of six recent animal hoarding cases in Manitoba. Can Vet J 50(10):1069–1073, 2009 20046607

Rynearson EK: Humans and pets and attachment. Br J Psychiatry 133:550–555, 1978 737392

Saldarriaga-Cantillo A, Rivas Nieto JC: Noah syndrome: a variant of Diogenes syndrome accompanied by animal hoarding practices. J Elder Abuse Negl 27(3):270–275, 2015 25397353

Slyne K, Tolin D, Steketee G, Frost R: Characteristics of animal owners among individuals with object hoarding. J Obsessive Compuls Relat Disord 2:466–471, 2013

Snowdon J, Halliday G, Elliott R, et al: Mental health of animal hoarders: a study of consecutive cases in New South Wales. Aust Health Rev 44(3):480–484, 2020 31693868

Steketee G, Gibson A, Frost RO, et al: Characteristics and antecedents of people who hoard animals: an exploratory comparative interview study. Rev Gen Psychol 15(2):114–124, 2011

Strong S, Federico J, Banks R, Williams C: A collaborative model for managing animal hoarding cases. J Appl Anim Welf Sci 22(3):267–278, 2019 30021473

Worth D, Beck AM: Multiple ownership of animals in New York City. Trans Stud Coll Physicians Phila 3(4):280–300, 1981 7043819

CHAPTER 13
Squalor

Distinguishing the features that are unique to hoarding disorder from those that overlap with other conditions is critical to both diagnosis (Chapter 2) and assessment (Chapter 3). In this chapter, we contrast hoarding disorder with squalor (also known as "severe domestic squalor") (Halliday et al. 2000; Snowdon et al. 2007). A challenge to this task is the lack of research on the relationship between the two. The DSM-5 work group commissioned a review to consider adding a third specifier to the diagnosis of hoarding disorder, relating to "a person's maintenance of cleanliness and hygiene within their domestic environment" (Snowdon et al. 2012, p. 417). Although this specifier was ultimately not added, the commission highlights the need for further study, because the reasons that someone accumulates items may vary from the reasons that someone lives in an unhygienic environment.

Squalor is characterized by an unhygienic environment to the extent that others of similar "culture and background would consider extensive clearing and cleaning to be essential" (Snowdon et al. 2012, p. 417). Squalid homes typically contain piles of soiled clothing and other debris, moldy/rotten food and food containers, urine-soaked floors and furniture, animal feces, insect and rodent infestation, and a suffocating odor. Neglect of personal hygiene usually accompanies the squalid conditions. Reports suggest that at least 1 in 1,000 elderly individuals lives in severe squalor (Snowdon and Halliday 2011). Hoarding disorder and squalor have a constellation of unique and overlapping features. For example, the accumulation of clutter can be seen in both hoarding disorder and squalor but is much less likely in squalor. At the same time, unhygienic conditions resulting from the accumulation of household waste and other rubbish—which are seen in squalor—are sometimes seen in hoarding disorder. In this chapter, we define squalor; describe the overlap between squalor and hoarding; provide case examples; outline squalor assessment tools, interventions, and trajectories of recovery; and highlight areas for future research.

Historical Terminology

Clark et al. (1975) coined the term "Diogenes syndrome" to refer to cases of severe domestic squalor, neglect of personal hygiene, and the hoarding of rubbish. Since then, the term has been used interchangeably to refer to both hoarding disorder and squalor. However, as noted in Chapter 11, the syndrome has been criticized as being poorly named (Cybulska 1998; Wrigley and Cooney 1992), given that Diogenes—a founder of the Greek philosophy of Cynicism, which rejects conventional desires for power, wealth, and fame in favor of virtuous self-sufficiency—did not exhibit the characteristics of extreme self-neglect or hoarding behavior described in the original case series (Clark et al. 1975). Others have noted that the various features of the syndrome do not coexist consistently enough to warrant a syndrome (Fontenelle 2008).

The term used by Clark and colleagues for the hoarding behavior aspect of Diogenes syndrome was "syllogomania," which refers to the hoarding of rubbish and trash (Clark et al. 1975). Syllogomania is reminiscent of the obsessive-compulsive personality disorder diagnostic criterion of the inability to "discard worn-out or worthless objects" (American Psychiatric Association 2013, p. 679). Yet it is unlike the type of difficulty discarding seen in hoarding disorder (see Chapter 2). Clark et al. (1975) suggested that syllogomania may be a distortion of an instinctive desire to collect things and may provide a feeling of security. Both Diogenes syndrome and syllogomania are loosely defined terms for behaviors (e.g., self-neglect and collecting of rubbish/trash, respectively) that are not currently included in DSM-5 diagnostic criteria for hoarding disorder. At the same time, aspects of these behaviors (e.g., neglect of personal hygiene and collecting of rubbish/trash) may be seen in cases of squalor.

Comparison of Phenomenological Features of Hoarding and Squalor

Squalor has phenomenological features that are both distinct from and common to those of hoarding disorder. In the absence of biomarkers or behavioral tests that can distinguish these features, careful attention to several aspects of the clinical phenotype can help in evaluation. Ten such features are described below and outlined in Table 13–1.

Clutter

Clutter and accumulation of objects can be seen in both hoarding disorder and squalor. Just as fever is an indicator of many diverse inflammatory conditions, clutter is a nonspecific finding. Indeed, clutter can be seen in mental disorders, neurological conditions, and physical or perceptual impairments that make it difficult to unclutter or remove unwanted material (e.g., fracture, retinal detachment, vertigo). However, clutter is a key feature of hoarding disorder that is required for hoarding disorder diagnosis, whereas it may not be present in the majority of squalor cases, as described in a study examining 115 referrals of older adults considered to be living in moderate to severe squalor (Snowdon and Halliday 2011). Snowdon and Halliday found that only 34% ($n=39$) of these individuals also had a large degree of clutter, while 66% ($n=76$) had some, little, or no accumulation of objects. Similarly, Lee et al. (2017) reported that 40% of 69 people living in squalor had significant hoarding behaviors. Based on these studies and the DSM-5 diagnostic criteria, squalid conditions in the absence of clutter exclude the diagnosis of hoarding disorder.

Intention for Accumulated Objects

Ascertaining the individual's intention for the accumulation can help inform the differential diagnosis. Purposeless accumulation that is the result of stereotypic or ritualistic behavior stemming from neuropsychiatric disorders is not considered hoarding disorder (Maier 2004; Snowdon et al. 2012). In the case of squalor, clutter may instead be the result of a wide range of conditions—physical, perceptual, or cognitive deficits—that lead to the inability to get rid of waste. In contrast, hoarding disorder involves the intentional and purposeful collection of possessions.

Parting With Objects

As previously described, a key driver of clutter in hoarding disorder is difficulty discarding due to attachment to objects. Individuals with squalor may be ambivalent about parting with possessions, whereas those with hoarding disorder will find parting with possessions difficult. For people with hoarding disorder, difficulty parting with objects is part of the diagnosis and therefore universal.

TABLE 13–1. Phenomenological features of squalor and hoarding disorder

Phenomenological feature	Squalor	Hoarding disorder
Clutter	Clutter is not present in the majority of cases	Clutter is a diagnostic criterion
Intention for accumulation of objects	Often purposeless (e.g., stereotypic or ritualistic behavior, no interest in item itself)	Purposeful (e.g., objects acquired and kept due to their usefulness, emotional value, or aesthetic qualities)
Parting with objects	Ranges from easy to ambivalent to difficult	Difficult; strong attachment to possessions
Condition of the home	Unhygienic, filthy environment	Typically clean—only a small percentage of people with hoarding disorder live in an unhygienic environment
Nature of objects	Wide range—can include rubbish, rotten food	Wide range, but rubbish and rotten food rarely seen
Self-neglect	Often	Seldom
Insight	Often poor to none	Ranges from good to poor
Time of onset and course of illness	May start suddenly in cases of brain injury or start later in life if due to a dementing process	Starts in childhood/ adolescence and increases in each decade
Diagnostic considerations	Physical, perceptual, or cognitive deficits that lead to inability to get rid of waste (e.g., broken arm, dementia, neuropsychiatric conditions other than hoarding disorder, animal hoarding)	Not due to other neuropsychiatric or medical conditions
Functional impairment in work, family, and/or social domains	Yes	Yes

Condition of the Home

The majority of hoarding disorder cases do not involve squalid conditions. Accumulation of objects and clutter, in and of itself, does not necessarily lead to a filthy environment. Research using volunteer participants indicates that only a small percentage of people with hoarding disorder live in unsanitary conditions (Snowdon et al. 2012). However, estimates of squalor in hoarding cases may be influenced by sampling issues. For instance, Woody et al. (2020) examined archival data from hoarding cases in the community and research populations and found that even after accounting for clutter volume, the homes of community-based clients were more likely to have squalor than homes of those who participated in research. Up to half of the community-based clients were judged to have significant squalor, while only 18% of volunteer research participants had significant squalor. Determination of hoarding status in community-based studies seldom involves careful diagnosis; thus, the higher frequency of squalor among community-based clients may have resulted from the tendency to conflate squalor and hoarding among agency personnel. As described in more detail in Chapter 12, nearly all cases involving animal hoarding are characterized by an unhygienic, squalid environment (Frost et al. 2000, 2011a). These unsanitary living conditions are significantly more common in animal hoarding cases than in situations of object hoarding (Frost et al. 2000). In more extreme cases, houses must be demolished as a result of the damage done by animal feces and urine in the home, which generate toxic levels of ammonia (Castrodale et al. 2010; Strong et al. 2019).

Nature of Objects, Self-Neglect, and Insight

Accumulated items in squalor can often include rotting food, whereas in hoarding disorder rotting food is uncommon (Pertusa et al. 2008). Self-neglect and poor insight are typical traits of those living in squalid conditions. Although self-neglect and poor insight are sometimes present in hoarding cases, they occur much less frequently in hoarding disorder than in cases of squalor (Snowdon et al. 2012).

Time of Onset and Course of Symptoms

Obtaining a careful psychiatric history is important to establishing the onset and time course of symptoms. In both hoarding disorder and cases of squalor, subsyndromal symptoms can start in adolescence. Hoarding disorder symptoms begin relatively early and worsen across the life span, with few cases starting after age 40 (Anderson et al. 2005; Dozier et al. 2016). However, the time of onset of symptoms in relation to brain damage can exclude diagnoses. For example, if the first evidence of hoarding symptoms or a sudden exacerbation of existing symptoms occurs after a head trauma, one should consider the possibility that the symptoms are induced by brain damage (Anderson et al. 2005; Cohen et al. 1999; Funayama et al. 2010; Hahm et al. 2001; Mendez and Shapira 2008; Nakaaki et al. 2007; Volle et al. 2002). Similarly, if accumulation of objects and squalor occur in the later years of life in the context of memory loss, functional decline, or self-neglect, one should consider a dementing process as a possible cause (Cipriani et al. 2012; Cooney and Hamid 1995). Individuals with dementia develop a progressive inability to care for themselves, including an inability to assess what is of value, leading to accumulation of trash (Radebaugh et al. 1987; Weiss 2010). Patients with self-neglect are typically diagnosed with dementia within 1–2 years of presentation (MacKnight 2001). Declining personal hygiene is one of the features in frontotemporal dementia (Neary et al. 1998), and self-neglect is one of the four clusters of behavioral symptoms in the frontotemporal behavioral scale (Lebert et al. 1998). In a sample of 30 patients with frontotemporal dementia, the prevalence of self-neglect was 93% ($n=28$), for conditions of squalor it was 93% ($n=28$), and for syllogomania it was 50% ($n=15$) (Lebert 2005). Of note, patients with frontotemporal dementia in this study—in contrast to reports by Clark et al. (1975) of Diogenes syndrome—did not exhibit suspicion, hostile attitude, and distrust (Lebert 2005), further underscoring the heterogeneous etiology of squalor.

Diagnostic Considerations

Physical, perceptual, or cognitive deficits in individuals (e.g., broken arm, dementia, neuropsychiatric conditions other than hoarding disorder, animal hoarding) may render them unable to get rid of waste, subsequently resulting in squalor. A comprehensive psychological evaluation is important to determine if there are other mental illnesses present that may be contributing to the squalid conditions.

The Snowdon et al. (2007) study described earlier examined 115 referrals of older adults considered to be living in moderate to severe squalor. After unstructured diagnostic interviews, 59% of the individuals with moderate to severe squalor and with moderate to severe clutter (23 of 39) had symptoms that met criteria for either neuropsychiatric disorders (10 dementia, 9 schizophrenia or psychotic disorder, 4 alcohol use disorder) or personality disorders (10 had paranoid or obsessive personality features). It is unknown how many of these individuals had symptoms that met criteria for hoarding disorder or obsessive-compulsive disorder (OCD). Of the other 76 individuals with squalor, who had only some, little, or no clutter, 87% (66 of 76) had a neuropsychiatric disorder (53 dementia, alcohol-related brain damage, or alcoholism; 9 schizophrenia or delusional disorder).

Evaluation of neuropsychological tasks may be informative regarding executive dysfunction (Gupta et al. 2017; Lee et al. 2014, 2016). In a community case series of 69 neuropsychological reports of patients living in squalor, frontal executive dysfunction was a prominent finding (Lee et al. 2017). Those patients with both hoarding and squalor were significantly older and more likely to have vascular or an Alzheimer's type of neurodegeneration, while those patients without hoarding showed more impairment in visuo-spatial reasoning, abstraction, planning, organization, problem-solving, and mental flexibility—with impaired mental flexibility showing the strongest association with squalor. Similarly, in a case series of six patients with squalor who were referred to an old-age psychiatry service, deficits in frontal executive function were found (Gregory et al. 2011). With this information in hand, referral for cognitive remediation and skill building occupational rehabilitation may be part of the treatment plan.

Individuals with hoarding have high comorbidity; thus, mood disorders are important to screen for (Frost et al. 2011b). For hoarding without squalor, comorbidity is high but is typically related to anxiety or depression, neither of which is seen as underlying the disorder. Similarly, information processing and executive function deficits appear to be compromised in patients with hoarding (Woody et al. 2014), but these are seen as vulnerability factors rather than underlying ones.

There are other psychiatric diagnoses that may account for squalid conditions (e.g., avoidance of touching rubbish due to contamination fears in OCD or avoidance of going outside to discard trash due to persecutory auditory hallucinations in schizophrenia). An accurate diagnosis is important given that current treatments differ and first-line medications for one condition may exacerbate the symptoms of the other (e.g., antipsychotics can exacerbate obsessive-compulsive symptoms, and serotonin reuptake inhibitors may exacerbate psychosis) (Poyurovsky et al. 2004; Rodriguez et al. 2010).

Functional Impairment

Both hoarding and squalor can lead to significant functional impairment in the work, family, and/or social domain (Snowdon et al. 2012). Among people with hoarding problems, higher levels of squalor are associated with greater functional impairment in the form of activities of daily living (Frost et al. 2013).

Assessments

Although the scientific review committee decided against adding a squalor specifier in the DSM-5 criteria for hoarding disorder (Snowdon et al. 2012), assessment of the degree of squalor in hoarding disorder is important in order to further understand its relationship with hoarding disorder and to assess outcomes of squalor interventions (McDermott and Gleeson 2009). Highlighted below are two squalor measures that have been developed for clinical use.

Environmental Cleanliness and Clutter Scale

The Environmental Cleanliness and Clutter Scale (ECCS; Halliday and Snowdon 2009) is a 10-item scale measuring the severity and uncleanliness in cases of severe domestic squalor. The scale lists items to be rated on a 4-point scale from 0 (none) to 3 (severe symptoms) to capture environmental conditions in the home, including accessibility due to clutter, clutter level, accumulation of garbage, cleanliness of living spaces, odor, and presence of vermin. The ECCS is reliable and valid and has a high internal consistency (Cronbach $\alpha=0.94$) (Halliday and Snowdon 2009). A total ECCS rating of greater than 12 indicates a person is living in squalor to such a degree that intervention is recommended (Snowdon et al. 2013). The ECCS has been shown to be useful for health agency officials regarding decisions on the timing and type of intervention (Tesauro et al. 2021).

Home Environment Index

The Home Environment Index (HEI; Rasmussen et al. 2014) is a 15-item scale focused on cleanliness in the home, personal hygiene, and daily cleaning behaviors. Situational items are rated from 0 (no squalor or symptoms) to 3 (severe symptoms), with specific descriptors for each response choice. Items in the cleaning behaviors section are also scored from 0 to 3 on the basis of the frequency of the behavior (nearly daily performance to never performed). The HEI has demonstrated good reliability and validity (Drury et al. 2014). It is highly correlated with hoarding severity and is associated to a lesser extent with nonhoarding psychopathology (depression and anxiety symptoms) and impairments in activities of daily living (Frost et al. 2013).

Intervention and Recovery

Although there are community-based approaches such as the partnerships and task forces described in Chapter 10 to address the needs of individuals with hoarding disorder (Bratiotis and Woody 2014), unfortunately, very little has been published regarding squalor interventions (Snowdon and Halliday 2009). Guidelines from a number of groups suggest that development of coordinated care services and case management may be helpful and that resources and interagency collaborations are especially needed (Congleton 2012; Guinane et al. 2019; Pelletier and Pollett 2000; Snowdon and Halliday 2009). The first step is typically a referral and assessment to determine the condition of the home, the factors that are causing or contributing to the squalor, and an intervention plan, which may include a number of treatments and services depending on the factors (Lacombe and Cossette 2018; Snowdon and Halliday 2009).

Not all clients are willing to engage in these types of assessments and interventions. In such situations, the next steps vary from country to country. Generally, the first step involves assessing capacity for self-care (Snowdon and Halliday 2009). An individual without capacity needs a guardian to be appointed who can help make decisions about treatment (Snowdon and Halliday 2009). If the client has the capacity but is unwilling to participate in treatment, a case manager can assist in reducing the potential for harm as a result of the hoarding. If this is unsuccessful, then an assessment of safety (e.g., fire hazard, pest infestation, property damage) may be necessary and might result in legal involvement (Freckelton 2012).

Regarding recovery, squalid conditions may improve with targeted treatment interventions for particular disorders, such as addiction treatment services when squalor is attributed to alcohol abuse (Gleason et al. 2015). Community case studies are helpful for gaining understanding in how to best support recovery (Raeburn et al. 2015). However, there is not yet robust evidence on outcomes of different interventions in cases of squalor, and obtaining more data is critical to understanding how best to intervene.

Case Examples

Case Example 1: Squalor as a Consequence of Hoarding Disorder and OCD

Kenneth was a 42-year-old white male construction worker who sought help when his landlord told him his neighbors had complained of pungent odors coming from his apartment. He described himself as an artist who was environmentally conscious. He was adamant about not being wasteful and, stemming from that, had high levels of discomfort when parting with items. For example, he did not throw away the cardboard tubes from toilet paper rolls, given that they could be used for a child's art project (even though he did not have children and did not have plans to donate them to a local school). This discomfort resulted in clutter that impaired his ability to use his bedroom and living room for their intended purposes. His insistence on not being wasteful extended to food in his kitchen. Kenneth admitted to drinking milk that was expired and making a sandwich that contained visible mold. He denied symptoms of mood disorders, psychosis, and substance abuse/dependence. Hoarding-specific rating scales were used to rate his current symptoms. His Hoarding Rating Scale—Interview (HRS-I) score was 25, which was well above the hoarding disorder cutoff of 14; and his Saving Inventory—Revised (SI-R) total score of 65 was also well above the recommended maximum of 39 for his age cohort. Kenneth's self-rated Clutter Image Rating (CIR) was 7 for the bedroom and living room and 4 for the kitchen. A CIR rating of 6 reflects clutter that would make any activity in the room extremely difficult. He denied that the conditions in his home might be causing a foul odor but was concerned that the neighbors' complaints might compel the landlord to enter his apartment and discover the clutter. Kenneth also endorsed intrusive thoughts of getting germs on his hands when he went outside, which contributed to anxiety about getting sick and to engaging in repetitive behaviors of washing his hands for hours under extremely hot water. Although he had had these thoughts since early adolescence, the thoughts had become worse after the death of his father the year prior. Most recently, he had begun feeling contaminated with germs when entering the bathroom, so he had stopped using the toilet and bathroom and had begun to put his urine and feces in jars in an effort to avoid the feelings of anxiety and contamination that arose from entering his bathroom.

Discussion

This case illustrates that a squalid, malodorous environment may have several origins. In this case, Kenneth's symptoms met DSM-5 criteria for both hoarding disorder and OCD. Odor was emanating both from rotten food in the pantry and refrigerator because of concerns of "waste" attributable to hoarding disorder and from urine/feces attributable to OCD avoidance of contamination. Concerns about waste and avoidance of it are among the most frequent rationales for saving and are the strongest predictors of hoarding severity (Dozier and Ayers 2014; Frost et al. 2015). The intense fear and avoidance of waste can become a moral imperative for people who hoard. Frost et al. (2018) refer to this phenomenon as "material scrupulosity," which they define as "an exaggerated sense of duty or moral/ethical responsibility for the care and disposition of possessions to prevent them from being harmed or wasted" (p. 20). This appears to be the case for Kenneth. For him, discarding rotten food leaves him feeling guilty and morally corrupt. Such a violation of his self image makes it difficult for him to change his behavior.

Case Example 2:
Squalor and Hoarding Disorder

Mary was a 70-year-old white female who cleaned houses and office buildings for a living. She sought help for hoarding disorder after seeing an advertisement for a research study. She reported having struggled with hoarding for most of her life, although she did not know what it was called. She recounted that her father used to refer to her as "my little garbage woman." At one point when her children were young, social services investigated her for possible neglect and threatened to remove the children. At the time of assessment, she had clutter piled nearly to the ceiling in some areas of her home. She needed to create walkways to get from her front door into her bedroom, and she had to move piles of papers and books from on top of her bed to sleep. Her toilet had clogged and overflowed, but she was too embarrassed to have a plumber enter her home, and eventually access to the bathroom had become blocked with clutter. She adored her cat and dog, but it was a challenge to clean up after them when they went to the bathroom behind the piles in her living room. A strong odor of mildew permeated her home. Each morning she would wake up with a headache. Although she made a decent living and got praise at her job working for a cleaning service, she was unable to clean her own apartment. She wanted to cook for herself rather than order takeout every night, but she felt as though she would not have time to clean the kitchen as perfectly as she would like.

Hoarding-specific rating scales were used to rate her current symptoms. Her HRS-I total score was 20, which was above the hoarding disorder cutoff of 14; and her SI-R total score of 65 was also above the recommended maximum of 33 for her age. Her self-rated CIR was 7 for the bedroom, living room, and kitchen. She had a history of depression, but on assessment, she denied all other psychiatric symptoms, and her presentation met DSM-5 criteria for hoarding disorder.

Discussion

This case illustrates that squalor can be seen in cases of hoarding disorder even when an individual has insight into their condition. In this case, embarrassment led to not calling a plumber, which resulted in mildew. Further, Mary likely would have cleaned up her pets' waste, but her piles of clutter impacted her ability to do so. Together, these factors resulted in squalid conditions. Most concerning is the toll they took on her health, as manifested by waking up with daily headaches. Ammonia can build up due to animal waste, and mold spores can also impact the quality of the air and the individual's health. Another issue was her perfectionism, which affected her ability to clean. Each time she tried to clean, the enormity of the task overwhelmed her, and she felt incapable of cleaning the home to her satisfaction. Attempts to do so made her feel inadequate and anxious, causing her to avoid cleaning her home. At the first attempt to work on the squalor in her kitchen with her therapist, she became agitated. "I should be in a loony bin." With the therapist's help, she was able not only to reduce the clutter but also to improve the level of sanitation of her home.

Case Example 3:
Neurological Injury and Squalor

Felipe, a 65-year-old Latinx male with no prior psychiatric or neurological diseases, was referred by his primary care doctor for psychiatric and neurological evaluation after 3 weeks of anxiety, sadness, and insomnia. On psychiatric evaluation, the patient was noted to be tearful and have psychomotor retardation. He endorsed low mood, anhedonia, fatigue, impaired concentration, difficulty falling asleep and waking up earlier than intended, feelings of worthlessness, and poor appetite. He denied suicidal ideation and prior history of suicide attempt. He denied symptoms of psychosis (no audio/visual hallucinations). Psychiatric review of symptoms was negative for other conditions, including substance use disorders, anxiety disorders, other mood disorders, eating disorders, and other OCD and related disorders. He was not taking medication. The neurological examination did not reveal any cranial nerve deficits, and neuropsychological testing demonstrated mild cognitive impairment, consistent with poor concentration and depressive symptoms. The diagnosis of major depression was made, fluoxetine was prescribed, and a routine computed tomography (CT) scan of the head was scheduled to rule out any other neurological conditions.

Surprisingly, the CT showed an anterior communicating artery aneurysm that required microsurgical clipping. By 2 weeks postsurgery, Felipe reported improvement in his symptoms—he no longer had low mood and anxiety and had improved sleep and energy. He continued to be asymptomatic for another year and then was lost to follow-up.

Three years later, Felipe presented with a rupture of an anterior communicating artery aneurysm that had triggered a subarachnoid hemorrhage that required urgent surgical clipping and caused damage to the right ventromedial caudate and adjacent white matter. After a few months in the hospital, he was discharged home but dealt with occasional difficulties with working memory, such as leaving food in the microwave. He remained asymptomatic for mood and anxiety symptoms; however, he began to accumulate a large number of objects in his home. When family members entered the home, they were overwhelmed by a foul odor, visible rotting food, and filth on most surfaces. Objects were stacked knee-high and consisted of a mixture of trash and new unopened purchases. Family members noted that he would not take a bath nor brush his teeth unless prompted. He acknowledged hygiene and clutter were problems and was accepting help; however, he maintained a nonchalant attitude about his living conditions. Psychiatric and neurological exams were both negative (no symptoms of depression, OCD, or hoarding disorder and no motor or sensory deficits). Repeat neuropsychological assessments showed normal executive function. A case manager was assigned and worked closely with the local hoarding task force (including the fire department) to reduce fire hazards in the home.

Discussion

This case illustrates that neurological damage can result in self-neglect and squalor and also that coordination with psychiatric and neurological consultation is critical to the diagnosis. The beginning of this case highlights how not all symptoms and behaviors can be attributed to purely psychiatric conditions; neurological processes (in this case an intracranial aneurysm) can be masqueraders. Although an unruptured aneurysm is rare, cases have been reported (Bunevicius et al. 2016). The second part of this case highlights how focal orbitofrontal damage can manifest in squalor, similar to another reported case (Funayama et al. 2010) of a high-functioning woman in her 40s who began to live in squalor after focal orbitofrontal damage without evidence of co-occurring dementia or mental disorders. The case of Felipe and Funayama et al.'s case also highlight that for these situations there seems to be a lack of both goal-directed acquisition of items and distress in parting with possessions, unlike what is seen in hoarding disorder. Rather, as is commonly seen in patients with frontal lobe damage, individuals may have an irrepressible desire to take nearby objects and store them (Volle et al. 2002) and then fail to remove useless items from the home (see Anderson et al. 2005 regarding a case involving damage to the mesial frontal cortex).

Case Example 4: Dementia and Squalor

Rosie, a 79-year-old Asian female, was brought to her primary care doctor by her concerned daughter. The daughter described how Rosie—who had previously been high-functioning and living independently—had slowly started to accumulate trash and filth in her home in the past year. Initially, Rosie had symptoms such as trouble differentiating between various kinds of vehicles. Then she developed a decreased interest in washing herself, cleaning, and eating, which led her daughter to think Rosie was mildly depressed. When Rosie began having trouble recognizing faces, her daughter became very worried, which led to the primary care appointment. The doctor gave Rosie a complete physical exam, ordered blood work (all negative), and conducted a preliminary psychiatric screen, which was negative for depression, anxiety, psychosis, and suicidal ideation. He ordered neuroimaging and a neuropsychological assessment, referring Rosie to a neurologist. On neurological examination, Rosie had an intact cranial nerve exam; however, testing showed Rosie had semantic and paraphasic errors, impoverished thought content, and loss of object knowledge. Neuroimaging revealed right anterior temporal lobe atrophy. Together with the patient's apathy, loss of insight, and difficulty with face recognition, the neurologist found Rosie's presentation suggestive of frontotemporal dementia and asked Rosie and her daughter to return to make a plan for management.

Discussion

This case illustrates how dementia can contribute to squalid conditions (Cipriani et al. 2012; Clark 1999; Radebaugh et al. 1987). Frontotemporal dementia is the third most common dementia for individuals age 65 and older (Brunnström et al. 2009) and affects brain regions associated with motivation, executive functioning, language, personality, and social cognition (Bott et al. 2014). Of the three variants of frontotemporal dementia, the semantic variant is characterized by anterior temporal lobe atrophy, which may result in behavioral presentations such as apathy, loss of insight, difficulty with face recognition, and social awkwardness (Bott et al. 2014; Thompson et al. 2003). These neurological impairments may contribute to squalid conditions through apathy (e.g., decreased inclination to wash oneself) and alteration of executive function (e.g., decreased capacity for cleaning, poor nutritional intake).

Conclusion

Squalor has features that are both distinct from and common to those of hoarding disorder. Both show significant functional impairment. Hoarding disorder, by definition, involves significant clutter, purposeful collecting, and difficulty parting with possessions, while these features only sometimes characterize people who live in squalor. Squalor, by definition, involves unhygienic conditions, while this feature is only sometimes associated with hoarding disorder. Self-neglect is often seen in squalor cases but is seldom seen in hoarding disorder. Insight appears to be poor more often in squalor cases. A number of other physical, neurological, or psychiatric disorders can lead to squalor, while hoarding disorder is not diagnosed if other disorders are deemed causal. Several new assessment scales are available to aide in intervention attempts. Finally, while there are existing treatments for hoarding disorder, there is no known effective treatment for squalor.

There are many unexplored areas of squalor, including the etiology (which may likely be heterogenous) and whether advancing age, living alone, and diminishing insight are risk factors. We also do not fully understand whether there are subdomains of squalor in which individuals also neglect their personal hygiene.

One intriguing line of inquiry involves the role of olfaction and insight. Anecdotally, individuals living in squalid conditions are not affected by the malodor stemming from rotting food or their own poor hygiene. Could this insensitivity to malodor be due to desensitization or damage to the olfactory bulb, and could this be a window into the neurobiology? As described in the context of squalor due to frontal cortex neurological injury, the olfactory cortex is on the ventral surface of the forebrain and thus may be affected as well. Olfactory perception may indeed play a role in the squalor observed in animal hoarding cases, as noted in Chapter 12. *Toxoplasma gondii* infection is a relatively widespread infection—affecting between 11% and 22% of the United States and United Kingdom (Flegr 2007)—which may stem from the relatively high prevalence of cat ownership. Seropositivity for *T. gondii* antibodies among cats removed in animal hoarding cases has been found to be exceptionally high (33.3%) (Cunha et al. 2019). Infection can have significant effects on olfactory perception. Olfactory perception changes in *T. gondii*–infected rodents appear to result in the loss of aversion to cat urine. Infected rodents stayed longer in areas infused with cat urine odor (Vyas et al. 2007). Even in humans, *T. gondii*–infected males rate the odor of diluted cat urine as more pleasant than noninfected males (Flegr 2007, 2013, 2015; Flegr et al. 2011). *T. gondii* infection–induced changes in olfaction might explain the absence of disgust in squalor cases where infected cats are present. Toxoplasmosis has been linked to related disorders, such as OCD. In a meta-analytic review of relevant studies including more than 9,000 cases, Nayeri Chegeni et al. (2019) found that over 25% of participants with OCD tested positive for *T. gondii*, while only 17% of participants without OCD did so. It is not clear whether hoarding status was assessed in these studies (Nayeri Chegeni et al. 2019).

Another question raised involves the psychological origins of behaviors around rotten food, particularly in the context of material deprivation, scrupulosity, and early-life trauma. The intense and rigid beliefs about waste seen in many hoarding cases have yet to be fully explored.

In addition to clarifying the boundaries of squalor, more research is needed to understand the heterogeneity and etiology of squalor and how best to personalize interventions based on this information.

KEY CLINICAL POINTS

- Squalor is characterized by an unhygienic environment to the extent that others from a similar culture would consider extensive cleaning to be vital.

- Squalid homes typically contain piles of soiled clothing and other debris, moldy or rotten food and food containers, urine-soaked floors and furniture, animal feces, insect and rodent infestation, and a suffocating odor.

- Neglect of personal hygiene usually accompanies the squalid conditions.

- The majority of hoarding cases do not involve squalid conditions; accumulation of objects and clutter, in and of itself, does not necessarily lead to a filthy environment.

- Squalor has phenomenological features that are both distinct from and common to those of hoarding disorder.

- Careful attention to several aspects of the clinical phenotype can help in evaluation of squalor versus hoarding disorder.

- Clutter may not be present in the majority of squalor cases, whereas clutter is a key feature of hoarding disorder that is required for diagnosis.

- In the case of squalor, the intention for accumulation of objects may be purposeless (e.g., stereotypic or ritualistic behaviors, no interest in the item itself). In contrast, hoarding disorder involves the intentional and purposeful collection of possessions (e.g., objects acquired and kept due to their usefulness, emotional value, or aesthetic qualities).

- Individuals with squalor may be ambivalent about parting with possessions, whereas those with hoarding disorder will find parting with possessions difficult.

- Self-neglect and poor insight are typical traits of those living in squalid conditions and occur much less frequently in hoarding disorder.

References

American Psychiatric Association: Diagnostic and Statistical Manual of Mental Disorders, 5th Edition. Arlington, VA, American Psychiatric Association, 2013

Anderson SW, Damasio H, Damasio AR: A neural basis for collecting behaviour in humans. Brain 128 (Pt 1):201–212, 2005 15548551

Bott NT, Radke A, Stephens ML, Kramer JH: Frontotemporal dementia: diagnosis, deficits and management. Neurodegener Dis Manag 4(6):439–454, 2014 25531687

Bratiotis C, Woody S: Community interventions for hoarding, in The Oxford Handbook of Hoarding and Acquiring. Edited by Frost RO, Steketee G. Oxford, UK, Oxford University Press, 2014, pp 316–328

Brunnström H, Gustafson L, Passant U, Englund E: Prevalence of dementia subtypes: a 30-year retrospective survey of neuropathological reports. Arch Gerontol Geriatr 49(1):146–149, 2009 18692255

Bunevicius A, Cikotas P, Steibliene V, et al: Unruptured anterior communicating artery aneurysm presenting as depression: a case report and review of literature. Surg Neurol Int 7 (suppl 18):S495–S498, 2016 27583172

Castrodale L, Bellay YM, Brown CM, et al: General public health considerations for responding to animal hoarding cases. J Environ Health 72(7):14–18, quiz 32, 2010 20235404

Cipriani G, Lucetti C, Vedovello M, Nuti A: Diogenes syndrome in patients suffering from dementia. Dialogues Clin Neurosci 14(4):455–460, 2012 23393422

Clark AN, Mankikar GD, Gray I: Diogenes syndrome: a clinical study of gross neglect in old age. Lancet 1(7903):366–368, 1975 46514

Clark J: Senile squalor syndrome: two unusual cases. J R Soc Med 92(3):138–140, 1999 10396262

Cohen L, Angladette L, Benoit N, Pierrot-Deseilligny C: A man who borrowed cars. Lancet 353(9146):34, 1999 10023949

Congleton M: The Fairfax County Hoarding Task Force. Age in Action 27(2):1–5, 2012

Cooney C, Hamid W: Review: diogenes syndrome. Age Ageing 24(5):451–453, 1995 8669353

Cunha G, Pellizzaro M, Marinelli Martins C, et al: Serological survey of Leptospira spp. and Toxoplasma gondii in companion animals rescued from hoarding behavior cases in Curitiba. Int J Dev Res 09:30683–30685, 2019

Cybulska E: Senile squalor: Plyushkin's not Diogenes' syndrome. Psychiatr Bull 22:319–320, 1998

Dozier ME, Ayers CR: The predictive value of different reasons for saving and acquiring on hoarding disorder symptoms. J Obsessive Compuls Relat Disord 3(3):220–227, 2014 32670784

Dozier ME, Porter B, Ayers CR: Age of onset and progression of hoarding symptoms in older adults with hoarding disorder. Aging Ment Health 20(7):736–742, 2016 25909628

Drury H, Ajmi S, Fernández de la Cruz L, et al: Caregiver burden, family accommodation, health, and well-being in relatives of individuals with hoarding disorder. J Affect Disord 159:7–14, 2014 24679383

Flegr J: Effects of Toxoplasma on human behavior. Schizophr Bull 33(3):757–760, 2007 17218612

Flegr J: How and why Toxoplasma makes us crazy. Trends Parasitol 29(4):156–163, 2013 23433494

Flegr J: Neurological and neuropsychiatric consequences of chronic Toxoplasma infection. Curr Clin Microbiol Rep 2:163–172, 2015

Flegr J, Lenochová P, Hodný Z, Vondrová M: Fatal attraction phenomenon in humans: cat odour attractiveness increased for Toxoplasma-infected men while decreased for infected women. PLoS Negl Trop Dis 5(11):e1389, 2011 22087345

Fontenelle LF: Diogenes syndrome in a patient with obsessive-compulsive disorder without hoarding. Gen Hosp Psychiatry 30(3):288–290, 2008 18433664

Freckelton I: Hoarding disorder and the law. J Law Med 20(2):225–249, 2012 23431842

Frost RO, Steketee G, Williams L: Hoarding: a community health problem. Health Soc Care Community 8(4):229–234, 2000 11560692

Frost RO, Patronek G, Rosenfield E: Comparison of object and animal hoarding. Depress Anxiety 28(10):885–891, 2011a 21608085

Frost RO, Steketee G, Tolin DF: Comorbidity in hoarding disorder. Depress Anxiety 28(10):876–884, 2011b 21770000

Frost RO, Hristova V, Steketee G, Tolin DF: Activities of Daily Living Scale in hoarding disorder. J Obsessive Compuls Relat Disord 2(2):85–90, 2013 23482436

Frost RO, Steketee G, Tolin DF, et al: Motives for acquiring and saving in hoarding disorder, OCD, and community controls. J Obsessive Compuls Relat Disord 4:54–59, 2015 25729641

Frost RO, Gabrielson I, Deady S, et al: Scrupulosity and hoarding. Compr Psychiatry 86:19–24, 2018 30041077

Funayama M, Mimura M, Koshibe Y, Kato Y: Squalor syndrome after focal orbitofrontal damage. Cogn Behav Neurol 23(2):135–139, 2010 20535064

Gleason A, Lewis M, Lee SM, Macfarlane S: A preliminary investigation of domestic squalor in people with a history of alcohol misuse: neuropsychological profile and hoarding behavior—an opportunistic observational study. Int Psychogeriatr 27(11):1913–1918, 2015 26076754

Gregory C, Halliday G, Hodges J, Snowdon J: Living in squalor: neuropsychological function, emotional processing and squalor perception in patients found living in squalor. Int Psychogeriatr 23(5):724–731, 2011 21108862

Guinane J, Bailey D, Fuge W, Lee SM: Analysis of patients referred for aged care assessment with concerns related to hoarding or squalor. Intern Med J 49(10):1313–1316, 2019 31602765

Gupta M, Bishnoi RJ, Schillerstrom JE: Neurobiological mediators of squalor-dwelling behavior. J Psychiatr Pract 23(5):375–381, 2017 28961667

Hahm DS, Kang Y, Cheong SS, Na DL: A compulsive collecting behavior following an A-com aneurysmal rupture. Neurology 56(3):398–400, 2001 11171910

Halliday G, Snowdon J: The Environmental Cleanliness and Clutter Scale (ECCS). Int Psychogeriatr 21(6):1041–1050, 2009 19589191

Halliday G, Banerjee S, Philpot M, Macdonald A: Community study of people who live in squalor. Lancet 355(9207):882–886, 2000 10752704

Lacombe MC, Cossette B: The role of public health in the development of a collaborative agreement with rural and semi-urban partners in cases of severe domestic squalor and hoarding. Community Ment Health J 54(6):766–772, 2018 29127561

Lebert F: Diogene syndrome, a clinical presentation of fronto-temporal dementia or not? Int J Geriatr Psychiatry 20(12):1203–1204, 2005 16315145

Lebert F, Pasquier F, Souliez L, Petit H: Frontotemporal behavioral scale. Alzheimer Dis Assoc Disord 12(4):335–339, 1998 9876962

Lee SM, Lewis M, Leighton D, et al: Neuropsychological characteristics of people living in squalor. Int Psychogeriatr 26(5):837–844, 2014 24495835

Lee SM, Lewis M, Leighton D, et al: A comparison of the neuropsychological profiles of people living in squalor without hoarding to those living in squalor associated with hoarding. Int J Geriatr Psychiatry 32(12):1433–1439, 2017 27911004

Lee SP, Ong C, Sagayadevan V, et al: Hoarding symptoms among psychiatric outpatients: confirmatory factor analysis and psychometric properties of the Saving Inventory—Revised (SI-R). BMC Psychiatry 16(1):364, 2016 27784281

MacKnight C: Taking the solitude out of self-neglect in the elderly. Canadian Alzheimer Disease Review 4(4):18–21, 2001

Maier T: On phenomenology and classification of hoarding: a review. Acta Psychiatr Scand 110(5):323–337, 2004 15458556

McDermott S, Gleeson R: Evaluation of the Severe Domestic Squalor Project: Final Report. Sydney, Social Policy Research Centre, University of New South Wales, 2009

Mendez MF, Shapira JS: The spectrum of recurrent thoughts and behaviors in frontotemporal dementia. CNS Spectr 13(3):202–208, 2008 18323753

Nakaaki S, Murata Y, Sato J, et al: Impairment of decision-making cognition in a case of frontotemporal lobar degeneration (FTLD) presenting with pathologic gambling and hoarding as the initial symptoms. Cogn Behav Neurol 20(2):121–125, 2007 17558256

Nayeri Chegeni T, Sarvi S, Amouei A, et al: Relationship between toxoplasmosis and obsessive compulsive disorder: a systematic review and meta-analysis. PLoS Negl Trop Dis 13(4):e0007306, 2019 30969961

Neary D, Snowden JS, Gustafson L, et al: Frontotemporal lobar degeneration: a consensus on clinical diagnostic criteria. Neurology 51(6):1546–1554, 1998 9855500

Pelletier R, Pollett G: Task Force on Senile Squalor—Final Report. London, Ontario, Middlesex-London Health Unit, 2000

Pertusa A, Fullana MA, Singh S, et al: Compulsive hoarding: OCD symptom, distinct clinical syndrome, or both? Am J Psychiatry 165(10):1289–1298, 2008 18483134

Poyurovsky M, Weizman A, Weizman R: Obsessive-compulsive disorder in schizophrenia: clinical characteristics and treatment. CNS Drugs 18(14):989–1010, 2004 15584769

Radebaugh TS, Hooper FJ, Gruenberg EM: The Social Breakdown Syndrome in the elderly population living in the community: the Helping Study. Br J Psychiatry 151:341–346, 1987 3501323

Raeburn T, Hungerford C, Escott P, Cleary M: Supporting recovery from hoarding and squalor: insights from a community case study. J Psychiatr Ment Health Nurs 22(8):634–639, 2015 26337594

Rasmussen JL, Steketee G, Frost RO, et al: Assessing squalor in hoarding: the Home Environment Index. Community Ment Health J 50(5):591–596, 2014 24292497

Rodriguez CI, Corcoran C, Simpson HB: Diagnosis and treatment of a patient with both psychotic and obsessive-compulsive symptoms. Am J Psychiatry 167(7):754–761, 2010 20595428

Snowdon J, Halliday G: How and when to intervene in cases of severe domestic squalor. Int Psychogeriatr 21(6):996–1002, 2009 19589194

Snowdon J, Halliday G: A study of severe domestic squalor: 173 cases referred to an old age psychiatry service. Int Psychogeriatr 23(2):308–314, 2011 20678298

Snowdon J, Shah A, Halliday G: Severe domestic squalor: a review. Int Psychogeriatr 19(1):37–51, 2007 16973099

Snowdon J, Pertusa A, Mataix-Cols D: On hoarding and squalor: a few considerations for DSM-5. Depress Anxiety 29(5):417–424, 2012 22553007

Snowdon J, Halliday G, Hunt GE: Two types of squalor: findings from a factor analysis of the Environmental Cleanliness and Clutter Scale (ECCS). Int Psychogeriatr 25(7):1191–1198, 2013 23561584

Strong S, Federico J, Banks R, Williams C: A collaborative model for managing animal hoarding cases. J Appl Anim Welf Sci 22(3):267–278, 2019 30021473

Tesauro M, Nunno L, Grappasonni I, et al: The Environmental Cleanliness and Clutter Scale (ECCS) in the management of sanitary risks in dwellings of hoarders in North Italy. J Public Health (Berl) (online), 2021

Thompson SA, Patterson K, Hodges JR: Left/right asymmetry of atrophy in semantic dementia: behavioral-cognitive implications. Neurology 61(9):1196–1203, 2003 14610120

Volle E, Beato R, Levy R, Dubois B: Forced collectionism after orbitofrontal damage. Neurology 58(3):488–490, 2002 11839860

Vyas A, Kim SK, Giacomini N, et al: Behavioral changes induced by Toxoplasma infection of rodents are highly specific to aversion of cat odors. Proc Natl Acad Sci USA 104(15):6442–6447, 2007 17404235

Weiss KJ: Hoarding, hermitage, and the law: why we love the Collyer brothers. J Am Acad Psychiatry Law 38(2):251–257, 2010 20542947

Woody SR, Kellman-McFarlane K, Welsted A: Review of cognitive performance in hoarding disorder. Clin Psychol Rev 34(4):324–336, 2014 24794835

Woody SR, Lenkic P, Bratiotis C, et al: How well do hoarding research samples represent cases that rise to community attention? Behav Res Ther 126:103555, 2020 32044474

Wrigley M, Cooney C: Diogenes syndrome: an Irish series. Ir J Psychol Med 9:37–41, 1992

CHAPTER 14
Conclusion and Future Directions

We have learned a tremendous amount about the phenomenology, etiology, and treatment of hoarding problems since the early 1990s. Advances in assessment and diagnosis have improved the estimates of age at onset and prevalence. Typical onset appears to be between ages 15 and 19 years. Severity and prevalence both increase with age, with an overall prevalence rate of around 2.5% (see Chapters 1 and 2). Prevalence of hoarding disorder appears to be equal for men and women, but women predominate in treatment-seeking and research samples. Hoarding appears across all countries and cultures for which there is research, though there may be some variation in the stated motives for saving (see Chapter 1). People with hoarding disorder are more likely to live alone—with higher rates of being divorced, widowed, or never married. They are more likely to have a lower socioeconomic status and have greater financial difficulties. Rates of comorbidity are high among people with hoarding disorder, with up to 75% comorbid for mood or anxiety disorders (Archer et al. 2019). Up to half of people with hoarding disorder have experienced significant trauma, and around half have comorbid major depressive disorder (Frost et al. 2011). Other common comorbidities include ADHD, obsessive-compulsive disorder (OCD), and eating disorders (see Chapter 2). Hoarding behaviors sometimes arise from other disorders—including depression, OCD, autism spectrum disorder, and dementia—but in these instances are not considered hoarding disorder.

Though originally thought to be a subtype of OCD, hoarding has been shown to have a number of phenomenological differences that indicate a distinct disorder. These include the ego-syntonic nature of hoarding symptoms, the existence of positive emotional states associated with symptoms, the absence of negative intrusive thoughts, and some features of neural activity (Mataix-Cols et al. 2010). Although a similar behavior has been used to diagnose obsessive-compulsive personality disorder (inability "to discard worn out or worthless objects even when they have no sentimental value" [American Psychiatric Association 2013, p. 679]), it is clear that this description does not match the behavior and experience of people with hoarding disorder. In hoarding disorder, saving behavior is not limited to worn out or worthless objects, and much of the saving *is* for sentimental reasons.

While we have made tremendous progress in understanding hoarding, what we have learned has also raised important questions that remain to be answered. The most fundamental question is whether we have captured the essence of the hoarding phenomena with our definition. The DSM-5 definition of hoarding disorder emphasizes difficulty discarding as the experience, attachments to possessions as its core, and clutter and dysfunction as the consequences. While the negative consequences have been clarified, the basic phenomenology and the role of attachments and other etiological factors have not.

For example, the DSM-5 definition downplays the role of excessive acquisition—something that is given a more prominent role in the ICD-11 classification of hoarding disorder. The DSM-5 definition includes excessive acquisition only as a specifier, since some people with hoarding problems deny acquiring excessively. But the research on this issue is far from clear. Our assessments of excessive acquisition in this context have all been self-reports, and there is reason to believe that recognition of excessive acquisition is sometimes limited in people who struggle with hoarding (Frost et al. 2009). We often see people who come to treatment for hoarding who deny having an acquisition problem, only to have it surface midway through treatment when they stop avoiding the places that cue acquiring. The motives that drive difficulty discarding also appear to drive acquisition—at least among people with hoarding disorder (Frost et al. 2015)—and acquisition is as strong a predictor of hoarding severity as difficulty discarding (Timpano et al. 2011). The existence of compulsive buying in the absence of hoarding has more experimental support and even some calls for a separate diagnosis (Müller et al. 2019). More detailed research on the acquiring behaviors of people who deny excessive acquisition is needed to determine whether it should be considered a core feature of hoarding.

The prevalence and severity of hoarding appear to increase with each decade of life. Perilous living conditions clearly pose greater health and safety risks for elderly people whose mobility and other functions may be impaired. Indeed, executive function and neurocognitive deficits are greater in elderly people who hoard than in people without hoarding problems, but it is not clear whether they are more prominent than in younger people who hoard. There is some evidence that elderly people who hoard experience more impairments in daily functioning than younger people with this disorder, and it makes sense that treatment may be more difficult for elderly people with hoarding disorder. These differences may be due to aging rather to than any qualitative differences in hoarding severity. It remains to be seen whether these differences require alterations in treatment.

It is rare to find a report of childhood hoarding in which the individual is free of other comorbidities. As a result, it is hard to distinguish what features are associated with childhood hoarding versus the comorbid disorders. The frequency of comorbid hoarding is high among a number of childhood disorders, including OCD (26%; Højgaard et al. 2019; Park et al. 2016), ADHD (29%; Hacker et al. 2016), autism (25%; Storch et al. 2016), anxiety disorders (22%; Hamblin et al. 2015), learning disabilities (16%; Testa et al. 2011), and Prader-Willi syndrome (80%; Dykens et al. 1996). Similar to hoarding in adults, hoarding in children is associated with anxiety, depression, indecisiveness, and other executive function deficits (Højgaard et al. 2019; Morris et al. 2016). The overlap of hoarding with ADHD has been the most thoroughly examined comorbidity, with some suggesting a correlated liabilities model, including genetic factors, executive function deficits, and other neurological problems (Lynch et al. 2015). Others have suggested that hoarding in childhood may be associated with an attachment disorder (Parker and Forrest 1993). Not surprisingly, several investigations indicate poor insight among children about their hoarding behaviors (Plimpton et al. 2009; Storch et al. 2007). Unfortunately, most of the research on hoarding in children has relied on OCD measures, which lack the precision to accurately assess hoarding. The one exception is the Children's Saving Inventory (Storch et al. 2011), a parental report of hoarding symptoms that has been shown to have good psychometric properties. In addition to assessment difficulties, questions remain about the manifestations of hoarding in children because they seldom have control over the resources to acquire possessions, and parents often control the amount of clutter in their living space. Without further research, few firm conclusions can be drawn about the nature and treatment of hoarding in children.

Another phenomenological feature that needs exploration concerns the focus on inanimate objects as targets for hoarding behavior. There are other problematic behaviors that look like hoarding disorder but do not involve inanimate objects. The most obvious is the hoarding of animals (see Chapter 12). DSM-5 suggests that "animal hoarding may be a specific manifestation of hoarding disorder" (American Psychiatric Association 2013, p. 249), but research on this topic is very limited (see Chapter 12). It remains to be seen whether the hoarding of animals should qualify as hoarding disorder, a subtype of hoarding disorder, or something else entirely.

A related question has been raised by the limited literature examining the saving of virtual or digital objects. van Bennekom et al. (2015) defined digital hoarding as "the accumulation of digital files to the point of loss of perspective, which eventually results in stress and disorganization" (p. 1). Early research on this topic suggests that digital hoarding has features in common with object hoarding, including strong emotional attachments—especially for digital images or videos (Thorpe et al. 2019)—and the saving of digital files "just in case" they may be needed in the future (Sweeten et al. 2018). There is some evidence, though weak, that digital hoarding is related to object hoarding (Luxon et al. 2018). This has led some to suggest that it should be considered a subtype of hoarding disorder (van Bennekom et al. 2015). It remains to be seen, however, whether the level of impairment from digital hoarding is significant enough to warrant consideration as a special subtype of hoarding disorder.

There may be other behaviors yet to be explored that qualify as hoarding. For example, one of us (R.F.) supervised the treatment of a gentleman who hoarded some inanimate objects but was most debilitated by his compulsion to attend every lecture/talk in his city. His report about the experience was that he needed to gather any and all information in the talks that might be in addition to what would be included in written reports. Virtually all of his time was consumed with this activity. This behavior has some of the characteristics of hoarding, including excessive acquisition of information deemed of significant importance. Consistent with this theme, Pushkarskaya et al. (2020) found that people with hoarding tendencies seek to acquire significantly more information before making a decision than people without hoarding tendencies.

A significant number of hoarding disorder cases involve unsanitary or squalid living conditions that pose health and safety risks. The presence of squalor in hoarding appears to vary based on level of insight or willingness to admit a problem (see Chapter 4). There are other possible explanations that have not yet been explored. For example, squalor in hoarding disorder may at times be a result of a rigid form of scrupulosity about avoiding waste. Or it may be related to deterioration of a person's olfactory functioning that interferes with their sensitivity to disgusting odors. This might be especially relevant for animal hoarding cases, in which the likelihood of *Toxoplasma gondii* infection is high. There are unanswered questions about the similarity of squalor in the absence of hoarding and squalor that is part of hoarding disorder. Given the serious problems associated with extremely unsanitary living conditions, research is critically needed on this topic.

The cognitive-behavioral model of hoarding (see Chapter 5) has driven much of the research on the phenomenology and etiology of hoarding. The model hypothesizes four basic features/deficits that contribute to the development of hoarding problems, including vulnerabilities (e.g., genetics, etc.), information processing deficits (e.g., attention), beliefs about and attachments to possessions (e.g., identity, etc.), and learning processes (e.g., negative reinforcement/avoidance conditioning). Research has substantiated a number of the factors in the model. Vulnerability factors—including genetics as well as personality characteristics such as perfectionism and intolerance of uncertainty—have been found in numerous studies to be associated with hoarding severity.

Information processing deficits, including executive function and emotion processing deficits, have been supported by some research. Research on the neurobiology of hoarding is in its infancy, but existing studies have highlighted networks associated with information processing, error monitoring, and salience detection, as well as abnormalities in cognitive control (see Chapter 6).

While we know that attachments to possessions seem to be what makes discarding difficult, we are only now seeing increasing research on the topic. But the research shows a wide variety of attachments, including opportunity and identity, comfort and safety, responsibility, and aesthetic appreciation (see Chapter 5 for more details). What we do not know is how all of these types of attachment relate to one another. Surely these types of attachment do not all separately lead to hoarding problems. There must be some underlying principle or feature they share. What do possessions contain or represent that would encompass all of these forms of attachment? One possible answer is that they hold information about the individual's engagement with the world around them. For each of the identified types of attachment, information relevant to the individual's place in the world is being preserved or generated. Perhaps the need to understand one's place in the world drives these attachments. For instance, growing research suggests that possessions play a role in one's sense of identity, one's view of future opportunities, and one's sense of comfort and security, and, in addition, how possessions are disposed of reflects one's moral code. Each of these roles reflects something about how individuals define themselves and engage with the world around them, similar to Erich Fromm's (1947) notion of a "hoarding orientation."

Fromm suggested that people with this orientation relate to the world around them through their possessions and gain a sense of security from acquiring and saving these items. Perhaps this orientation is the core feature that ties all four types of motives or attachments together. For most people, possessions carry limited information. But for people with hoarding disorder, each possession carries a richness of meaning and information. Considering this in combination with the apparent need among people who hoard for excessive amounts of information before they are able to make a decision (Pushkarskaya et al. 2020), possessions are put at the center of interactions with the world.

Another possible explanation is that these motives or attachments are simply artifacts of some more primal need to save things. Perhaps there is a sense of incompleteness driving this urge—similar to some theories related to OCD—and the attachments we have identified are simply after-the-fact explanations for the urge. Incompleteness or not-just-right experiences are closely associated with hoarding severity, more so than other OCD symptoms (Mataix-Cols et al. 2010). Whether this explanation is accurate or not, patients report that the attachments are what make discarding so difficult. Consequently, they must be directly addressed in treatment.

Both positive and negative reinforcement paradigms contribute to the development and maintenance of hoarding behaviors. Beliefs about and attachments to possessions lead people to overvalue possessions and find it rewarding to acquire and save them. At the same time, forgoing acquiring and letting go of possessions are emotionally taxing efforts, leading people with such strong attachments to avoid nonacquiring and discarding. Our knowledge of these reinforcement patterns has yet to be fully utilized in our treatment paradigms.

Many of the advancements in knowledge about hoarding have been facilitated by adequate assessment strategies. A plethora of assessment devices for hoarding disorder have been developed and tested. Four types of hoarding disorder measures include measures of risk, diagnostic interviews, symptom severity measures, and measures of motives/attachments/beliefs related to possessions. Other measures of related constructs, such as perfectionism, are also useful adjuncts to a complete case evaluation. For the most part, these measures are well established (see Chapter 3). However, assessment of several important constructs has yet to be developed. In particular, measures of insight and motivation are greatly needed. Insight (see Chapter 4) is a complicated construct, because many patients come to treatment with the recognition that there is a problem but have little idea of what that means or how it relates to their attachment to possessions. Several types of assessments would be useful for understanding and treating hoarding, including measures of the amount of discomfort necessary to endure during treatment and the client's understanding of the cognitive-behavioral model of hoarding on which treatment is based. This information would be valuable for matching treatment session content with what is needed for progress.

To date, little progress has been made on possible medications for hoarding disorder (see Chapter 8). There have been no randomized controlled trials, and only a few open trials have been conducted. In contrast, a great deal of progress has been made in the development and testing of cognitive-behavioral treatments for hoarding disorder. Both individual and group cognitive-behavioral therapy (CBT) for hoarding disorder have been shown to be effective in randomized controlled trials. In addition, peer-facilitated groups following highly scripted regimens based on the *Buried in Treasures* self-help book have been found to be effective compared with wait-list controls and have comparable effectiveness to group CBT with a trained therapist. Existing follow-up data from treatment trials suggest good maintenance of gains among treated clients. More such research is needed.

Despite this progress, many clients still suffer from significant symptoms at the end of treatment, and the degree of improvement in symptom severity is still far below that seen among patients treated for OCD. Clearly more work is needed to identify and test new and improved forms of treatment for hoarding disorder. Predictors of treatment outcomes offer some clues for avenues to pursue to improve hoarding disorder treatment. Among the predictive factors examined to date are the number of home visits during treatment, amount of homework completed, and levels of perfectionism as a preexisting condition. Also, it would be helpful to have a clearer understanding of how the treatment causes changes in symptoms. To date, few studies have identified mediators of treatment outcome. The exception is research that indicates that changes in the nature of attachment to possessions mediate change in symptoms (see Chapter 7).

Several variations of or additions to CBT for hoarding disorder have shown some promise, but none of these have been subjected to direct comparison with existing CBT (see Chapter 7). These include compassion-focused therapy, inference-based treatment, contingency management, and virtual reality. None of these variations have shown dramatically more significant improvements than the original CBT for hoarding disorder. Undoubtedly, more research on these promising strategies will continue. It may be that a different paradigm for treatment is needed. Some investigators have suggested a more primary focus on self-concept and identity.

Cross-fertilization of successful interventions in other fields, such as substance abuse, may be helpful for targeting hoarding behavior. Acquisition of objects generates pleasure, which positively reinforces hoarding behaviors. These behaviors can be difficult to overcome, but the addiction literature has several evidence-based strategies. One of these areas is contingency management, which involves giving patients tangible rewards (e.g., voucher-based or prize incentives) to reinforce positive behaviors such as abstinence (Budney et al. 2006; Petry et al, 2005; Prendergast et al. 2006). At least one study (Worden et al. 2016) has demonstrated the potential of contingency management in the treatment of hoarding. Another important treatment for substance abuse—motivational interviewing—has been incorporated into CBT for hoarding disorder. As of yet, there are no data on how much motivational interviewing facilitates treatment for hoarding disorder. Although hoarding disorder and substance use disorders have different symptoms, finding treatments that address the dysfunctional processes that are shared across diagnoses (e.g., reward processing, motivation) may be helpful.

Making advances in translational approaches—such as refining mouse models of hoarding behaviors and conducting neuroimaging of circuits underlying attachment to objects and decision-making—will help us understand how neural substrates are linked to symptom reduction (see Chapter 6). Exciting avenues for future work include precision psychiatry (see Williams and Hack 2022), in which patients with specific, definable clinical and/or neurobiological characteristics could be prescribed tailored treatments based on their predicted treatment response. We know little about how our treatments work at the level of the nervous system. Although we are starting to understand the neurobiological activation of various brain circuits in hoarding disorder, much more research needs to be done to elucidate the etiology and pathophysiology of these circuits and how they interface with other research frameworks (e.g., National Institute of Mental Health Research Domain Criteria [RDoC] such as threat reactivity; www.nimh.nih.gov/research/research-funded-by-nimh/rdoc/about-rdoc).

Promising directions include the combination of neuromodulation with neuroimaging, which may lead to inroads toward next-generation treatments and further elucidate neural mechanisms of hoarding disorder. Indeed, in a case study of repetitive transcranial magnetic stimulation, right dorsolateral prefrontal cortex neuromodulation improved hoarding symptoms and altered functional connectivity of the dorsolateral and ventromedial prefrontal cortex and amygdala—regions important in goal-directed choices during value-based decision-making (Diefenbach et al. 2015). Neuromodulation also allows for experimental manipulation of brain activity via stimulation and inhibition that opens a powerful pathway in understanding causal relationships (rather than purely correlative understanding).

Untapped potential exists in community interventions and implementation of evidence-based CBT strategies. Community engagements through hoarding task forces and public-academic partnerships improve the lives of clients and their communities (see Chapter 10). Further, for individuals with poor insight, harm reduction (see Chapter 9) can be an effective tool. Burgeoning technologies, like virtual reality, are being developed to allow therapists to treat clients by practicing sorting and discarding of their items in safe spaces. Increased interest In and attention to mobile mental health apps have led to more content development; yet at the same time, there is an urgent need to generate an evidence base for efficacy, engagement, and reach for these options (Ng et al. 2019; Wasil et al. 2020). Virtual and web/app-based technologies may be good options for those elders with hoarding symptoms who have limited mobility or access to care (see Chapter 11).

To date, phenomenological research studies on hoarding behaviors have captured largely Caucasian samples from the United States and Europe, which raises the question: How can we better understand and reach underrepresented groups? Cross-cultural research is an emerging area for hoarding disorder (see Chapter 1) (Fernández de la Cruz et al. 2016; Nordsletten et al. 2018; Timpano et al. 2015; Tsuchiyagaito et al. 2017), and there are many questions to be explored. For example, are there cultural differences in symptom expression that lead to a lack of identification of hoarding symptoms? How can we enhance recruitment efforts to reach underrepresented groups and across global ethnicities? How can we foster clinical research that is inclusive, diverse, and equitable? How can we assess the impact of biological and social factors related to culture, ethnicity, and race on clinical outcomes in hoarding disorder? Given that hoarding disorder is thought to affect individuals across the globe (see Chapter 1), translation and validation of hoarding scales into non-English languages represent an important first step in increasing the availability and reach of clinical research studies (see Chapter 3). Continued research on hoarding behaviors through a broader cultural lens is needed to identify the linguistic and cultural factors that may contribute to differences in phenomenology, vulnerability, and treatment response across groups.

Finally, informed patients are both allies and partners in this work. Investing in resources on hoarding through organizations that provide publicly accessible content—like the American Psychiatric Association (available at: www.psychiatry.org/patients-families/hoarding-disorder/what-is-hoarding-disorder) and the International OCD Foundation (IOCDF; https://hoarding.iocdf.org)—provides avenues for education, referrals, hoarding-specific conferences, and training for providers.

KEY CLINICAL POINTS

- Though hoarding disorder was originally thought to be a subtype of obsessive-compulsive disorder, research on hoarding has revealed a number of phenomenological differences—including symptoms and neural correlates—that indicate a distinct disorder.

- More detailed research is needed on whether we have captured the essence of the hoarding phenomena, including whether excessive acquisition should be considered a core feature of hoarding.

- Both individual and group cognitive-behavioral therapy (CBT) for hoarding have been shown to be effective in randomized controlled trials.

- To date, little progress has been made on possible medications for hoarding disorder; there have been no randomized controlled trials, and only a few open trials have been conducted.

- Untapped potential exists in community engagement and implementation of evidence-based CBT strategies through hoarding task forces and public-academic partnerships.

- Emerging areas in hoarding disorder include translational approaches, technology (mental health apps and virtual reality), and cross-cultural research.

- Informed patients are both allies and partners in this work.

References

American Psychiatric Association: Diagnostic and Statistical Manual of Mental Disorders, 5th Edition. Arlington, VA, American Psychiatric Association, 2013

Archer CA, Moran K, Garza K, et al: Relationship between symptom severity, psychiatric comorbidity, social/occupational impairment, and suicidality in hoarding disorder. J Obsessive Compuls Relat Disord 21:158–164, 2019

Budney AJ, Moore BA, Rocha HL, Higgins ST: Clinical trial of abstinence-based vouchers and cognitive-behavioral therapy for cannabis dependence. J Consult Clin Psychol 74(2):307–316, 2006 16649875

Diefenbach GJ, Tolin DF, Hallion LS, et al: A case study of clinical and neuroimaging outcomes following repetitive transcranial magnetic stimulation for hoarding disorder. Am J Psychiatry 172(11):1160–1162, 2015 26575452

Dykens EM, Leckman JF, Cassidy SB: Obsessions and compulsions in Prader-Willi syndrome. J Child Psychol Psychiatry 37(8):995–1002, 1996 9119946

Fernández de la Cruz L, Nordsletten A, Mataix-Cols D: Ethnocultural aspects of hoarding disorder. Curr Psychiatry Rev 12:115–123, 2016

Fromm E: Man for Himself: An Inquiry Into the Psychology of Ethics. New York, Rinehart, 1947

Frost RO, Tolin DF, Steketee G, et al: Excessive acquisition in hoarding. J Anxiety Disord 23(5):632–639, 2009 19261435

Frost RO, Steketee G, Tolin DF: Comorbidity in hoarding disorder. Depress Anxiety 28(10):876–884, 2011 21770000

Frost RO, Steketee G, Tolin DF, et al: Motives for acquiring and saving in hoarding disorder, OCD, and community controls. J Obsessive Compuls Relat Disord 4:54–59, 2015 25729641

Hacker LE, Park JM, Timpano KR, et al: Hoarding in children with ADHD. J Atten Disord 20(7):617–626, 2016 22923782

Hamblin RJ, Lewin AB, Salloum A, et al: Clinical characteristics and predictors of hoarding in children with anxiety disorders. J Anxiety Disord 36:9–14, 2015 26407051

Højgaard DRMA, Skarphedinsson G, Ivarsson T, et al: Hoarding in children and adolescents with obsessive-compulsive disorder: prevalence, clinical correlates, and cognitive behavioral therapy outcome. Eur Child Adolesc Psychiatry 28(8):1097–1106, 2019 30656432

Luxon A, Hamilton E, Bates S, Chasson G: Pinning our possessions: associations between digital hoarding and symptoms of hoarding disorder. J Obsessive Compuls Relat Disord 21:60–68, 2018

Lynch F, McGillivray J, Moulding R, Byrne L: Hoarding in attention deficit hyperactivity disorder: understanding the comorbidity. J Obsessive Compuls Relat Disord 4:37–46, 2015

Mataix-Cols D, Frost RO, Pertusa A, et al: Hoarding disorder: a new diagnosis for DSM-V? Depress Anxiety 27(6):556–572, 2010 20336805

Morris SH, Jaffee SR, Goodwin GP, Franklin ME: Hoarding in children and adolescents: a review. Child Psychiatry Hum Dev 47(5):740–750, 2016 26597114

Müller A, Brand M, Claes L, et al: Buying-shopping disorder—is there enough evidence to support its inclusion in ICD-11? CNS Spectr 24(4):374–379, 2019 30604662

Ng MM, Firth J, Minen M, Torous J: User engagement in mental health apps: a review of measurement, reporting, and validity. Psychiatr Serv 70(7):538–544, 2019 30914003

Nordsletten AE, Fernández de la Cruz L, Aluco E, et al: A transcultural study of hoarding disorder: insights from the United Kingdom, Spain, Japan, and Brazil. Transcult Psychiatry 55(2):261–285, 2018 29508639

Park JM, Samuels JF, Grados MA, et al: ADHD and executive functioning deficits in OCD youths who hoard. J Psychiatr Res 82:141–148, 2016 27501140

Parker KC, Forrest D: Attachment disorder: an emerging concern for school counselors. Elementary School Guidance & Counseling 27(3):209–215, 1993

Petry NM, Peirce JM, Stitzer ML, et al: Effect of prize-based incentives on outcomes in stimulant abusers in outpatient psychosocial treatment programs: a National Drug Abuse Treatment Clinical Trials Network study. Arch Gen Psychiatry 62(10):1148–1156, 2005 16203960

Plimpton EH, Frost RO, Abbey BC, Dorer W: Compulsive hoarding in children: six case studies. Int J Cogn Ther 2(1):88–104, 2009

Prendergast M, Podus D, Finney J, et al: Contingency management for treatment of substance use disorders: a meta-analysis. Addiction 101(11):1546–1560, 2006 17034434

Pushkarskaya H, Stern E, Tolin D, Pittenger C: Excessive acquisition of information during simple judgments in individuals with hoarding disorder. J Obsessive Compuls Relat Disord 24:100505, 2020

Storch EA, Lack CW, Merlo LJ, et al: Clinical features of children and adolescents with obsessive-compulsive disorder and hoarding symptoms. Compr Psychiatry 48(4):313–318, 2007 17560950

Storch EA, Rahman O, Park JM, et al: Compulsive hoarding in children. J Clin Psychol 67(5):507–516, 2011 21381027

Storch EA, Nadeau JM, Johnco C, et al: Hoarding in youth with autism spectrum disorders and anxiety: incidence, clinical correlates, and behavioral treatment response. J Autism Dev Disord 46(5):1602–1612, 2016 26749256

Sweeten G, Sillence E, Neave N: Digital hoarding behaviours: underlying motivations and potential negative consequences. Comput Hum Behav 85:54–60, 2018

Testa R, Pantelis C, Fontenelle LF: Hoarding behaviors in children with learning disabilities. J Child Neurol 26(5):574–579, 2011 21303763

Thorpe S, Bolster A, Neave N: Exploring aspects of the cognitive behavioural model of physical hoarding in relation to digital hoarding behaviours. Digit Health 5:2055207619882172, 2019 31636918

Timpano KR, Exner C, Glaesmer H, et al: The epidemiology of the proposed DSM-5 hoarding disorder: exploration of the acquisition specifier, associated features, and distress. J Clin Psychiatry 72(6):780–786, quiz 878–879, 2011 21733479

Timpano KR, Çek D, Fu ZF, et al: A consideration of hoarding disorder symptoms in China. Compr Psychiatry 57:36–45, 2015 25483851

Tsuchiyagaito A, Horiuchi S, Igarashi T, et al: Factor structure, reliability, and validity of the Japanese version of the Hoarding Rating Scale-Self-Report (HRS-SR-J). Neuropsychiatr Dis Treat 13:1235–1243, 2017 28533685

van Bennekom MJ, Blom RM, Vulink N, Denys D: A case of digital hoarding. BMJ Case Rep 2015:bcr2015210814, 2015 26452411

Wasil AR, Gillespie S, Shingleton R, et al: Examining the reach of smartphone apps for depression and anxiety. Am J Psychiatry 177(5):464–465, 2020 32354266

Williams LM, Hack LM (eds): Precision Psychiatry: Using Neuroscience Insights to Inform Personally Tailored, Measurement-Based Care. Washington, DC, American Psychiatric Association Publishing, 2022

Worden B, Bowe W, Tolin D: An open trial of cognitive behavioral therapy with contingency management for hoarding disorder. J Obsessive Compuls Relat Disord 12:78–86, 2016

Appendices

Appendix A: Structured Interview for Hoarding Disorder (SIHD)

Appendix B: Clutter Image Rating (CIR)

Appendix C: Saving Inventory—Revised (SI-R)

Appendix D: Hoarding Rating Scale (HRS)

Appendix E: Activities of Daily Living—Hoarding Scale (ADL-H)

APPENDIX A

Structured Interview for Hoarding Disorder (SIHD)

Instructions for the rator

The questions contained in this interview relate to each of the six criteria needed to evaluate the presence of hoarding disorder and its two specifiers. These questions appear in bold print and should be asked during the course of the interview, whereas the text in italics is present only to assist the rater. For a diagnosis of hoarding disorder all six criteria must be endorsed. If any of the criteria are not met, the diagnosis can be ruled out. The specifiers are only relevant for individuals endorsing all diagnostic criteria.

It is important to carefully distinguish hoarding disorder from nonpathological collecting, as well as from the general medical and DSM-5 conditions that may result in the accumulation of possessions (e.g., brain injury, obsessive-compulsive disorder, autism spectrum disorder). Therefore, this interview should ideally be used as a complement to a more comprehensive assessment of the patient's medical history and psychopathology. If in doubt about the endorsement of a specific criterion, the rater should complete the interview and consider all available information before rendering a diagnosis. Special sections are provided at the end of this document to assist with some of the most common differential diagnoses.

Ideally, the interview should be conducted directly with the sufferer and in the person's home. If the individual of interest is not available or refuses to be interviewed, this interview may be administered to a reliable informant. This approach may also be employed for cases presenting with poor or absent insight, where the subject's responses may significantly conflict with the reality of the hoarding behavior. In cases where there is a strong clinical suspicion of hoarding disorder (e.g., based on familial or legal reports), paired with poor insight on the part of the hoarding individual, the interviewer should use his or her clinical judgment to determine the relevance of each criterion.

If a home visit is not possible, photographs of the person's home environment may be helpful to assess the presence of clinically significant clutter (Criterion C). The presence of clutter may also be quantified with other available instruments such as the Clutter Image Rating Scale (Frost RO, Steketee G, Tolin DF, Renaud S: "Development and Validation of the Clutter Image Rating." *Journal of Psychopathology and Behavioral Assessment* 30(3):193–203, 2008). On the Clutter Image Rating Scale, a room score greater than 4 is usually indicative of clinically significant clutter; however, this is only for guidance and all available information needs to be taken into account.

Criterion A

Persistent difficulty discarding or parting with possessions, regardless of their actual value.

Do you experience difficulty discarding or parting with possessions?

This may include throwing away, selling, giving away, recycling, and so on.

- ☐ **YES** → go to **next question**
- ☐ **NO** → *hoarding disorder not present*

How long have you had this problem? _____ months/years.

*If hoarding is a persistent problem that has been present for a long period of time → CRITERION A is present → go to **next question***

If hoarding has been present for a relatively short period of time (i.e., only a few weeks or months), inquire about temporary factors that may account for the difficulties discarding (e.g., recent inheritance of a large number of possessions, moving to a different home). If the hoarding behavior can be entirely explained by these circumstances → hoarding disorder not present

What items do you find most difficult to discard?
Please list items below (both valuable and worthless items should be taken into account for the diagnosis).

_____

_____

_____

_____

_____

If **CRITERION A** is present,
place a check in the circle and go to CRITERION **B**   ⟳

Criterion B

This difficulty is due to a perceived need to save items and to distress associated with discarding them.

Do you intentionally keep these items (are they important/useful for you)?

Do you generally feel distressed or upset when discarding possessions?

These questions are intended to evaluate whether the accumulation of objects is intentional/active and whether the discarding process causes distress (or would cause distress, in cases where discarding is entirely avoided). Where the accumulation is due to passive accumulation, or where the discarding process does not cause distress, the hoarding may be subclinical or attributable to an alternative psychopathology.

- ☐   If **YES** to both of the above questions → **CRITERION B is present**
- ☐   If **NO** to any of the above questions → *hoarding disorder not present*

If **CRITERION B** is present,
place a check in the circle and go to CRITERION **C**   ○

Criterion C

The difficulty discarding possessions results in the accumulation of possessions that congest and clutter active living areas and substantially compromise their intended use. If living areas are uncluttered, it is only because of the interventions of third parties (e.g., family members, cleaners, authorities).

Do you have a large number of possessions that congest and clutter the main rooms in your home? *Note that "clutter" refers to the presence of a large number of items that are lying about in a disorganized way. The question refers to the key living spaces such as bedrooms, kitchen, or living room. Here exclude garages, attics, lofts, basements, and other areas that may commonly be cluttered in the homes of nonhoarding individuals.*

To meet Criterion C, active living spaces that are necessary for every-day life must be cluttered to the extent that their use is substantially compromised. If unclear, ask about the level of obstruction for particular rooms or domestic activities:

Because of the clutter or number of possessions, how difficult is it for you to use the rooms in your home?

- **Kitchen (sink, fridge, worktop, etc.):**

  _____

  _____

- **Bathroom (sink, toilet, shower/bathtub, etc.):**

  _____

  _____

- **Bedroom (bed, wardrobe, drawers, etc.):**

  _____

  _____

- **Living room (sofa, chairs, table, floor, etc.):**

  _____

  _____

- **Other (halls/corridors/stairs; difficult to walk through due to piles of items):**

  _____

  _____

  ☐   If **YES** → *CRITERION C is present*
  ☐   If **NO** → *go to* **next question**

Have other people (such as family members or local authorities) helped you to remove (or forcibly removed) some of your possessions? If so, how cluttered was your house/room before their intervention?
Explore to what extent the living spaces are currently clutter free because of the intervention of other people. If this is the case, the criterion can be endorsed in the absence of significant clutter.

  ☐   If **YES** → *CRITERION C is present*
  ☐   If **NO** → *hoarding disorder not present*

If **CRITERION C** is present,
place a check in the circle and go to CRITERION **D**   ◯

Criterion D

The hoarding causes clinically significant distress or impairment in social, occupational, or other important areas of functioning (including maintaining a safe environment for self and others).

Do the difficulties discarding or the clutter cause you distress? *Note that some individuals with poor insight may not acknowledge being distressed, though any attempts to discard possessions by third parties will result in distress or anger.*

Do the difficulties discarding or the clutter interfere with your family life, friendships, or ability to perform well at home or work? *Note that the impairment may only be apparent to those around an individual with poor insight.*

- ☐ If **YES** to one or both of the above questions →
  CRITERION D is present
- ☐ If **NO** to both questions → *hoarding disorder not present*

If **CRITERION D** is present,
place a check in the circle and go to CRITERION **E**   ○

Criterion E

The hoarding is not attributable to another medical condition (e.g., brain injury, cerebrovascular disease, Prader-Willi syndrome).

Do you have any general medical conditions, a history of head injury, or cerebrovascular disease? *Review past medical history for neurological disorders and inquire about history of severe head trauma. Some relevant conditions include traumatic brain injury, surgical resection for the treatment of a tumor or seizure control, cerebrovascular disease, infections of the central nervous system (e.g., herpes simplex encephalitis), or neurogenetic conditions such as Prader-Willi syndrome. If appropriate and available, additional investigations (e.g., EEG, CT, MRI, neuropsychological assessment) may be useful to help confirm the presence of brain damage.*

- ☐ **YES** → *go to **next question***
- ☐ **NO** → *hoarding disorder not present*

Did you have difficulties with discarding/clutter before you became ill?
Try to establish whether there is a clear temporal link between the medical condition and the onset of the hoarding behavior.

☐ **YES** → *CRITERION E is present*

☐ **NO** → *if hoarding clearly preceded by a general medical condition* → *hoarding disorder not present*

If **CRITERION E** is present,
place a check in the circle and go to CRITERION **F**　　　　〇

Criterion F

The hoarding is not better explained by the symptoms of another mental disorder (e.g., obsessions in obsessive-compulsive disorder, decreased energy in major depressive disorder, delusions in schizophrenia or another psychotic disorder, cognitive deficits in major neurocognitive disorder, restricted interests in autism spectrum disorder).

Ideally, this interview should be administered in the context of a full psychopathological assessment. If this is not available, ask the interviewee or informant about current or past psychiatric diagnoses. Note current and lifetime mental disorders here:

_____　_____

_____　_____

_____

_____　_____

The presence of another mental disorder does not preclude the diagnosis of hoarding disorder. However, hoarding disorder is not diagnosed if the symptoms are judged to be secondary to or a direct consequence of another mental disorder, such as:

- *Obsessions or compulsions in obsessive-compulsive disorder*
- *Special or circumscribed interests in autism spectrum disorder or intellectual disability.*
- *Decreased energy, psychomotor retardation, or fatigue in major depressive disorder.*
- *Delusions or negative symptoms in schizophrenia spectrum or other psychotic disorders.*
- *Cognitive deficits in a neurocognitive disorder such as frontotemporal lobar degeneration or Alzheimer's disease.*

If another mental disorder is present, it is useful to establish the temporal relation with the onset of hoarding symptoms.

PLEASE SEE APPENDIX FOR FURTHER GUIDANCE ON THE DIFFERENTIAL DIAGNOSIS WITH OBSESSIVE-COMPULSIVE DISORDER AND AUTISM SPECTRUM DISORDER.

If **CRITERION F** is present, place a check in the circle   ◯

If all six criteria are met, the diagnosis of **hoarding disorder** should be coded.

If **hoarding disorder is present,**
please place a check mark in the circle   ◯

Specifiers

If hoarding disorder has been diagnosed, assess the presence of Excessive Acquisition and determine the Degree of Insight.

Excessive Acquisition Specifier

If the difficulty discarding possessions is accompanied by excessive acquisition of items that are not needed or for which there is no available space.

Do you often acquire free items that you don't need or for which you have no available space at home?

- ☐ **YES**
- ☐ **NO**

Do you often buy items that you don't need, you can't afford, or for which you have no available space at home?

- ☐ **YES**
- ☐ **NO**

Do you sometimes steal things that you don't need, you can't afford, or for which you have no available space at home?

- ☐ **YES**
- ☐ **NO**

If YES *to **any** of the above 3 questions,* **With Excessive Acquisition** *should be coded.*

Please place a check mark in the circle   ◯

Insight Specifier

With good or fair insight: The individual recognizes that hoarding-related beliefs and behaviors (pertaining to difficulty discarding items, clutter, or excessive acquisition) are problematic.

With poor insight: The individual is mostly convinced that hoarding-related beliefs and behaviors (pertaining to difficulty discarding items, clutter, or excessive acquisition) are not problematic despite evidence to the contrary.

With absent or delusional insight: The individual is completely convinced that hoarding-related beliefs and behaviors (pertaining to difficulty discarding items, clutter, or excessive acquisition) are not problematic despite evidence to the contrary.

To what extent do you think that your saving behavior (including your difficulties discarding, the resulting clutter, and the excessive acquisition) is problematic? *If in doubt, refer back to information provided by the subject during the interview. If a reliable informant is present, check for discrepancies between the subject's and the informant's report and assess degree of insight accordingly.*

- ☐ **Good/Fair** insight
- ☐ **Poor** insight
- ☐ **Absent/Delusional** insight

Risk Assessment

This section helps the rater document any possible risks associated with problematic hoarding behavior. Please check whether the following are present:

Fire hazard

- ☐ *Are there flammable materials near a heat source?*
- ☐ *Are there electrical hazards?*

Blocked exits

- ☐ *Is the door that allows entry and exit to the house clear?*
- ☐ *Are there additional doors within the property that are blocked?*

Risk of falling

- ☐ Is there a lack of clear pathways, impeding movement throughout the property?
- ☐ Is it necessary to climb piles of objects in order to move between rooms or access objects?

Insects, infestations

- ☐ Is there any evidence of insects (visible individuals, swarms, cobwebs, droppings)?
- ☐ Are there any rodents or other infestations present?

Unhygienic conditions

- ☐ Is there human or animal waste/vomit in the property?
- ☐ Is there moldy or rotten food or dirty food containers in the kitchen or other areas of the property?
- ☐ Is the sink, washbasin, bathroom, shower, or bathtub clogged or notably dirty?
- ☐ Is there standing water anywhere in the property (sink, tub, basement, other)?
- ☐ Does the property emit a strong odor?

Neglect of children, elders, or disabled people

- ☐ If there are children, elders, or disabled people present, is there sufficient space to permit routine care and activities (e.g., a functioning kitchen, a place to eat meals, access to a shower or bathtub)?
- ☐ If there are children present, is there sufficient space for them to sleep, play, or do school homework?

Animal hoarding

- ☐ Are there starving, neglected, or maltreated animals on the premises?

Additional notes (please write any additional information that may be useful for risk assessment)

APPENDIX: DIFFERENTIAL DIAGNOSIS ASSISTANT

Hoarding as a Symptom of Obsessive-Compulsive Disorder

This section will assist the rater in assessing whether the hoarding behavior is better conceptualized as a symptom of obsessive-compulsive disorder (OCD). First, establish whether OCD is present (independently of the hoarding). If there is an established diagnosis of OCD, then ask the following questions:

Are your discarding difficulties caused by a specific obsession or fear?

☐　**YES** (more likely in OCD)

☐　**NO**

If hoarding is mainly driven by prototypical obsessions → hoarding disorder probably not present (hoarding likely to be a symptom of OCD)

Some examples of obsessions include:

- *Not discarding for fear of contaminating self or others.*
- *Superstitious thoughts about discarding, for example, fear of something bad happening to a loved one if certain items are discarded.*
- *Intense feelings of incompleteness.*
- *Saving to maintain a record of all life experiences.*

Is it difficult for you to discard things because this triggers endless rituals (e.g., washing or checking rituals)?

☐　**YES** (more likely in OCD)

☐　**NO**

If hoarding is the result of persistent avoidance of onerous compulsions → hoarding disorder probably not present (hoarding likely to be a symptom of OCD)

Do you enjoy/find it comforting to acquire possessions and being around them?

☐　**YES**

☐　**NO** (more likely in OCD)

Are you emotionally attached to most of the items you save?

☐　**YES**

☐　**NO** (more likely in OCD)

Do you save items mainly because they are valuable/beautiful or they may come in handy in the future?

☐ **YES**

☐ **NO** (more likely in OCD)

Do you keep body products (feces, urine, nails, hair, used diapers) or rotten food?

☐ **YES** (more likely in OCD)

☐ **NO**

Individuals with hoarding disorder are more likely to report that their hoarding behavior is pleasurable/comforting, that they are emotionally attached to their saved objects, or that they save due to a belief that their items will prove handy in the future. The retention of body products or rotten food is, conversely, more often seen in OCD.

REMEMBER *that both OCD and hoarding disorder may be diagnosed at the same time when severe hoarding symptoms appear concurrently with other typical symptoms of OCD but are judged to be independent from these symptoms. In case of diagnostic uncertainty, we recommend diagnosing OCD only.*

Hoarding as a Symptom of Autism Spectrum Disorder

This section will assist the rater in assessing whether the hoarding behavior is better conceptualized as a symptom of autism spectrum disorder (ASD). First, establish whether ASD is present (independently of the hoarding). If there is an established diagnosis of ASD, then ask the following questions:

Are the objects you save generally confined to a single, specific (circumscribed) area of interest?

A circumscribed interest, as seen in ASD, is typified by an intense interest in a specific, narrow, and often unusual topic. These interests may result in the accumulation of many similar objects, which are unified as exemplars of this area of interest. Individuals with hoarding disorder are more likely to accumulate a wide range of objects (e.g., not confined to a single area of interest, or unified by a highly specific characteristic). A lack of organization is, furthermore, more typical in hoarding disorder.

☐ **YES** (more likely in ASD)

☐ **NO**

If **YES** *to the preceding question:* **What is the area of interest?**

Do the objects you save largely share a particular physical characteristic (e.g., material, texture, or shape)?

☐ **YES** (more likely in ASD)

☐ **NO**

In ASD, the gathering of many like objects may signal an unusual sensory preoccupation.

Examples of such preoccupations include intense fascinations with:

- *Visual stimuli (e.g., shiny objects, blinking lights, the motion of liquid—such as the rotation of water being flushed).*
- *Auditory stimuli (e.g., the sound of a vacuum cleaner).*
- *Tactile stimuli (e.g., smooth surfaces).*

Do you enjoy organizing and classifying your possessions?

☐ **YES** (more likely in ASD)

☐ **NO**

If **YES** *to the preceding question:* **Could you tell me a bit about your organizing system?**

A focus on uniformity and order with one's possessions is common to ASD. Unlike with OCD, in ASD this organization process should be ego-syntonic and pleasurable.

If hoarding is primarily the result of a circumscribed interest, sensory preoccupation, or a desire to save/classify information → hoarding disorder probably not present (hoarding likely to be a symptom of ASD)

REMEMBER *that both ASD and hoarding disorder may be diagnosed at the same time when severe hoarding symptoms appear concurrently with other typical symptoms of ASD but are judged to be independent from these symptoms. In case of diagnostic uncertainty, we recommend diagnosing ASD only.*

APPENDIX B
Clutter Image Rating (CIR)

For details on development and validation, see Frost R, Steketee G, Tolin D, Renaud S: "Development and Validation of the Clutter Image Rating." *Journal of Psychopathology and Behavioral Assessment* 30(3):193–203, 2008.

Clutter Image Rating: Bedroom
Please select the photo below that most accurately reflects the amount of clutter in your room.

Clutter Image Rating: Kitchen
Please select the photo below that most accurately reflects the amount of clutter in your room.

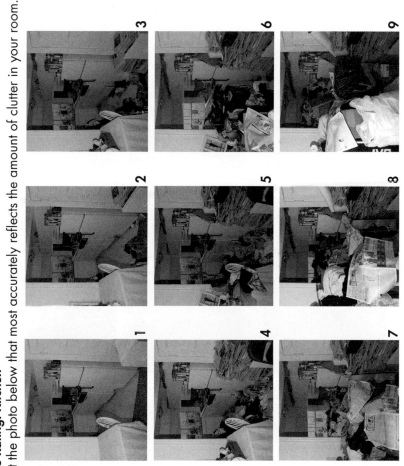

Clutter Image Rating: Living Room
Please select the photo below that most accurately reflects the amount of clutter in your room.

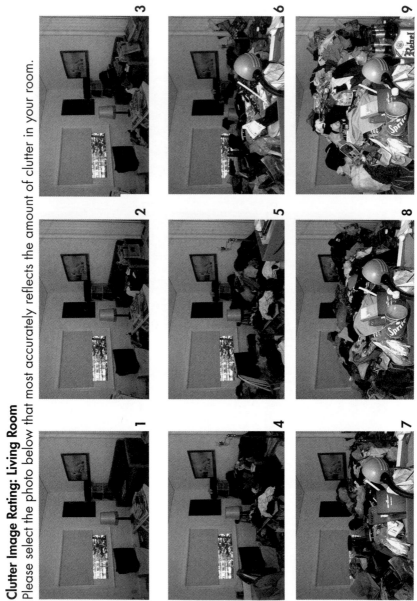

APPENDIX C
Saving Inventory— Revised (SI-R)

Reprinted from Frost RO, Steketee G, Grisham J: "Measurement of Compulsive Hoarding: Saving Inventory—Revised." *Behaviour Research and Therapy* 42:1163–1182, 2004. Used with permission.

For each question below, circle the number that corresponds most closely to your experience **DURING THE PAST WEEK.**

0	1	2	3	4
None	A little	A moderate amount	Most/ Much	Almost all/ Complete

1. How much of the living area in your home is cluttered with possessions? (Consider the amount of clutter in your kitchen, living room, dining room, hallways, bedrooms, bathrooms, or other rooms.)   0   1   2   3   4

2. How much control do you have over your urges to acquire possessions?   0   1   2   3   4

3. How much of your home does clutter prevent you from using?   0   1   2   3   4

4. How much control do you have over your urges to save possessions?   0   1   2   3   4

5. How much of your home is difficult to walk through because of clutter?   0   1   2   3   4

For each question below, circle the number that corresponds most closely to your experience **DURING THE PAST WEEK.**

0	1	2	3	4
Not at all	Mild	Moderate	Considerable/ Severe	Extreme

6. To what extent do you have difficulty throwing things away?   0   1   2   3   4

7. How distressing do you find the task of throwing things away?   0   1   2   3   4

8. To what extent do you have so many things that your room(s) are cluttered?   0   1   2   3   4

For each question below, circle the number that corresponds most closely to your experience **DURING THE PAST WEEK.**

0	1	2	3	4
Not at all	Mild	Moderate	Considerable/ Severe	Extreme

9. How distressed or uncomfortable would you feel if you could not acquire something you wanted?	0	1	2	3	4
10. How much does clutter in your home interfere with your social, work, or everyday functioning? Think about	0	1	2	3	4
things that you don't do because of clutter.	0	1	2	3	4
11. How strong is your urge to buy or acquire free things for which you have no immediate use?	0	1	2	3	4
12. To what extent does clutter in your home cause you distress?	0	1	2	3	4
13. How strong is your urge to save something you know you may never use?	0	1	2	3	4
14. How upset or distressed do you feel about your acquiring habits?	0	1	2	3	4
15. To what extent do you feel unable to control the clutter in your home?	0	1	2	3	4
16. To what extent has your saving or compulsive buying resulted in financial difficulties for you?	0	1	2	3	4

For each question below, circle the number that corresponds most closely to your experience **DURING THE PAST WEEK.**

0	1	2	3	4
Never	Rarely	Sometimes/ Occasionally	Frequently/ Often	Very often

17. How often do you avoid trying to discard possessions because it is too stressful or time-consuming?	0	1	2	3	4
18. How often do you feel compelled to acquire something you see (e.g., when shopping or offered free things)?	0	1	2	3	4
19. How often do you decide to keep things you do not need and have little space for?	0	1	2	3	4
20. How frequently does clutter in your home prevent you from inviting people to visit?	0	1	2	3	4
21. How often do you actually buy (or acquire for free) things for which you have no immediate use or need?	0	1	2	3	4
22. To what extent does the clutter in your home prevent you from using parts of your home for their intended purpose (e.g., cooking, using furniture, washing dishes, cleaning)?	0	1	2	3	4
23. How often are you unable to discard a possession you would like to get rid of?	0	1	2	3	4

SI-R (Modified) Scoring Subscales:

Clutter Subscale (9 items):
Sum items: 1, 3, 5, 8, 10, 12, 15, 20, 22

Difficulty Discarding/Saving Subscale (7 items):
Sum items: 4 (reverse score), 6, 7, 13, 17, 19, 23

Acquisition Subscale (7 items):
Sum items: 2 (reverse score), 9, 11, 14, 16, 18, 21

Total Score = Sum of all items

APPENDIX D
Hoarding Rating Scale (HRS)

Reprinted from Tolin DF, Frost RO, Steketee G: "A Brief Interview for Assessing Compulsive Hoarding: The Hoarding Rating Scale—Interview." *Psychiatry Research* 178:147–152, 2010. Used with permission.

1. Because of the clutter or number of possessions, how difficult is it for you to use the rooms in your home?

0	1	2	3	4	5	6	7	8
No problem		Mild a few of the living spaces are difficult to use, but most spaces are usable		Moderate some of the living spaces are difficult to use		Severe most of the living spaces are difficult to use		Extreme nearly all of the living spaces are difficult or impossible to use

2. To what extent do you have difficulty discarding (or recycling, selling, giving away) ordinary things that other people would get rid of?

0	1	2	3	4	5	6	7	8
No problem		Mild occasionally (less than weekly) has difficulty discarding, or saves a few unneeded items		Moderate regularly (once or twice weekly) has difficulty discarding, or saves some unneeded items		Severe frequently (several times per week) has difficulty discarding, or saves many unneeded items		Extreme very often (daily) has difficulty discarding, or saves large numbers of unneeded items

3. To what extent do you currently have a problem with collecting free things or buying more things than you need, or can use, or can afford?

0	1	2	3	4	5	6	7	8
No problem		**Mild** occasionally (less than weekly) acquires items not needed or affordable, or acquires a few unneeded items		**Moderate** regularly (once or twice weekly) acquires items not needed or affordable, or acquires some unneeded items		**Severe** frequently (several times per week) acquires items not needed or affordable, or acquires many unneeded items		**Extreme** very often (daily) acquires items not needed or affordable, or acquires large numbers of unneeded items

4. To what extent do you experience emotional distress because of clutter, difficulty discarding, or problems with buying or acquiring things?

0	1	2	3	4	5	6	7	8
No problem		**Mild** occasionally (less than weekly) feels distressed, or feels mildly distressed but generally OK		**Moderate** regularly (once or twice weekly) feels distressed, or feels moderately distressed		**Severe** frequently (several times per week) feels distressed, or feels severely distressed with a noticeable intensity		**Extreme** very often (daily) feels distressed, or feels extremely distressed to point of being completely unable to cope

5. To what extent do you experience impairment in your life (daily routine, job/school, social activities, family activities, financial difficulties) because of clutter, difficulty discarding, or problems with buying or acquiring things?

0	1	2	3	4	5	6	7	8
No problem		Mild slight impairment in work, social or family activities, and/or finances, but for the most part functioning is intact		Moderate noticeable impairment in work, social or family activities, and/or finances, but many areas of functioning are intact		Severe substantially reduced capacity to work, and/or have good social or family activities, and/or significant financial problems due to hoarding		Extreme virtually unable to perform any work, virtually no social or family activities, and/or severe financial problems due to hoarding

Criteria for clinically significant hoarding

A score of 4 or greater on questions 1 and 2, and a score of 4 or greater on either question 4 or question 5.

APPENDIX E

Activities of Daily Living—Hoarding Scale (ADL-H)

Reprinted from Frost RO, Hristova V, Steketee G, Tolin DF: "Activities of Daily Living Scale in Hoarding Disorder." *Journal of Obsessive Compulsive and Related Disorders* 2:85–90, 2013. Used with permission.

<u>Activities of Daily Living</u>: Sometimes clutter in the home can prevent you from doing ordinary activities. For each of the following activities, please circle the number that best represents the degree of difficulty you experience in doing this activity <u>because of the clutter or hoarding problem</u>. If you have difficulty with the activity for other reasons (for example, unable to bend or move quickly due to physical problems), do not include this in your rating. Instead, rate only how much difficulty you would have due to hoarding. If the activity is <u>not relevant</u> to your situation (for example, you don't have laundry facilities or animals), circle Not Applicable (NA).

Activities affected by clutter or hoarding problem	Can do it easily	Can do it with a little difficulty	Can do it with moderate difficulty	Can do it with great difficulty	Unable to do	NA
1. Prepare food	1	2	3	4	5	NA
2. Use refrigerator	1	2	3	4	5	NA
3. Use stove	1	2	3	4	5	NA
4. Use kitchen sink	1	2	3	4	5	NA
5. Eat at table	1	2	3	4	5	NA
6. Move around inside the house	1	2	3	4	5	NA
7. Exit home quickly	1	2	3	4	5	NA
8. Use toilet	1	2	3	4	5	NA
9. Use bath/shower	1	2	3	4	5	NA
10. Use bathroom sink	1	2	3	4	5	NA
11. Answer door quickly	1	2	3	4	5	NA
12. Sit in sofa/chair	1	2	3	4	5	NA
13. Sleep in bed	1	2	3	4	5	NA
14. Do laundry	1	2	3	4	5	NA
15. Find important things (such as bills, tax forms, etc.)	1	2	3	4	5	NA
16. Care for animals	1	2	3	4	5	NA

Scoring key:
Sum items 1–16, excluding items with NA (not applicable) ratings.
Divide by the number of items that are given a numerical rating to yield an average score that ranges from 1.0 to 5.0. An average score in the 3 range is likely to indicate substantial problems with functioning due to clutter.

Index

*Page numbers printed in **boldface** type refer to tables and figures.*

Academic-public partnerships, 187–190
Accumulation, squalor and, 235, **236**
Acquisition
  of animals, 217
  assessment of, 64
  as comorbidity of hoarding disorder, 41
  denial of excessive, 34
  excessive, 41, 104, 130
  of free things, 34, 56, 103
  of possessions, 32, 33
  strength of the urge to acquire, 130
  triggers, 130
Activities of Daily Living—Hoarding Scale (ADL-H), 49, **52,**134, 169, 184
  sample of, 293–294
ADHD
  as comorbidity of hoarding disorder, 38–39
  comorbidity with hoarding disorder, 132
  hoarding and, 93–94
ADL-H. *See* Activities of Daily Living—Hoarding Scale
Adolescents, hoarding in, 15–16
Adult Protective Services (APS), 167–168, 170, 185–186
Age. *See* Adolescents; Children; Elders
Alighieri, Dante, 4
Amphetamine salts, 154
Animal hoarding
  breeders and, 222
  case example of, 223
  criminal proceedings with, 219

criminal prosecution for animal abuse, 225
  culture and, 220
  definition of, 215–216
  demographics and course of, 220–221
  DSM-5 and, 216–218, 228
  etiology, 222–224
  exploiters, 222, 228
  features of hoarding behaviors, 118–119, 120, 218–220
  interventions, 225–227
  mouse models, 260
  overview, 215–216
  parasitic infection as conduit for, 224
  recognition of, 226–227
  rescuers, 221–222, 224, 228
  subtypes, 221–222, 228
  translational animal models, 119
  types of animals, 220
Anorgasmia, 158
Anosognosia, 70–76, **71**
Anthropomorphism Questionnaire (AQ), 60–61
Antisocial personality disorder, with animal hoarding, 222
APS. *See* Adult Protective Services
AQ. *See* Anthropomorphism Questionnaire
Aristotle, 3, 8
Atomoxetine, for treatment of hoarding disorder, 153
Attachments
  animal hoarding and, 223–224
  deficits and, 92–93
  to possessions, 57–58, 257–258

Augmentation treatments, for treatment of hoarding disorder, 154
Australian Twin Registry, 15
Avaricious Man, 3–4
Avoidance, experiential, 92, 102

Behavior
  consequence of, 193
  features of animal and human hoarding behaviors, 118–119
  hoarding, 182
  hoarding behaviors attributable to another medical condition vs. hoarding disorder, 112–113
BIT. *See* Buried in Treasures (BIT) Workshop
"Black box" warning, 159
Bleak House, 4
Board of Health, 183, 191
Boston University School for Social Work, 189
Bulimia, as comorbidity of hoarding disorder, 39
Buried in Treasures (BIT) Workshop, 133–134, 143, 188, 189

CAS. *See* Compulsive Acquisition Scale
Case examples
  of animal hoarding, 223
  of community approach to hoarding, 191–192
  of comorbid hoarding disorder and inattention, 159–160
  of comorbid hoarding disorder and mild major depression, 156–157
  of comorbid hoarding disorder and severe major depression, 157–159
  of fluoxetine, 158
  of harm reduction, 172–176
  of hoarding, 61–62
  of methylphenidate extended-release, 159–160
  of paroxetine, 156–157
  of squalor, 241–246
  of venlafaxine, 158

CAS-Free. *See* Compulsive Acquisition Scale—Free
Categorization, difficulties with, 94–95
CBM-I. *See* Cognitive bias modification of interpretation
CBT. *See* Cognitive-behavioral therapy, for hoarding
CFT. *See* Compassion-focused therapy
CGI. *See* Clinical Global Impression—Improvement scale
CGI-I. *See* Clinical Global Impression—Improvement scale; Clinical Global Impression Severity of Illness
Child Protection Services, 167–168, 185–186
Children
  hoarding in, 15–16, 255
    assessment, 56
    guardian ad litem for, 185
  pets and, 223
Children's Saving Inventory (CSI), **52,** 56, 255
Chronic disorganization, definition of, 186
CIR. *See* Clutter Image Rating
City of Vancouver Hoarding Action Response Team (HART), 185
Clinical Global Impression—Improvement (CGI-I) scale, 152
Clinical Global Impression (CGI) Severity of Illness, 135–136
Clutter. *See also* Home
  severity of, 38
  squalor and, 235, **236,** 248
"Clutter blindness," 73–74, 95
Clutter Image Rating (CIR), 48–49, **50, 52,** 72–73, 134, 150, 169, 183–184, 188, 190, 242
  sample of, 281, **282–284**
Clutter Scale from the Saving Inventory—Revised, 48
Cognition
  deficits in, 94, 209, 210
Cognitive-behavioral model of hoarding, **90,** 257
  aesthetics, 101–102
  anxiety sensitivity and, 91
  comfort and safety, 99

contributing factors, 104
features of, 91
impulsivity and, 92
information processing deficits, **91,**
    93–96, 104, 120
opportunity and identity, 96–99
overview, 89
possessions, meaning of, **91,** 96, 104
reinforcement patterns, **91,** 102–103
responsibility, 99–101
vulnerabilities to development of,
    89–93, **91,** 104,
Cognitive-behavioral therapy (CBT),
    for hoarding, 259, 262. *See also*
    Pharmacotherapy, for treatment
    of hoarding disorder
evidence base, 133–136
follow-up findings, 136–137
improvements in, 143
in-home assistance for, 135
overview, 127–133
peer group and, 133, 135
personality variables and, 137
randomized controlled trials and,
    133, 143
treatment
    difficulty with, 130
    goals, 129
    inference-based therapy,
        139–140
    mediators of treatment
        response, 138
    motivational interviewing,
        128–129
    motivation for, 129–130, 143
    predictors of treatment
        outcome, 137–138
    therapeutic promise, 127–128
    visualization exercise, 129
    variations in and additions to,
        138–142
Cognitive bias modification of inter-
    pretation (CBM-I), 131
Cognitive Rehabilitation and Expo-
    sure/Sorting Therapy (CREST),
    132–133, 135
Collecting
    vs. hoarding, 9–10, 20
    without hoarding, 50

Collyer, Homer, 4–6
Collyer, Langley, 4–6
Collyer Brothers Park, 6
COMMIT, 141
Community partnerships, 190
    case example of, 191–192
    public health officials, 183
Compassion-focused therapy (CFT),
    138
Compensatory cognitive training,
    132
Compulsive Acquisition Scale (CAS),
    52, 56–57,
Compulsive Acquisition Scale—Free
    (CAS-Free), 57
Compulsive buying, 34, 254–255
Compulsive Cognitions Working
    Group, 137
Concept formation, difficulties with,
    94–95
Copro-symbols, 8
Critical time intervention (CTI;
    CTI-HD), 188
CSI. *See* Children's Saving Inventory
CTI. *See* Critical time intervention
CTI-HD. *See* Critical time inter-
    vention
Culture, of hoarding
    American, 17
    animal hoarding, 220
    Asian, 17
    Chinese, 17
    hoarding and, 16–19
    Indian, 17–18
    Iranian, 18
    Japanese, 17
    Latin American, 18
    lost objects and, 16–17
    Manusians of Papua New Guinea,
        16–17
    Portuguese-speaking countries, 18
    Spanish-speaking countries, 18
    Tasaday of the Philippines, 17
    television shows about, 19
    Turkish, 18
CYP. *See* Cytochrome P450 (CYP)
    isoenzyme system
Cytochrome P450 (CYP) isoenzyme
    system, 159

Dead Souls, 4
Decision-making, impaired, 95
Dementia
    MRI studies in patients with co-
        occurring OCD, dementia,
        and other neurological
        disorders, 113–114
    squalor and, 245–246
Depression
    case example of comorbid hoarding
        disorder and mild major
        depression, 156–157
    comorbid hoarding disorder and
        severe major depression,
        157–159
    as comorbidity of hoarding
        disorder, 38
    hoarding symptoms and, 16
    treatment for, 61–62
*Diagnostic and Statistical Manual of
    Mental Disorders*, 3rd Edition,
    Revised (DSM-III-R)
    hoarding-like behavior as diagnostic
        criterion for OCPD in, 28–29
*Diagnostic and Statistical Manual of
    Mental Disorders*, 4th Edition, Text
    Revision (DSM-IV-TR)
    hoarding as a form of OCD, 27
    hoarding as a form of OCPD, 27
*Diagnostic and Statistical Manual of
    Mental Disorders*, 5th Edition
    (DSM-5)
    adoption of hoarding disorder, 3
    animal hoarding and, 216–218, 228
    definition of definition of hoarding,
        254
    diagnostic criteria for hoarding, 10,
        13–14
    diagnostic criteria for hoarding
        disorder, 30–35
    functional MRI studies using
        DSM-5 hoarding criteria,
        116–117
    hoarding before, 27–29
    hoarding in, 29–35
Dickens, Charles, 4
Difficulty Discarding subscale, 59
Dimensional Yale-Brown Obsessive
    Compulsive Scale (DY-BOCS), 16

Diogenes syndrome, 203–204
Discarding
    avoidance of, 104
    as cause of impairment in social,
        occupational, or other impor-
        tant areas of functioning, 32
    consequences of difficulty of, 32
    criterion, 29
    "difficulty" of, 31, 57–58, 130–131
    distress associated with, 31
    parting with objects, 235
Doyle, Sir Arthur Conan, 4
DSM-III-R. *See Diagnostic and Statisti-
    cal Manual of Mental Disorders*. 3rd
    Edition, Revised
DSM-IV-TR. *See Diagnostic and Statis-
    tical Manual of Mental Disorders*,
    4th Edition
DSM-5. *See Diagnostic and Statistical
    Manual of Mental Disorders*, 5th
    Edition
DY-BOCS. *See* Dimensional Yale-
    Brown Obsessive Compulsive
    Scale

ECCS. *See* Environmental Cleanliness
    and Clutter Scale
Education. *See also* Public-academic
    partnerships
    community partners and, 189
Effexor, for treatment of depression,
    61–62
Elders
    abuse prevention services, 185
    changes in social context of,
        202–203
    death of spouse, 203
    financial stability, 203
    functional impairments associated
        with late-life hoarding,
        202–205
    hoarding behavior in, 199
    hoarding prevalence and severity in,
        199–202
    interventions for hoarding and,
        207–209
    medical comorbidities in elders who
        hoard, 205–207
    mobility, 210

prevalence in, 210
psychiatric comorbidity and
    associated features of late-life
    hoarding, 207
social isolation, 206
Eliot, George, 4
Emergency medical team, 184–185
Emotions, dysfunctions in regulation
    of, 90
Environmental Cleanliness and
    Clutter Scale (ECCS), 57, 240
Essentialism, 96
Eviction, 182, 187
Experiential avoidance, 92, 102

Fair Housing Act, 183
Family
    effect of hoarding on, 172–174
    hoarding and, 12, 90
FDA. *See* U.S. Food and Drug Admin-
    istration
Fluoxetine, case example of, 158
Fluvoxamine, for treatment of hoard-
    ing disorder, 153–154
Freud, Sigmund, 8
Fromm, Erich, 8
Furby, Lita, 7–8

GAD. *See* Generalized anxiety disorder
Gambling, as comorbidity of hoarding
    disorder, 39
GATS. *See* Graves Anthropomorphism
    Task Scale
Gender, hoarding disorder and, 37
Generalized anxiety disorder (GAD),
    as comorbidity of hoarding
    disorder, 39
Genetics, 109–112
Gogol, Nikolai, 4
"Good home syndrome," 101
Graves Anthropomorphism Task Scale
    (GATS), 61
guardian ad litem, 185

HARC. *See* Hoarding of Animals
    Research Consortium
Harm reduction
    case examples of, 172–176
    description of, 176

features of the process
    assessment, 169–170
    engagement, 168–169
    harm reduction plan, 170–171
    harm reduction team, 170, 176
    initiation, 167–168
    maintenance, home visits, and
        agreement failures,
        171–172
    goals, 165, 176
    model, 166–167
    overview, 165–166
    personal safety, 169–170
    phases of, 167, 176
    principles, 166–167, 168–169
HART. *See* City of Vancouver Hoard-
    ing Action Response Team
HAS. *See* Hoarding Assessment Scale
HD-D. *See* Hoarding Disorder—
    Dimensional Scale
Health. *See also* Medical conditions;
    Mental illness
    hoarding and, 11
Health Insurance Portability and
    Accountability Act (HIPAA),
    170
HEI. *See* Home Environment Index
HIPAA. *See* Health Insurance Portabil-
    ity and Accountability Act
Hoarders, 19
Hoarders: Buried Alive, 19
Hoarding. *See also* Cognitive-
    behavioral model of hoarding;
    Cognitive-behavioral therapy;
    Culture; MRI studies; PET
    studies
    ADHD and, 93–94
    admission of, 76–77, 82
    anal fixation and, 8
    assessment
        Activities of Daily Living—
            Hoarding Scale, 49
        Anthropomorphism Question-
            naire, 60–61
        of attachments to and beliefs
            about possessions, 57–58
        Children's Saving Inventory, 56
        Clutter Image Rating, 48–49, **50**
        Clutter Rating Scale, 48

Hoarding (*continued*)
    assessment (*continued*)
        Compulsive Acquisition Scale,
            56–57
        Environmental Cleanliness and
            Clutter Scale, 57
        Graves Anthropomorphism
            Task Scale, 61
        Hoarding Assessment Scale, 56
        Hoarding Disorder—
            Dimensional Scale, 54
        Hoarding Rating Scale, 53–54, **55**
        Home Environment Index, 57
        HOMES Multi-disciplinary
            Hoarding Risk Assessment,
            49–50
        home visits, 64
        informal observations, 47–48
        measure of areas of overlap to
            assess relationship to
            possessions, 60
        Measure of Material Scrupulosity,
            59
        Object Attachment Scale, 59
        overview, 47
        Possessions Comfort Scale,
            59–60
        Possessions in View, 60
        protocol, 64
        Saving Cognitions Inventory,
            58, **59**
        Saving Inventory—Revised,
            52–53, **54**
        Structured Interview for Hoard-
            ing Disorder, 51
        of symptom severity, 51, **52,** 120
        UCLA Hoarding Severity Scale,
            55
    behavior in minority groups, 18–19
    behaviors, 28
    case example of, 61–62
    characteristics of, 80–81
    in childhood and adolescence, 15–16
    vs. collecting, 9–10, 20
    comorbidities with, 11, 38–40, 90,
        239
    comparison of phenomenological
        features and squalor, 234–239,
        236

"compulsions," 13
consequences of, 71
course of, 35–37
demographics, 37–38
depression and, 16
before DSM-5, 27–29
in DSM-5, 29–35
DSM diagnostic criteria for, 10,
    13–14
early measures of, 61
examples of, 4–7
in families, 90
family and, 12, 172–174
features of animal and human
    hoarding behaviors, 118–119
finance management and, 11
financial costs of, 11–12
health and, 11
history of, 3–7
hoarding-like behavior as diagnos-
    tic criterion for OCPD in
    DSM-III-R, 28
    description of, 28
hoarding-like behaviors in other
    disorders, 40–41
of inanimate objects, 256
interference of life and, 10–11
involvement of legal system in,
    182–184
isolation and, 38
language and, 78–79
as life-threatening, 10
in literature, 4, 20
in mental health, 7
mental illness and, 193
neural correlates of, 28
obesity and, 90
onset of, 35–37, 41
"orientation," 8
ownership and, 8
as ownership of objects, 7–8
perfectionism and, 77–78, 92
in popular media, 4–5
prevalence of, 12–16, 20, 53, 255
    among older adults, 200–201
    epidemiological studies, 13–16
public-academic partnerships,
    187–190
public attention to, 181

quality of life and, 11
range of, 20
reinforcement of, 258
rejecting attitudes toward people
    with, 78
responsibility of, 99–100
screening, 39
self-identified, 35–36
severity of, 10–12, 97, 255
    life events and, 36
social aspects of, 81
squalor measures, 57
stigma of, 82
symptoms of, 7, 20, 51, **52,** 81
    changes in, 143
    in the elderly, 210
    trauma and, 36
time of onset and course of symp-
    toms, 237–238
trauma and, 36–37
in twins, 14, 200
violence and, 36–37
Hoarding Assessment Scale (HAS), **52,**
    56
Hoarding disorder. *See also* Obsessive-
    compulsive disorder; Pharmaco-
    therapy, for treatment of hoarding
    disorder
admission vs. recognition of, 76–79
assessment phase, 128
case studies
    of comorbid hoarding disorder
        and inattention, 159–160
    of comorbid hoarding disorder
        and mild major depression,
        156–157
    of comorbid hoarding disorder
        and severe major depres-
        sion, 157–159
community and, 179–180
comorbidities with, 41, 132
    ADHD, 132
demographics of, 10, 37–38
description in ICD-11, 29–30
description of, 138
diagnosis of, 18, 216–217
DSM-5 diagnostic criteria for,
    30–35, 254
future directions of, 253–261

harm reduction and, 176
ideation, overvaluation of, 79–82
included in DSM-5, 3
included in ICD-11, 3
insight into, 70–76, **71**
MRI studies in patients with hoard-
    ing disorder, 114
neuroimaging and, 260
phenomenological differences
    between other mental disor-
    ders and, 109, 254
poor problem recognition of, 70–76,
    71
self-identity and, 140
support group, 141
symptoms of, 35, 41
treatment for, 62–64, **65,** 193
    contingency management, 260
    motivation, 80–81
    overview, 69
Hoarding Disorder—Dimensional
    Scale (HD-D), 54
Hoarding of Animals Research Con-
    sortium (HARC), 215–216
Hoarding Rating Scale (HRS), 14–15,
    16, 48, **52,** 53–54, **55,** 134, 150, 200,
    sample of, 289–292
Hoarding Rating Scale—Interview
    (HRS-I), 53–54, 156
Hoarding Referral Sheet, 184
Hoarding task force intervention
    model, 180–181
Home. *See also* Clutter
    age-related changes in, 203
    in-home assistance, 141
    level of clutter in, 72, 73
    professional organizers in work and
        home, 186–187
    squalor in, **236, 237**
    unsanitary, 204
    visits, 64, 72, 141, 170, 171–172
Home Environment Index (HEI), 57,
    169, 184, 240
Homelessness, 182
HOMES (Health Obstacles Mental
    Health, Endangerment, and
    Structure & Safety) Multi-
    disciplinary Hoarding Risk
    Assessment, 49–50, **52**

HOMES Multi-disciplinary Hoarding
    Risk Assessment, 169
HRS. *See* Hoarding Rating Scale
HRS-I. *See* Hoarding Rating Scale
    Interview
HRS-Self-Report, 15
Humane Care for Animals Act, 225

IBT. *See* Inference-based therapy
ICD. *See* Institute for Challenging
    Disorganization
ICD-11. *See International Classification
    of Diseases*, 11th Revision
ICD Clutter-Hoarding Scale, 184
Ideation
    of hoarding, 79–82
    of OCD, 79–80
Identity, 96–97
Impulsivity, 92
Inference-based therapy (IBT),
    139–140
The Inferno, 4
Information processing
    deficits, **91,** 93–96, 104, 120, 257
Inspections Hoarding Referral Tool,
    184
Institute for Challenging Disorganiza-
    tion (ICD), 184
International Classification of Diseases,
    11th Revision (ICD-11). *See also*
    World Health Organization
    description of hoarding disorder,
    29–30
    included in, 3
International OCD Foundation
    (IOCD), 150
IOCD. *See* International OCD Foun-
    dation
Isolation, hoarding and, 38

James, William, 8
Jones, Ernest, 8

Language, of hoarding, 78–79
Legal system. *See also* Adult Protective
    Services; Child Protection
    Services
    criminal proceedings for animal
    hoarding, 219

criminal prosecution for animal
    abuse, 225
Guardian ad litem, 185
involvement in hoarding cases,
    182–184
private property, 183
Legislation
    Fair Housing Act, 183
    Health Insurance Portability and
    Accountability Act, 170
    Humane Care for Animals Act, 225
A Life of Grime, 6
London Field Trial for Hoarding Dis-
    order, 72

Major depressive disorder (MDD), as
    comorbidity of hoarding disorder,
    38
"Material scrupulosity," 100–101
MCHEC. *See* Montreal Compulsive
    Hoarding Enlarged Committee
MCMI-III. *See* Millon Clinical Multi-
    axial Inventory—III
MDD. *See* Major depressive disorder
Measure of Material Scrupososity
    (MOMS), 59
Medical conditions. *See also* Mental
    illness
    dementia and squalor, 245–246
    hoarding behaviors attributable to
    another medical condition vs.
    hoarding disorder, 112–113, 120
    medical comorbidities in elders who
    hoard, 205–207
    neurological injury and squalor,
    244–245
Medication. *See also* Pharmacotherapy,
    for treatment of hoarding disorder
    drug-drug interactions, 161
    side effects of, 155, 161
Memory
    difficulties with, 94
    triggers for, 98
Men, hoarding disorder in, 37, 41
Mental illness. *See also* Health
    hoarding behavior and, 193
    psychiatric comorbidity and associ-
    ated features of late-life hoard-
    ing, 207

Methylphenidate extended-release
case example of, 159–160
for treatment of hoarding disorder,
153
Metropolitan Boston Housing Partnership, 189
Metropolitan Fire Brigade study, 10, 11
Millon Clinical Multiaxial Inventory—
III (MCMI-III), 40
Minocycline, 154
Models. *See also* Cognitive-behavioral
model of hoarding
cognitive-behavioral model of
hoarding, 257
of harm reduction, 166–167
HART's model of community-
based intervention, 185, 193
hoarding task force intervention
model, 180–181
mouse models of hoarding behaviors, 260
of rodents hoarding, 118–119, 120
translational animal models, 119
MOMS. *See* Measure of Material Scrupulosity
Montreal Compulsive Hoarding Enlarged Committee (MCHEC), 190
Motivational interviewing, 128–129,
168–169
MRI studies
functional MRI studies using
DSM-5 hoarding criteria,
116–117, 120
in patients with co-occurring OCD,
dementia, and other neurological disorders, 113–114
in patients with hoarding disorder,
114
PET and MRI studies in OCD
patients with and without
hoarding symptoms, 114–115
Museum of Modern Art, 7

NAPO. *See* National Association of
Productivity and Organizing
Professionals
National Association of Productivity
and Organizing Professionals
(NAPO), 186

National Comorbidity Survey
Replication, 13, 205
National Epidemiologic Survey on
Alcohol Related Conditions, 13
Netherlands Twin Registry, 15, 200
Neurobiology
classification of hoarding disorder
and, 120
features of animal and human
hoarding behaviors,
118–119
functional neuroanatomy, 114–117,
120
functional MRI studies using
DSM-5 hoarding criteria,
116–117
PET and MRI studies in OCD
patients with and without
hoarding symptoms,
114–115
genetics, 109–112
hoarding behaviors attributable to
another medical condition vs.
hoarding disorder, 112–113
neuropsychological studies,
117–118
phenomenological differences
between hoarding disorder
and other mental disorders,
109
structural abnormalities, 113–114
MRI studies in patients with co-
occurring OCD, dementia,
and other neurological disorders, 113–114
MRI studies in patients with
hoarding disorder, 114
translational animal models, 119
Neuroimaging, 260
Neuropsychological studies, 117–118
New York Daily News, 6
New York State Office of Mental
Health (OMH) Policy Scholars
program, 187 –188
Notice to Cure, 174

OAS. *See* Object Attachment Scale
Obesity, hoarding and, 90, 205
Object Attachment Scale (OAS), 59

Obsessive-compulsive disorder
    (OCD), 3, 10. *See also* Hoarding
    disorder
  as comorbidity of hoarding
        disorder, 39–40
  in DSM-IV-TR, 27
  hoarding-like behavior with, 40–41
  MRI studies in patients with
        co-occurring OCD, dementia,
        and other neurological
        disorders, 113–114
  overvalued ideation in, 79–80
  PET and MRI studies in OCD
        patients with and without
        hoarding symptoms, 114–115
Obsessive-compulsive personality
    disorder (OCPD), 3, 8
  criterion, 13
  in DSM-IV-TR, 27
  hoarding-like behavior as diagnos-
        tic criterion in DSM-III-R, 28
OCD. *See* Obsessive-compulsive
    disorder
OCPD. *See* Obsessive-compulsive per-
    sonality disorder
OMH. *See* New York State Office of
    Mental Health Policy Scholars
    program
Organization
  grouping "like with like," 95
  professional organizers, 186–187
  skills for decluttering, 131–132
Ownership
  definition of, 8
  hoarding and, 8

"The Palace of Junk," 6
Paroxetine
  case example of, 156–157
  for treatment of hoarding disorder,
        151–152
PCS. *See* Possessions Comfort Scale
Penurious Man, 3–4
Perfectionism, 143, 258
  dimension of, 95–96
  hoarding and, 77–78, 92
  squalor and, 244
Personality disorders, as comorbidity
    of hoarding disorder, 40

PET studies, PET and MRI studies in
    OCD patients with and without
    hoarding symptoms, 114–115
Pharmacodynamics
  description of, 156
  studies with psychopharmacology, 161
Pharmacokinetics, description of,
    155–156
Pharmacotherapy, for treatment of
    hoarding disorder, 259, 262.
    See also Case examples; Cognitive-
    behavioral therapy, for hoarding;
    Medication
  atomoxetine, 153
  augmentation treatments, 154
  efficacy studies, 151–155
  fluvoxamine, 153–154
  interactions with other drugs and
        warnings, 155–156
  management of side effects, 155
  methylphenidate extended-release,
        153
  overview, 149
  paroxetine, 151–152
  risperidone, 154
  shared decision-making, 161
  strength of evidence, 154–155
  treatment goals, 150
  venlafaxine extended-release, 152
Phobias, "mirror image" of, 18
PIV. *See* Possessions in View
Plato, 8
Possessions
  acquisition of, 32, 33
  attachments to, 57–58
  beliefs about, 57–58
  "churning" through, 93
  decisions to save, 28
  emotional attachment to, 139
  insight into value of, 80
  meaning of, **91**, 96, 104
  measure of areas of overlap to assess
        relationship to possessions, 60
  motives to save, 58, 64
  overvalued ideas about, 82
Possessions Comfort Scale (PCS), 59–60
Possessions in View (PIV), 60
Prader-Willi syndrome, 32–33, 255
Private property, 183

Proust, Marcel, 98
"Proust effect," 98
Public-academic partnerships,
    187–190
Public health officials, 183
"A Putative Link Between Compulsive
    Hoarding and Homelessness:
    A Pilot Study," 182

Quality of life, hoarding and, 11

Randomized controlled trials (RCTs),
    for CBT, 133, 143
RCTs. *See* Randomized controlled
    trials
Receiver operating characteristic
    (ROC), 54, **54**
Risperidone, for treatment of hoarding
    disorder, 154
ROC. *See* Receiver operating
    characteristic
Rodents, hoarding in, 118–119, 120

Safety. *See also* Harm reduction; Squalor
    emergency medical team, 184–185
    fire response, 184–185
    personal, 169–170, 193
    personnel, 184–185
    risks, 193
Salvation Army, 182
Sartre, Jean-Paul, 8
Saving Cognitions Inventory (SCI), 58,
    59
Saving Inventory—Revised (SI-R), 14,
    16, 39, **52**, 52–53, **54**, 64, 131,
    134, 150, 188, 242
    sample of, 285–288
SCI. *See* Saving Cognitions Inventory
Self
    ambivalence about, 92–93
    "authentic," 140
    future of, 97–98, 103
    identity and, 140
    neglect, 204, **236**, 246
    "ought self," 140
    personal hygiene, 248
    "possible future self," 140
Serotonin reuptake inhibitors, abrupt
    discontinuation of, 161

Sherlock Holmes stories, 4
SIHD. *See* Structured Interview for
    Hoarding Disorder
Silas Marner, 4
SI-R. *See* Saving Inventory—Revised
SMART (specific, measurable, attain-
    able, relevant, and time-bound)
    goals, 171
Song Dong, 6–7, 17
Soteria, 99
"Soteric neurosis," 99
Squalor, 184, 204. *See also* Safety
    accumulated objects and, 235, **236**
    from animal hoarding, 228
    assessment measures, 57
    case examples of, 241–246
    characterization of, 248
    clutter and, 235, **236**, 248
    comparison of phenomenological
        features of hoarding and,
        234–239, **236**
    dementia and, 245–246
    diagnostic considerations, 238–239
    etiology, 247
    executive dysfunction and, 239
    food and, 247
    functional impairment in work,
        family, and/or social domains,
        236
    health and safety risks, 256–257
    history of, 234
    intervention and recovery, 240–241
    neurological injury and, 244–245
    olfaction and, 247
    overview, 233–234
    parting with objects, 235
Structured Interview for Hoarding
    Disorder (SIHD), 14, 51, 64
    sample of, 267–279
Study of the Epidemiology of Mental
    Disorders, 13

Tenancy Preservation Program, 189
Theophrastus, 3
Toxoplasma gondii, 224, 247
Trauma, hoarding and, 36–37
Trebus, Edmund, 6–7
Twins, 14, 200
    hoarding in, 14

UCLA Hoarding Severity Scale
    (UHSS), **52**, 55, 136, 152
UHSS. *See* UCLA Hoarding Severity
    Scale
Uniform Inspection Checklist,
    191–192
University of Rhode Island Change
    Assessment questionnaire, 137
U.S. Food and Drug Administration
    (FDA), "black box" warning, 159

Vallejo-Nágera, Juan Antonio, 18, 99
Venlafaxine
    case example of, 158
    management of sexual side effects,
        158
    for treatment of hoarding disorder,
        153
Violence, hoarding and, 36–37
Visualization exercise, 129

Waste, avoidance of, 100–101
Waste Not, 6 7, 17
Western Massachusetts Hoarding
    Resource Network, 181
WHO. *See* World Health
    Organization
Women, hoarding disorder in, 37, 41
World Health Organization (WHO).
    *See also International Classification
    of Diseases,* 11th Revision
    Composite International
        Diagnostic Interview, 13
    World Mental Health Survey
        Initiative, 94

Yale-Brown Obsessive Compulsive
    Scale (Y-BOCS) checklist, 18, 19,
    27, 70
Y-BOCS. *See* Yale-Brown Obsessive
    Compulsive Scale checklist